Body MRI Cases

William E. Brant, MD, FACR
Professor of Radiology
Director, ThoracoAbdominal Imaging Division
Department of Radiology and Medical Imaging
University of Virginia
Charlottesville, Virginia

Eduard E. de Lange, MD
Professor of Radiology
Director, Body MRI
Department of Radiology and Medical Imaging
University of Virginia
Charlottesville, Virginia

OXFORD
UNIVERSITY PRESS

OXFORD
UNIVERSITY PRESS

Oxford University Press is a department of the University of Oxford. It furthers the University's objective of excellence in research, scholarship, and education by publishing worldwide.

Oxford   New York
Auckland   Cape Town   Dar es Salaam   Hong Kong   Karachi
Kuala Lumpur   Madrid   Melbourne   Mexico City   Nairobi
New Delhi   Shanghai   Taipei   Toronto

With offices in
Argentina   Austria   Brazil   Chile   Czech Republic   France   Greece
Guatemala   Hungary   Italy   Japan   Poland   Portugal   Singapore
South Korea   Switzerland   Thailand   Turkey   Ukraine   Vietnam

Oxford is a registered trade mark of Oxford University Press in the UK and certain other countries.

Published in the United States of America by
Oxford University Press
198 Madison Avenue, New York, NY 10016

Library of Congress Cataloging-in-Publication Data
Brant, William E.
    Body MRI cases / William E. Brant, Eduard E. de Lange.
        p.; cm.—(Cases in radiology)
    Includes bibliographical references and index.
    ISBN 978-0-19-974071-0 (pbk.: alk. paper)
    I. De Lange, Eduard E.   II. Title.   III. Series: Cases in radiology.
    [DNLM: 1. Magnetic Resonance Imaging—Case Reports.   2. Image Interpretation, Computer-Assisted—Case Reports. WN 185]
    LC Classification not assigned
    616.07′548—dc23
    2012012774

9 8 7 6 5 4 3 2 1
Printed in China
on acid-free paper

To my daughter, Rachel, who brings tremendous joy,
graciousness, strength, and humor to our lives, and
to my wife, Barbara, whose patience and support
grants me many hours working at my desk.
W. E. B.

To Cesca, Mabet, and Sacha
E. E. d. L.

Body MRI Cases

Preface

Body MRI Cases provides the student with 143 cases of common and uncommon conditions encountered in the daily practice of body MRI. The book was written for the student to practice interpretation and improve the diagnostic skills when reviewing MR images of the heart, abdomen, and pelvis. It serves as a companion study guide to our *Essentials of Body MRI* textbook, also published by Oxford University Press, which provides the "essential" background of knowledge required for understanding the principles of the modality and the appearance of disease when performing body MRI.

The cases in *this book* are presented in random order instead of by specific organ or disease, to mimic the diagnostic challenges that typically occur when reading the daily worklist of cases in a routine clinical body MR practice. The front page of each case includes a brief clinical history and multiple, carefully selected images that best show the important findings of the disease or entity that is being discussed. When turning the page the key imaging findings that lead to the diagnosis are highlighted, followed by a brief discussion emphasizing the differential diagnostic considerations and important teaching points as well as the pertinent literature.

To facilitate the learning process, the text is written in bullet format and the discussions are kept short. For most clinical cases the diagnosis was pathologically proven. The Index by Topic provides a guide to review the cases by organ system or topic for those who may wish to study the cases in a specific order rather than randomly. This case book can also be used to further illustrate the principles and many of the disease states discussed in our *Essentials* text.

As with the *Essentials* text, all authors of this book are, or have been, affiliated with the University of Virginia as faculty, fellows, or residents in the Department of Radiology and Medical Imaging. Each case has been carefully reviewed and edited for accuracy. We hope the book will become a valuable tool for learning about Body MRI.

William E. Brant, MD, FACR
Eduard E. de Lange, MD

Contents

Contributors

Body MRI Cases

William E. Brant and Eduard E. de Lange

List of Contributors

Talissa A. Altes, M.D.
Associate Professor and Vice Chairman of
    Research
Director, Pediatric Radiology Division
Department of Radiology and Medical
    Imaging
University of Virginia School of Medicine
Charlottesville, Virginia

Matthew J. Bassignani, M.D.
Associate Professor, Radiology
ThoracoAbdominal Imaging Division
Department of Radiology and Medical
    Imaging
University of Virginia School of Medicine
Charlottesville, Virginia

Matthew R. Bernhard, M.D.
Resident, Diagnostic Radiology
Department of Radiology and Medical
    Imaging
University of Virginia School of Medicine
Charlottesville, Virginia

Scott G. Book, M.D.
Fellow, ThoracoAbdominal Imaging
    Division
Department of Radiology and Medical
    Imaging
University of Virginia School of Medicine
Charlottesville, Virginia

William E. Brant, M.D., FACR
Professor, Radiology
Director, ThoracoAbdominal Imaging
    Division
Department of Radiology and Medical
    Imaging
University of Virginia School of Medicine
Charlottesville, Virginia

Gia A. DeAngelis, M.D.
Associate Professor, Radiology
ThoracoAbdominal Imaging Division
Department of Radiology and Medical
    Imaging
University of Virginia School of Medicine
Charlottesville, Virginia

Eduard E. de Lange, M.D.
Professor, Radiology
Director, Body MRI
Department of Radiology and Medical
    Imaging
University of Virginia School of Medicine
Charlottesville, Virginia

Nicholas A. Demartini, M.D.
Resident, Diagnostic Radiology
Department of Radiology and Medical
    Imaging
University of Virginia School of Medicine
Charlottesville, Virginia

R. Michael DeWitt, M.D.
Fellow, ThoracoAbdominal Imaging
    Division
Department of Radiology and Medical
    Imaging
University of Virginia School of Medicine
Charlottesville, Virginia

Rebecca E. Gerber, M.D.
Resident, Diagnostic Radiology
Department of Radiology and Medical
    Imaging
University of Virginia School of Medicine
Charlottesville, Virginia

Jennifer E. Gillis, M.D.
Resident, Diagnostic Radiology
Department of Radiology and Medical
    Imaging
University of Virginia School of Medicine
Charlottesville, Virginia

Jean-Martin M. Gingras, M.D.
Resident, Diagnostic Radiology
Department of Radiology and Medical
    Imaging
University of Virginia School of Medicine
Charlottesville, Virginia

Brandon A. Howard, M.D., Ph.D.
Resident, Diagnostic Radiology
Department of Radiology and Medical
    Imaging
University of Virginia School of Medicine
Charlottesville, Virginia

Sean D. Kalagher, M.D.
Resident, Diagnostic Radiology
Department of Radiology and Medical
    Imaging
University of Virginia School of Medicine
Charlottesville, Virginia

Minhaj S. Khaja, M.D., M.B.A.
Resident, Diagnostic Radiology
Department of Radiology and Medical
    Imaging
University of Virginia School of Medicine
Charlottesville, Virginia

Hannes Kroll, M.D.
Resident, Diagnostic Radiology
Department of Radiology and Medical
    Imaging
University of Virginia School of Medicine
Charlottesville, Virginia

Sean J. Lyman, M.D., Ph.D.
Resident, Diagnostic Radiology
Department of Radiology and Medical
    Imaging
University of Virginia School of Medicine
Charlottesville, Virginia

David M. Mauro, M.D.
Resident, Diagnostic Radiology
Department of Radiology and Medical
    Imaging
University of Virginia School of Medicine
Charlottesville, Virginia

Sara Moshiri, M.D.
Assistant Professor, Radiology
ThoracoAbdominal Imaging Division
Department of Radiology and Medical
    Imaging
University of Virginia School of Medicine
Charlottesville, Virginia

John P. Mugler, III, Ph.D.
Professor, Radiology and Biomedical
  Engineering
Chair for Research
Department of Radiology and Medical
  Imaging
University of Virginia School of Medicine
Charlottesville, Virginia

Patrick T. Norton, M.D.
Assistant Professor, Radiology, Medicine,
  Pediatrics
Non-invasive Cardiovascular Imaging
  Division
Director, Advanced Visualization Lab
Department of Radiology and Medical
  Imaging
University of Virginia School of Medicine
Charlottesville, Virginia

Juan M. Olazagasti, M.D.
Associate Professor, Radiology
ThoracoAbdominal Imaging Division
Department of Radiology and Medical
  Imaging
University of Virginia School of Medicine
Charlottesville, Virginia

Nicholas Said, M.D., M.B.A.
Resident, Diagnostic Radiology
Department of Radiology and Medical
  Imaging
University of Virginia School of
  Medicine
Charlottesville, Virginia

John R. Scheel, M.D., Ph.D.
Resident, Diagnostic Radiology
Department of Radiology and Medical
  Imaging
University of Virginia School of Medicine
Charlottesville, Virginia

Stephen D. Scotti, M.D.
Assistant Professor, Radiology
Department of Radiology and Medical
  Imaging
University of Virginia School of Medicine
Charlottesville, Virginia

Peter O. Simon, Jr., M.D.
Resident, Diagnostic Radiology
Department of Radiology and Medical
  Imaging
University of Virginia School of Medicine
Charlottesville, Virginia

Brian M. Trotta, M.D.
Resident, Diagnostic Radiology
Department of Radiology and Medical
  Imaging
University of Virginia School of Medicine
Charlottesville, Virginia

Nebayosi Twahirwa, M.D.
Fellow, ThoracoAbdominal Imaging
  Division
Department of Radiology and Medical
  Imaging
University of Virginia School of Medicine
Charlottesville, Virginia

Antoine Wadih, M.D.
Fellow, ThoracoAbdominal Imaging
  Division
Department of Radiology and Medical
  Imaging
University of Virginia School of Medicine
Charlottesville, Virginia

Universal Abbreviations

2D	2-dimensional
3D	3-dimensional
CT	Computed Tomography
ERCP	Endoscopic Retrograde Cholangiopancreaticography
FSE/TSE	Fast/Turbo Spin Echo
GRE	Gradient Echo
LGE	Late Gadolinium Enhancement
MIP	Maximum Intensity Projection
MR	Magnetic Resonance
MRA	Magnetic Resonance Angiography
MRCP	Magnetic Resonance Cholangiopancreaticography
MPGRE	Magnetization Prepared Gradient Echo
PSI	Phase Sensitive Inversion Recovery
RF	Radiofrequency
SNR	Signal to Noise
SSFP	Steady State Free Precession

History

► 75-year-old man with chronic renal insufficiency presents with a mediastinal abnormality detected during workup of emphysema.

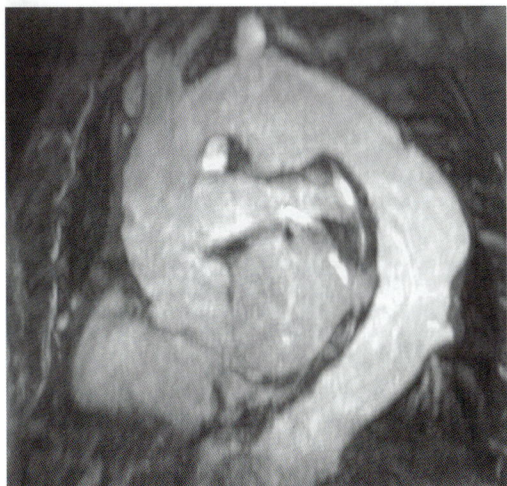

A

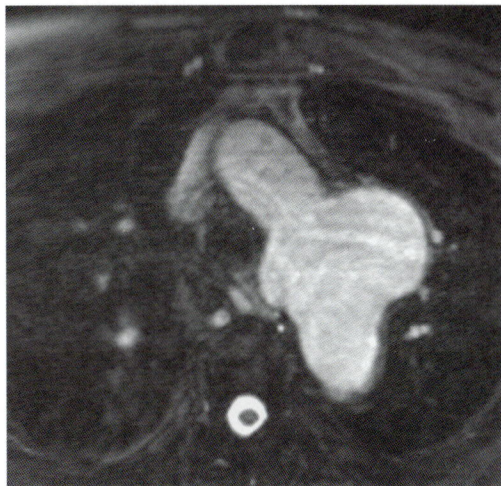

B

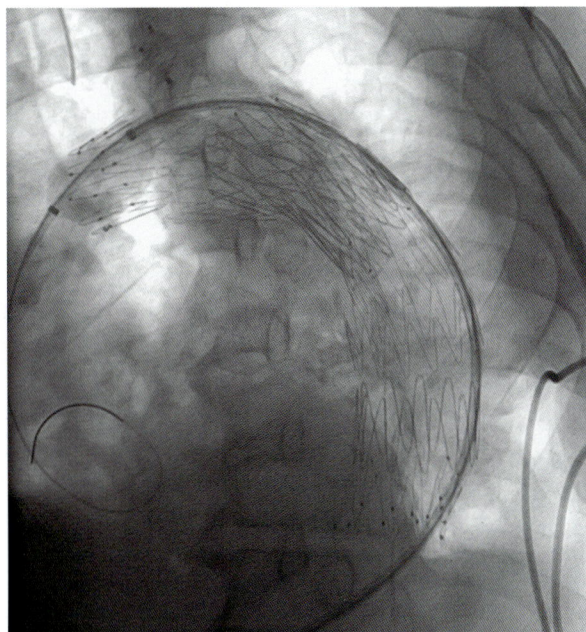

C

Sagittal (**A**) and axial (**B**) reconstructed MRA image of the thoracic aorta generated from 3D respiratory-gated balanced SSFP.
C. Radiograph of the thoracic aorta after stent-graft deployment

Case 1   Multiple Pseudo-Aneurysms from Penetrating Ulcers

Findings

- ► Saccular aneurysmal dilatation of the proximal thoracic aorta (A)
- ► Shallow saccular aneurysm of the mid-thoracic aorta and small penetrating ulcer of the distal thoracic aorta (**B**)
- ► Common trunk of the innominate and left common carotid arteries (**A**)
- ► Treatment of aortic aneurysm with aortic endograft. Deployment of endograft required occlusion of left subclavian artery and covering of the vessel origin with the endograft (**C**).

Differential diagnosis

Pseudo-aneurysm resulting from thoracic trauma

Teaching points

- ► Penetrating aortic ulcers result when luminal blood enters into the subintimal aortic wall via an ulcerated atherosclerotic plaque. Medial degeneration associated with atherosclerosis results in regional wall weakness, allowing for pseudo-aneurysm formation.
- ► MR sequences without the use of gadolinium-based contrast agents such as SSFP are effective and reliable for use as the sole imaging method before endovascular treatment of aortic pathology.
- ► Surgical or endovascular treatment is recommended when the diameter at the level of the ascending aorta exceeds 49 mm and when the caliber of the aortic arch or the descending aorta exceeds 45 mm in diameter. In patients with Marfan syndrome, treatment is recommended when the aortic diameter exceeds 43 mm.
- ► Surgical therapy of descending aortic aneurysm with prosthetic graft repair is associated with a perioperative mortality rate ranging from 5% to 20%, depending on the clinical condition of the patient.
- ► Endovascular repair of a thoracic aortic aneurysm is associated with a mortality rate of 0% to 20% and a periprocedural stroke rate of 0% to 7%.
- ► A landing zone for stent placement of 20 mm between the left subclavian and the origin of the aneurysm is preferred, unless occlusion of the left subclavian artery is planned.
- ► Major complications of endovascular repair include stroke, spinal cord ischemia, endoleak, and retrograde aortic dissection.

Management

Conventional surgical repair or endovascular stent graft placement.

Further reading

1. Atar E, Belenky A, Hadad M, et al. MR angiography for abdominal and thoracic aortic aneurysms: assessment before endovascular repair in patients with impaired renal function. AJR Am J Roentgenol 2006;186:386–393.
2. Fanelli F, Dake MD. Standard of practice for the endovascular treatment of thoracic aortic aneurysms and type B dissections. Cardiovasc Intervent Radiol 2009;32:849–860.
3. Norton P, Hagspiel K. Vascular MR imaging. In: Brant WE, de Lange EE (Eds), Essentials of Body MRI. New York: Oxford University Press, 2012.

History

▶ 56-year-woman with left upper quadrant pain.

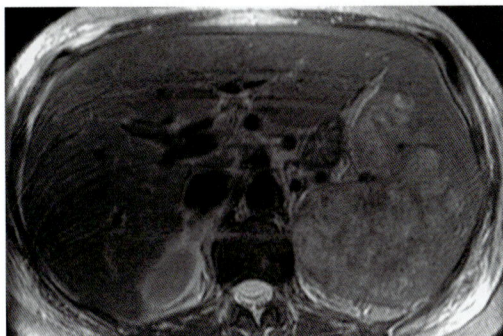

A

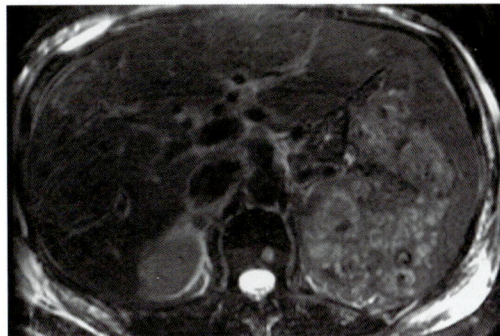

B

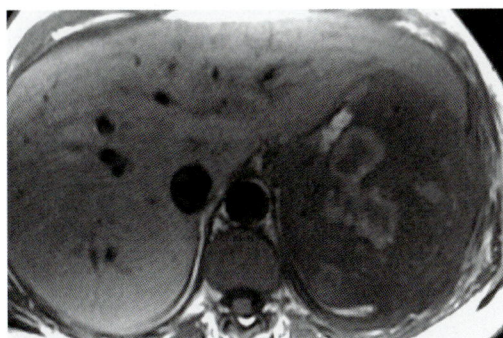

C

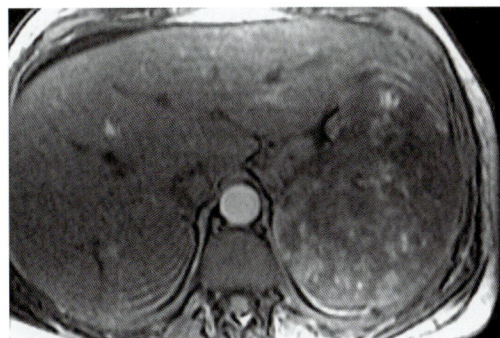

D

A. T2-weighted FSE/TSE. **B**. T2-weighted FSE/TSE with fat saturation. **C**. T1-weighted gradient-echo. **D**. T1-weighted post-gadolinium contrast-enhanced gradient-echo.

Case 2 Angiosarcoma of the Spleen

Findings

- The spleen is enlarged and its parenchyma is largely replaced by a heterogeneous mass.
- The mass shows foci of high and low signal intensity on T1- and T2-weighted images consistent with blood products and necrosis.
- Following intravenous gadolinium-based contrast material administration, the mass shows heterogeneous enhancement indicating a vascular necrotic solid mass.

Differential diagnosis

- Large splenic hemangiomas may be associated with splenomegaly and present as a heterogenous mass with cystic and solid components. Hemangiomas are typically hypo- to isointense to normal spleen on T1-weighted images and hyperintense to spleen on T2-weighted images. Post-gadolinium contrast-enhanced images show peripheral enhancement with progressive fill-in centrally. Large lesions frequently have a central non-enhancing scar. Large hemangiomas are frequently complicated by infarction, hemorrhage, and thrombosis, giving them a more variable appearance.
- Splenic hamartomas tend to compress rather than replace splenic parenchyma. They are well circumscribed and nodular in contour. Hamartomas are isointense on T1-weighted images and heterogeneously hyperintense on T2-weighted images. While early enhancement may be heterogeneous, delayed images show more uniform enhancement.
- Splenic lymphangioma is a predominantly cystic lesion with enhancing septations.

Teaching points

- Primary splenic angiosarcoma is rare but nonetheless is the most common non-hematopoietic malignant tumor of the spleen.
- Patients are rarely under 40 years of age.
- Splenomegaly is usually clinically apparent.
- Up to 30% of patients present with acute hemoperitoneum caused by spontaneous rupture of the spleen.
- Metastases are often widespread at presentation involving the liver, lungs, bone marrow, and lymph nodes.

Management

Diagnosis and treatment are surgical with splenectomy, optimally performed prior to splenic rupture.

Further reading

1. Abbott RM, Levy AD, Aguilera NS, et al. Primary vascular neoplasms of the spleen: radiologic-pathologic correlation. RadioGraphics 2004;24:1137–1163.
2. Brant WE, Lambert D. Gastrointestinal tract, peritoneal cavity, and spleen MR imaging. In: Brant WE, de Lange EE (eds.), Essentials of Body MRI. New York: Oxford University Press, 2012.

Case 3

History

► Presented are six consecutive images of the abdomen obtained using the same pulse sequence. Images are shown from cranial (**A**) to caudal (**F**) and are displayed with same window and center settings. Explain the change in signal intensity going from cranial to caudal.

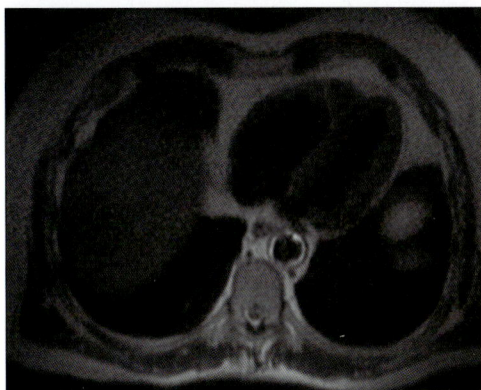

A

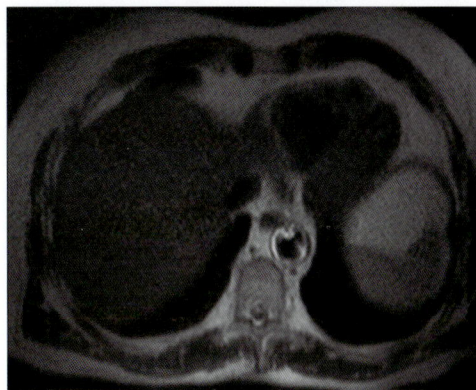

B

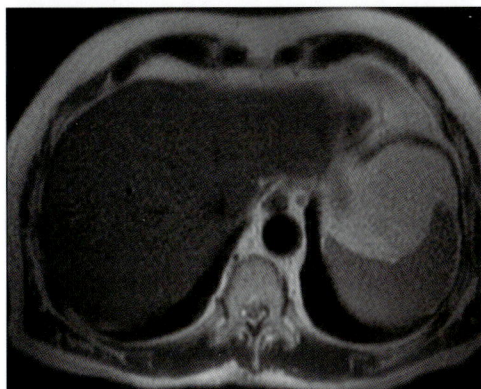

C

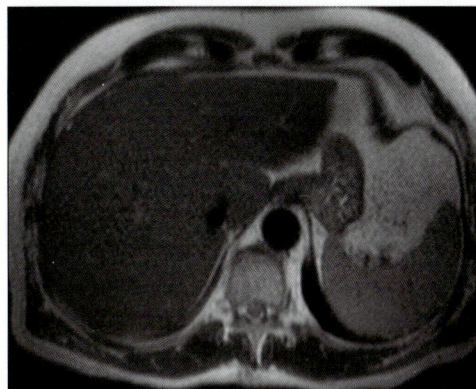

D

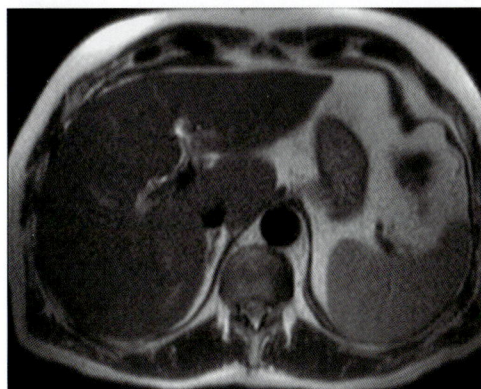

E

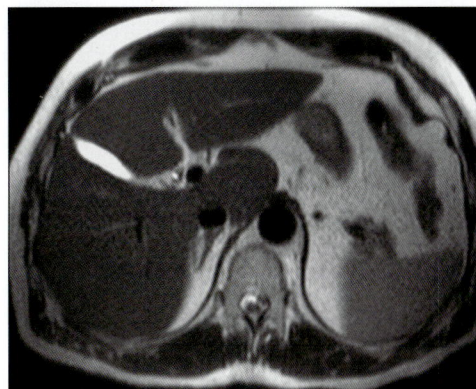

F

A–F. Axial single-shot FSE/TSE.

Case 3   Improper Positioning of the Phased/Body Array Coil Over the Abdomen with Respect to the Desired Tissue Volume

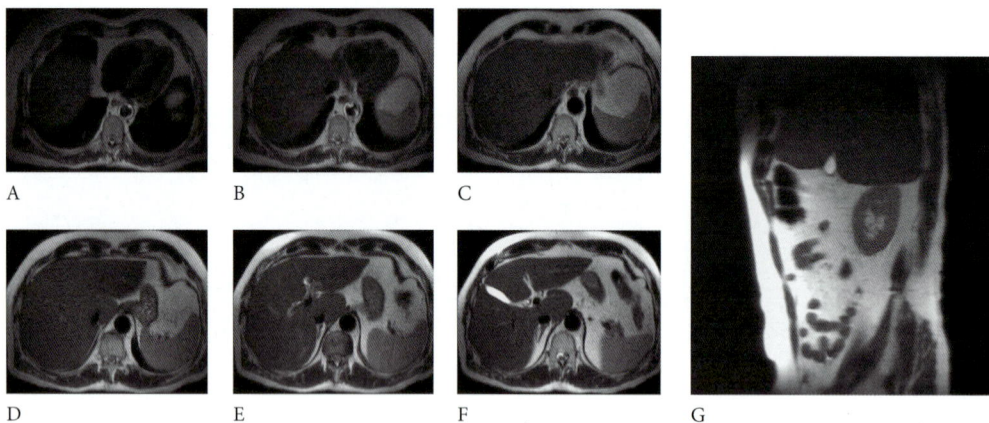

A

B

C

G

D

E

F

Findings

Image brightness increases from cranial to caudal.

Teaching points

▶ The phased/body array coil was positioned too low (i.e., too much toward the feet) with respect to the upper margin of the abdomen (**G**). As a result, the tissues in the upper abdomen are not within the volume for which the coil yields high signal-to-noise ratio (SNR). Because of the increased distance between the coil the SNR for the most upper abdominal tissues is reduced and they appear relatively grainy and dark compared to tissues lower in the abdomen. Images obtained from the tissues within the coil volume show higher SNR.

▶ Other causes for relatively low SNR:
   – Image obtained using the body coil of the MR scanner
   – Image obtained at low field strength

▶ The field of view of the phased/body array coil is limited by the overall coil dimensions. Hence, tissues that fall far outside the coil volume are not "seen" by the coil and therefore yield no signal. Signals from tissues just outside the coil volume are still received, but to a lesser degree, and these tissues therefore appear relatively dark.

▶ When using a phased/body array coil for abdominal imaging it is important to place the coil a few centimeters beyond the expected outer margin of tissues to be imaged. This allows for variations in breath holding, which may sometimes move a portion of the tissues outside of the coil volume, leading to decreased signal.

▶ In normal individuals, a relatively large portion of the upper abdomen is behind the ribcage. Thus, for upper abdominal imaging, the coil should include the lower portion of the chest as the inferior margin of the rib cage cannot be used to determine the junction between chest and abdomen.

▶ The body RF coil of the MR scanner covers essentially the entire tissue volume within the bore of the scanner. As a result, the body coil does not need positioning over a particular volume of interest, and with this coil there is usually no darkening of the images from signal drop-off at the most outer cranial or caudal slices.

History

▶ 14-year-old girl with primary amenorrhea after normal onset of puberty.

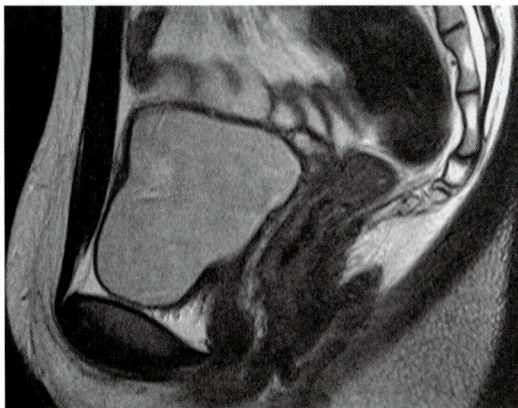

A

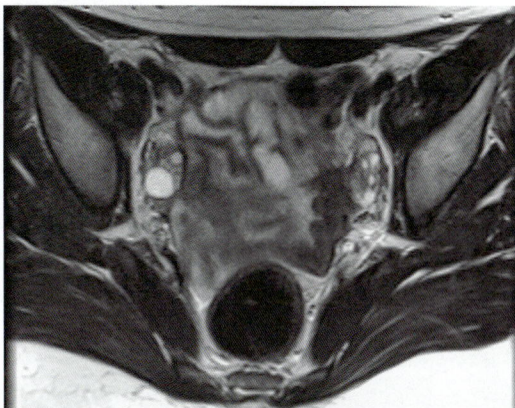

B

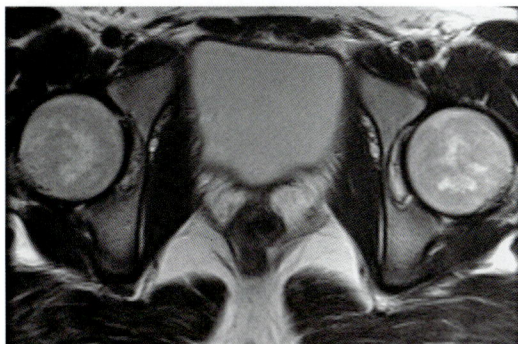

C

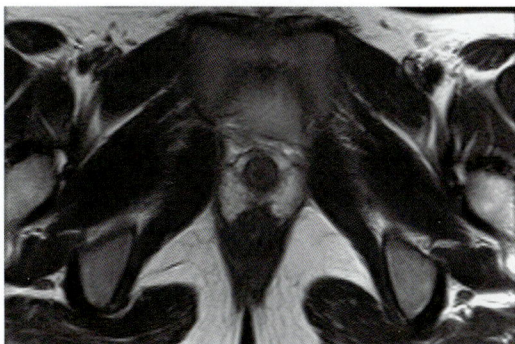

D

A. Sagittal T2-weighted FSE/TSE. **B.** Axial T2-weighted FSE/TSE obtained at the level of the acetabula, (**C**) of the hip joints, and (**D**) of the symphysis.

Case 4   Agenesis of the Uterus and Vagina

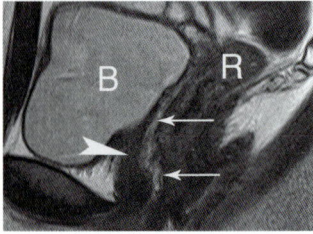
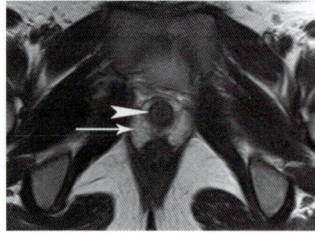
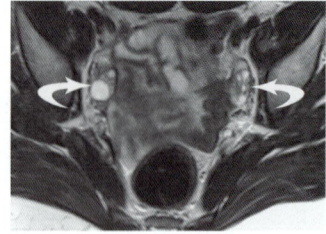

E   F   G

Findings

- Absence of the uterus and vagina. Only fat is seen where the uterus and vagina should be (*arrows* in **E** and **F**).
- The urethra (*arrowheads*), bladder (*B*), and rectum (*R*) are normal.
- Normal-appearing ovaries (*curved arrows* in **G**) are present bilaterally.

Differential diagnosis

- Hermaphroditism
- Turner syndrome

Teaching points

- Absence of the uterus and the upper two thirds of the vagina results from bilateral agenesis of the müllerian ducts. This entity has been termed the Mayer-Rokitansky-Küster-Hauser syndrome. The uterus and cervix, fallopian tubes, and most or all of the vagina are absent. The ovaries are present and function normally, resulting in the normal onset of puberty. This condition is the second most common cause of primary amenorrhea, following gonadal failure. The syndrome affects approximately 1 in 4,500 women. The cause is unknown. There is no genetic predisposition.
- The vulva, labia majora, labia minor, and clitoris are normal.
- Unilateral renal agenesis or dysplasia and skeletal malformations may be associated.

Management

The use of vaginal dilators or surgical creation of an artificial vagina will allow sexual intercourse. There is no treatment that will allow pregnancy.

Further reading

1. DeAngelis G. Gynecologic MR imaging. In: Brant WE, de Lange EE. Essentials of Body MR Imaging. New York: Oxford University Press, 2012.
2. Saleem SN. MR imaging diagnosis of uterovaginal anomalies: current state of the art. RadioGraphics 2003;23:e13 online only 10.1148/rg.e13.
3. Sultan C, Biason-Lauber A, Phililbert P. Mayer-Rokitansky-Küster-Hauser syndrome: recent clinical and genetic findings. Gynecol Endocrinol 2009;25:8–11.

History

▶ 46-year-old man in good health volunteered to test out new MR imaging protocols.

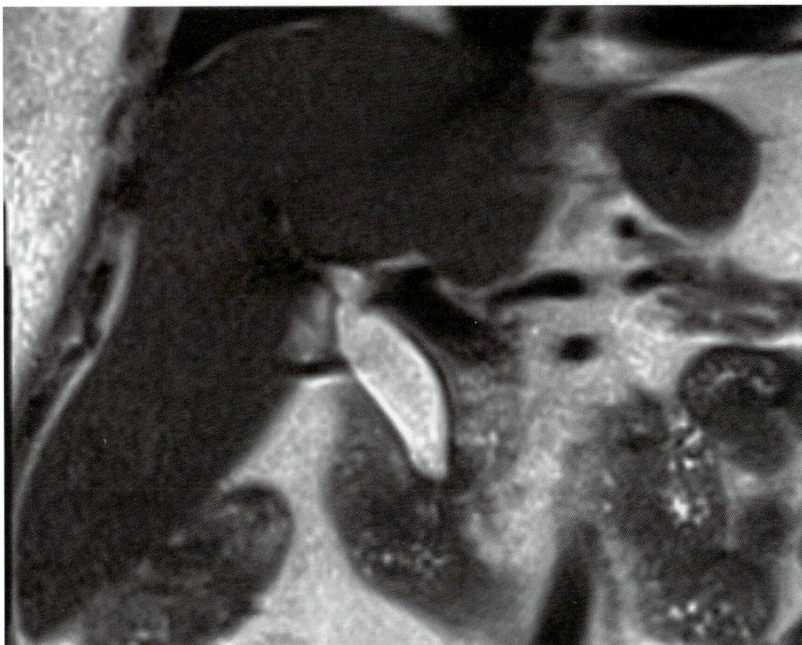

A

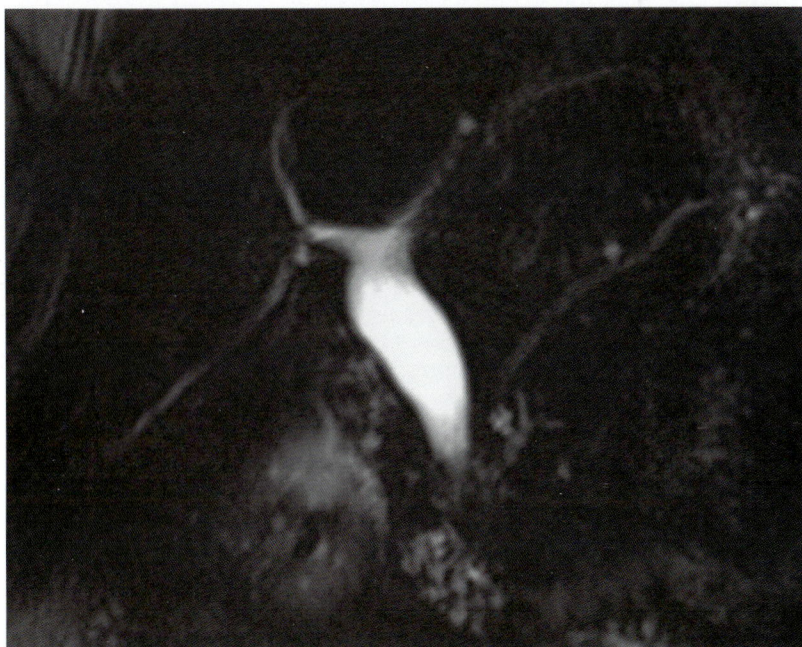

B

A. Coronal T2-weighted single shot FSE/TSE. **B**. Thick-slice MRCP obtained with single-shot FSE/TSE with fat saturation.

Case 5 Choledochal Cyst, Type Ic

Findings
▸ Fusiform dilatation of the common hepatic and common bile duct without stricture or abnormal-appearing intrahepatic bile ducts

Differential diagnosis
▸ Distal common bile duct stricture
▸ Distal common bile duct neoplasm
▸ Primary sclerosing cholangitis

Teaching points
▸ Most commonly used classification system of choledochal cysts is based on the Todani system of 1977. Choledochal cysts are uncommon congenital anomalies of the bile ducts involving cystic dilatation of the intrahepatic bile ducts, the extrahepatic bile ducts, or both.
▸ Type 1 choledochal cyst is the most common, occurring in 85% of cases, and is confined to the extrahepatic biliary ducts.
▸ Type I choledochal cyst is further subdivided into three types:
  – Type Ia—saccular dilatation of the entire extrahepatic biliary duct, both common hepatic and common bile duct
  – Type Ib—focal segmental dilatation of the common bile duct between the cystic duct and the ampulla. The common hepatic and intrahepatic bile ducts are normal.
  – Type Ic—fusiform dilatation of the common bile duct; normal common hepatic duct
▸ Predisposition to malignancy is believed to be related to bile stasis and pancreatic fluid reflux. Cholangiocarcinoma occurs in 9% to 28% of patients with choledochal cysts. Asian ancestry, especially Japanese, carries an increased risk.
▸ Most patients develop symptoms in childhood and are diagnosed prior to age 10 years. Some patients remain asymptomatic until the condition is discovered incidentally in adulthood.

Management
▸ Because of risk of development of cholangiocarcinoma surgical resection of the choledochal cyst is usually recommended.

Further reading
1. de Vries JS, de Vries S, Aronson DC, et al. Choledochal cysts: age of presentation, symptoms, and late complications related to Todani's classification. J Pediatr Surg 2002;37:1568–1573.
2. Irie H, Honda H, Jimi M. Value of MR cholangiopancreatography in evaluating choledochal cysts. AJR Am J Roentgenol 1998;171:1381–1385.
3. Kim OH, Chung HJ, Choi BG. Imaging of the choledochal cyst. RadioGraphics 1995;15:69–88.

History

▶ 46-year-old man with recurrent episodes of abdominal pain.

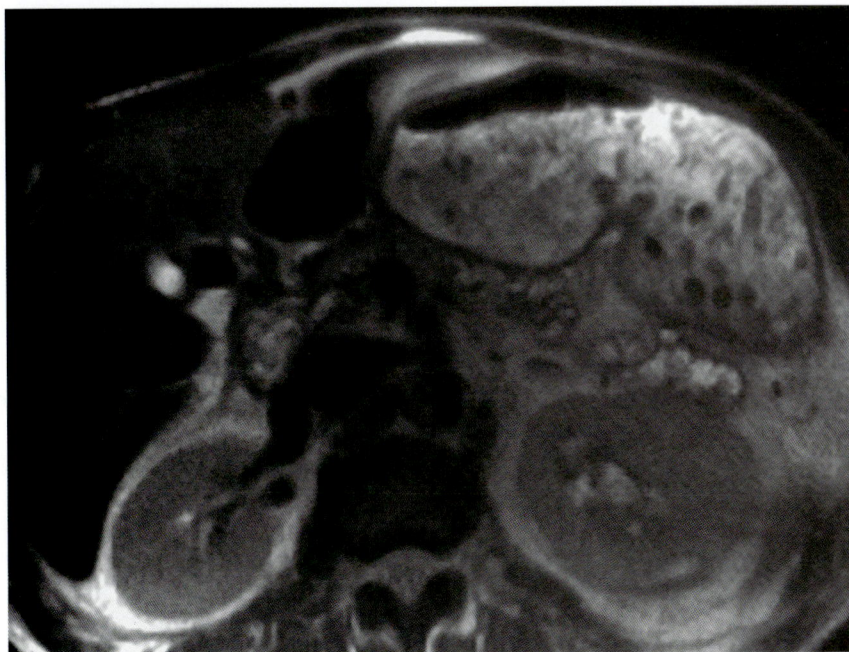

A

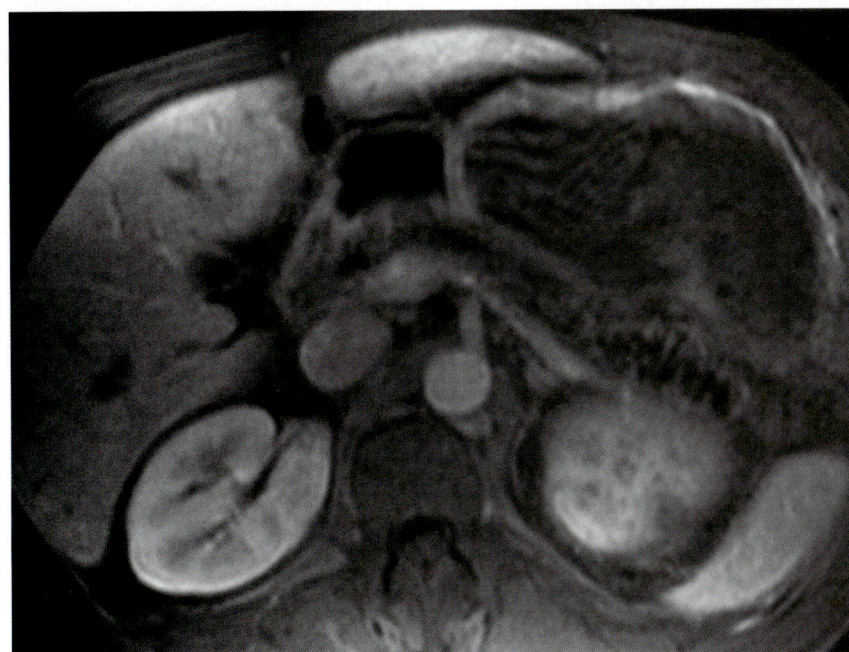

B

A. Axial T2-weighted single shot FSE/TSE. **B**. T1-weighted post-gadolinium contrast-enhanced gradient echo with fat saturation.

Case 6 Chronic Calcific Pancreatitis

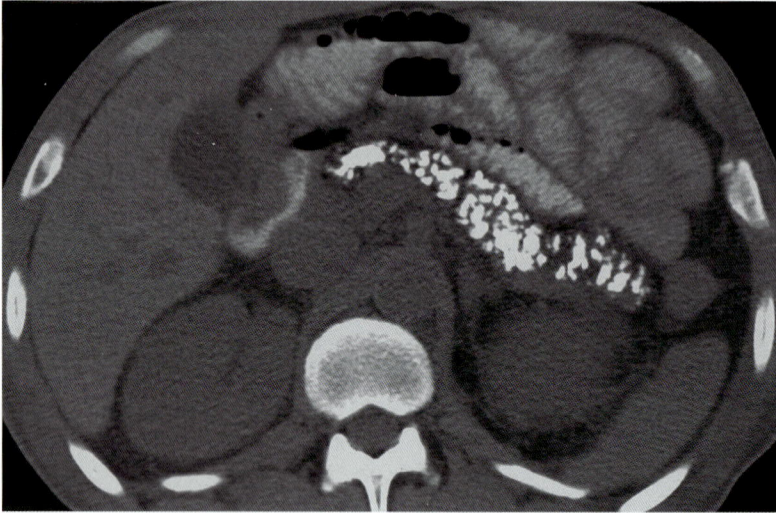

C

Findings

▶ MR demonstrates pancreatic atrophy and a tortuous, irregular, and dilated pancreatic duct characteristic of chronic pancreatitis.

▶ The prominent calcifications evident on the non-contrast-enhanced CT images (C) are difficult to appreciate on MR images.

Differential diagnosis

None

Teaching points

▶ Chronic pancreatitis is caused by a variety of conditions including biliary disease, smoking, alcohol abuse, and a variety of hereditary and autoimmune factors.

▶ The presence of prominent calcifications in association with characteristic findings of chronic pancreatitis limits the likely causes of chronic pancreatitis to alcohol abuse, hereditary chronic pancreatitis, and tropical calcific pancreatitis.

▶ Hereditary chronic pancreatitis refers to a heterogeneous group of genetic disorders most commonly inherited as an autosomal dominant trait. Early presentation in childhood and gradual progression of disease are typical.

▶ Tropical calcific pancreatitis typically presents in patients from developing countries. It carries a high risk of pancreatic adenocarcinoma.

Management

▶ Findings of chronic pancreatitis on MR warrant examination of conventional radiographs or CT scans for the presence of pancreatic calcifications.

▶ Abstinence from alcohol and pain management are the mainstays of treatment.

Further reading

1. Sunnapwar A, Prasad SR, Menias CO, et al. Nonalcoholic, Nonbiliary pancreatitis: cross sectional imaging spectrum. AJR Am J Roentgenol 2010;195:67–75.

History

▶ 57-year-old man with rectal cancer. Assess right adrenal mass.

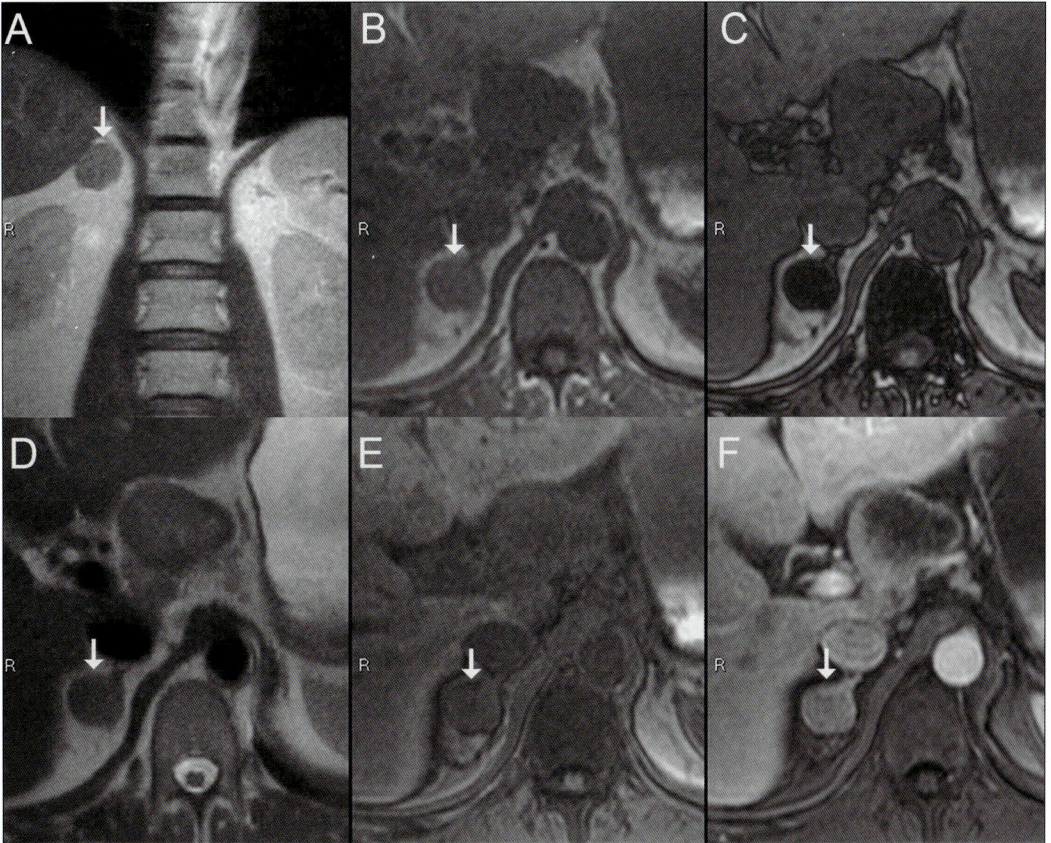

A. Coronal T2-weighted single shot FSE/TSE. **B**. Axial in-phase and (**C**) opposed-phase T1-weighted gradient echo. **D.** Axial T2-weighted FSE/TSE. **E**. Pre- and (**F**) post-contrast-enhanced axial T1-weighted gradient echo with fat saturation.

Case 7 Benign Lipid-Rich Adrenal Adenoma

Findings

- 2-cm mass (*arrows*) arises from right adrenal gland (**A**).
- In-phase image (**B**) compared with opposed-phase image (**C**) shows visible decrease in signal in C indicating the presence of intracellular fat.
- The mass displays intermediate signal intensity on T2-weighted images (**D**).
- The mass enhances with gadolinium-based contrast agent (**E, F**).

Teaching points

- The drop in signal on opposed-phase gradient-echo image compared with in-phase image is diagnostic of a lipid-rich adrenal adenoma with very high accuracy. Most (70% to 80%) adrenal adenomas contain sufficient intracellular lipid to be characterized by in-phase/opposed-phase gradient-echo MR imaging.
- The small size (<3 cm) and homogeneous signal intensity of the lesion on all sequences are good indicators that this lesion is benign.
- Most adrenal adenomas show significant enhancement following intravenous contrast material administration.

Management

- A follow-up cross-sectional imaging study between 3 months to 1 year is often recommended to confirm the stability of adrenal adenomas.
- Endocrinologic evaluation may be indicated to exclude pheochromocytoma and subclinical Cushing syndrome. Exclusion of pheochromocytoma can be done on clinical grounds (is there hypertension with bouts of diaphoresis, headaches, and palpitations?) or biochemically (serum resting catecholamine levels, 24-hour urine collection to assay for catecholamine metabolites). Exclusion of subclinical Cushing syndrome is done using the dexamethasone suppression test.

Further reading

1. Bassignani MJ. Adrenal and retroperitoneal MR. In: Brant WE, de Lange EE (eds), Essentials of Body MR Imaging. New York: Oxford University Press, 2012.
2. Boland GW, Blake MA, Hahn PF, Mayo-Smith WW. Incidental adrenal lesions: principles, techniques, and algorithms for imaging characterization. Radiology 2008;249:756–775.
3. Elsayes KM, Mukundan G, Narra VR, et al. Adrenal masses: MR imaging features with pathologic correlation. RadioGraphics 2004;24:S73–S86.
4. Gross MD, Korobkin M, Bou Assaly W, Dwamena B, Djekidel M. Contemporary imaging of incidentally discovered adrenal masses. Nature Reviews Urology 2009;6:363–373.
5. Grumbach MM, Biller BM, Braunstein GD, et al. Management of the clinically inapparent adrenal mass ("incidentaloma"). Ann Intern Med 2003;138:424–429.
6. Krebs TL, Wagner BJ. MR imaging of the adrenal gland: radiologic-pathologic correlation. RadioGraphics 1998;18:1425–1440.

History

▶ 40-year-old woman, who had hysterectomy for uterine leiomyomas, presents with a pelvic mass discovered on routine physical examination.

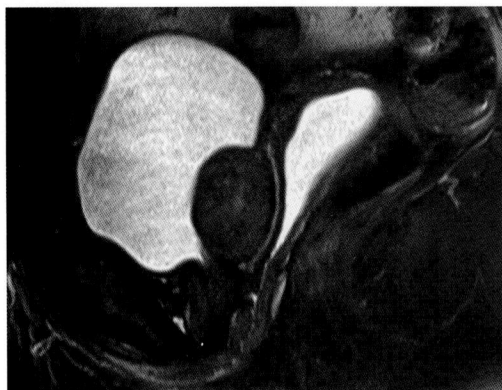

A

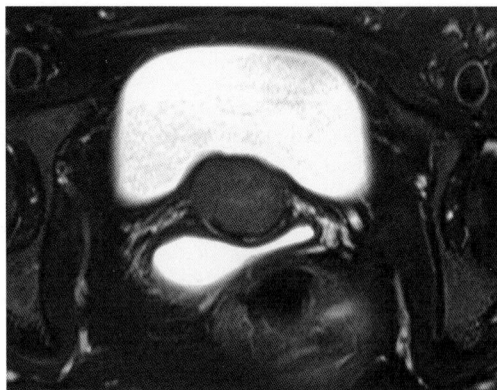

B

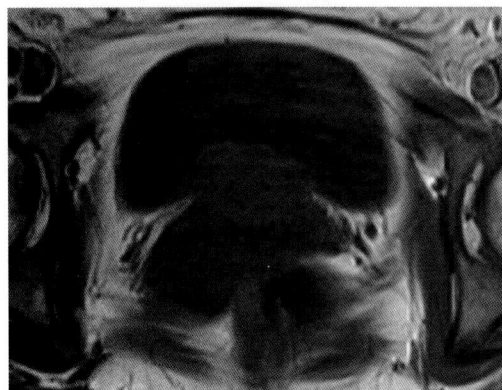

C

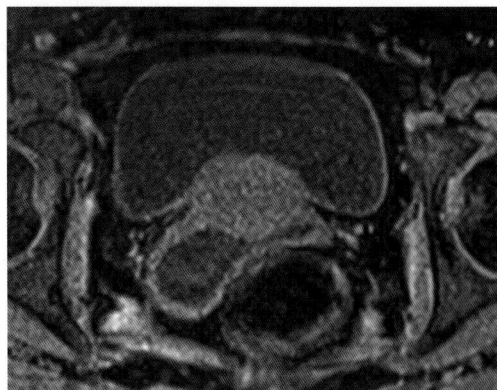

D

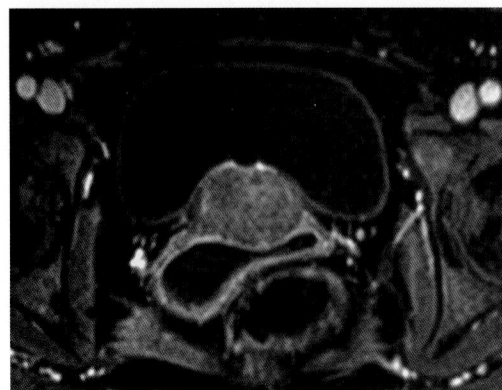

E

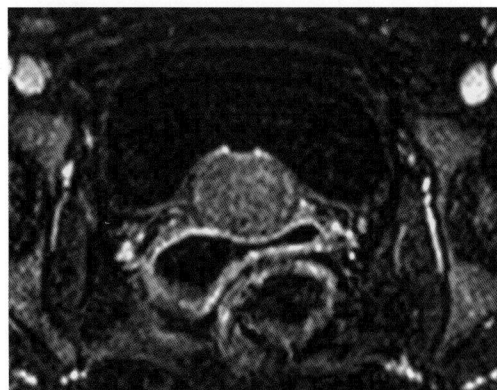

F

A. Sagittal and (**B**) axial T2-weighted FSE/TSE. **C**. Axial T1-weighted spin echo. **D**. Axial pre- and (**E**) post-gadolinium contrast-enhanced T1-weighted gradient echo. **F**. Axial post-contrast-enhanced subtraction image.

Case 8 Leiomyoma Arising from the Bladder Wall Near the Trigone

Findings

- A well-defined oval solid mass arises from the posterior bladder wall causing mass effect on the anterior vaginal wall. A distinct fat plane separates the bladder wall from the vaginal wall.
- The mass shows mild enhancement on post-gadolinium contrast-enhanced images.

Differential diagnosis

- Pheochromocytoma
- Urothelial cancer
- Leiomyosarcoma/rhabdomyosarcoma

Teaching points

- Leiomyoma of the bladder is a rare tumor occurring predominantly (75%) in women and accounting for only 0.4% of bladder neoplasms. Imaging shows a smooth, homogeneous, well-defined solid mass. Cystoscopy, needed to exclude a bladder mucosal tumor, showed normal bladder epithelium covering the tumor.
- Typical MR findings show the lesion with intermediate signal intensity on T1-weighted images, low signal intensity on T2-weighted images, and variable contrast enhancement.
- Leiomyomas have no malignant potential but must be differentiated from leiomyosarcomas and rhabdomyosarcomas. Necrosis, absence of sharply defined borders, and heterogeneity on T2-weighted and post-gadolinium contrast-enhanced images are suggestive of malignancy. Rhabdomyosarcomas are the most common bladder tumor of children under 10, and occur rarely in adults.

Management

Symptomatic leiomyomas are removed by simple enucleation, avoiding radical surgery.

Further reading

1. Brant WE, Williams JL. Computed tomography of bladder leiomyoma. J Comput Assist Tomogr 1984;8:562–563.
2. Wong-You-Cheong JJ, Woodward PJ, Manning MA, Davis CJ. Inflammatory and nonneoplastic bladder masses: radiologic-pathologic correlation. RadioGraphics 2006;26:1847–1868.
3. Wong-You-Cheong JJ, Woodward PJ, Manning MA, Sesterhenn IA. Neoplasms of the urinary bladder: radiologic-pathologic correlation. RadioGraphics 2006;26:553–580.

History

50-year-old woman complaining of nausea, vomiting, and abdominal pain following laparoscopic cholecystectomy.

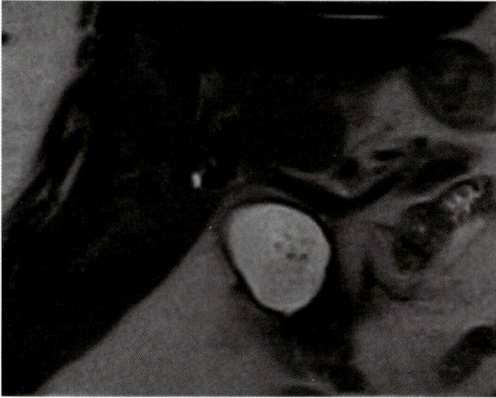

A

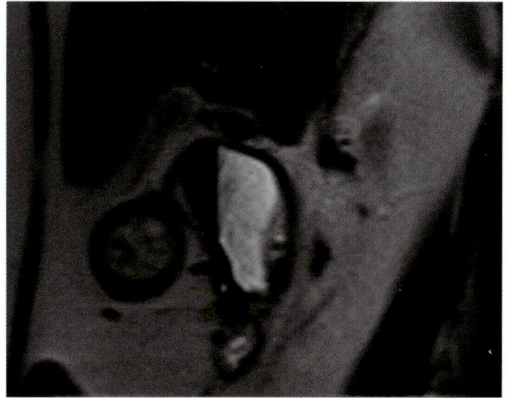

B

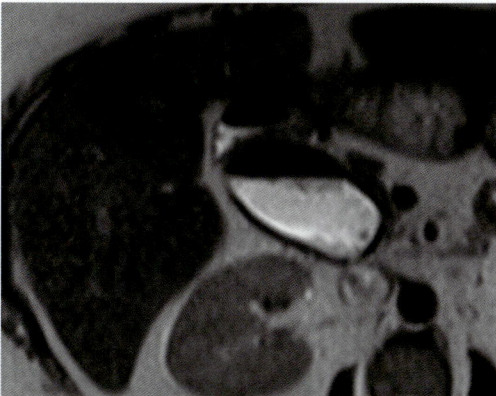

C

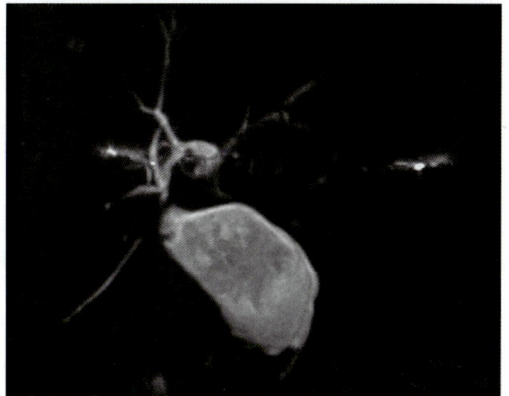

D

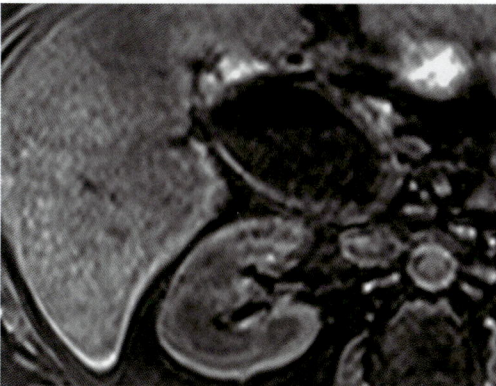

E

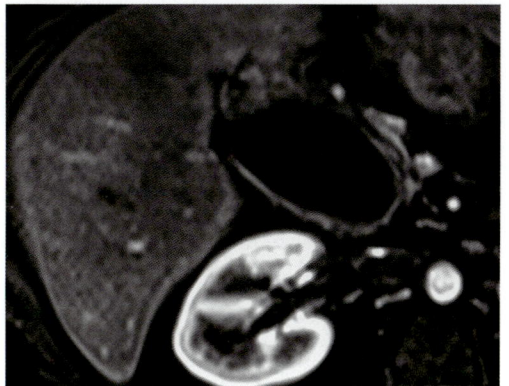

F

A. Coronal and (**B**, **C**) sagittal T2-weighted single shot FSE/TSE. **D**. Maximum intensity projection MRCP generated from 3D FSE/TSE. **E**. Axial pre-contrast and (**F**) early phase post-gadolinium contrast-enhanced T1-weighted gradient echo with fat saturation.

Case 9 Choledochal Cyst, Type Ib, with Acute and Chronic Inflammation Confirmed at Histology

Findings

- The common bile duct shows diffuse saccular dilatation.
- Air, debris, and stones are evident within the dilated duct. The presence of air is the result of a previously performed sphincterotomy.
- The wall of the dilated bile duct enhances but there is no evidence of an enhancing mass within the dilated duct.

Differential diagnosis

- Biliary stricture with proximal dilatation

Teaching points

- Choledochal cysts most commonly involve the common bile duct (type I), though the term applies to congenital cystic dilatations of any portion of the biliary tree. Choledochal cysts of the common bile duct are believed to arise from anomalous union of the common bile duct and the pancreatic duct just proximal to the sphincter of Oddi and just outside the wall of the duodenum.
- Choledochal cysts type I may present in childhood or remain asymptomatic and undiscovered until adulthood. They may be identified as an incidental finding on imaging obtained for other reasons. Clinical presentation of choledochal cyst includes pancreatitis, biliary sepsis, abdominal pain, or painless jaundice.
- Complications associated with choledochal cysts type I include biliary stone formation within the cyst, cholangitis, biliary stricture, pancreatitis, sepsis, liver abscess, and cholangiocarcinoma.
- Postoperative complications following surgical repair of choledochal cysts type I are relatively common (up to 30%). Biliary stricture is the most troublesome complication, reported in 6% to 7% of patients. Additional complications include anastomotic leak, fistula formation, cholangitis, biliary stone formation, and cholangiocarcinoma.

Management

- Complete surgical excision of the cyst and creation of a Roux-en-Y hepatico-jejunostomy to restore continuity of bile flow

Further reading

1. Cha SW, Park MS, Kim KW, et al. Choledochal cyst and anomalous pancreaticobiliary ductal union in adults: radiological spectrum and complications. J Comput Assist Tomogr 2008;32:17–22.
2. Lee HK, Park SJ, Yi BH, et al. Imaging features of adult choledochal cysts: a pictorial review. Korean J Radiol 2009;10:71–90.
3. Olazagasti J. Biliary system MR imaging. In: Brant WE, de Lange EE (eds), Essentials of Body MRI. New York: Oxford University Press, 2012.
4. Singham J, Yoshida EM, Scudamore CH. Choledochal cysts—Part 3 of 3: management. Can J Surg 2010;53:51–56.

History

► Follow-up of bilateral adrenal lesions.

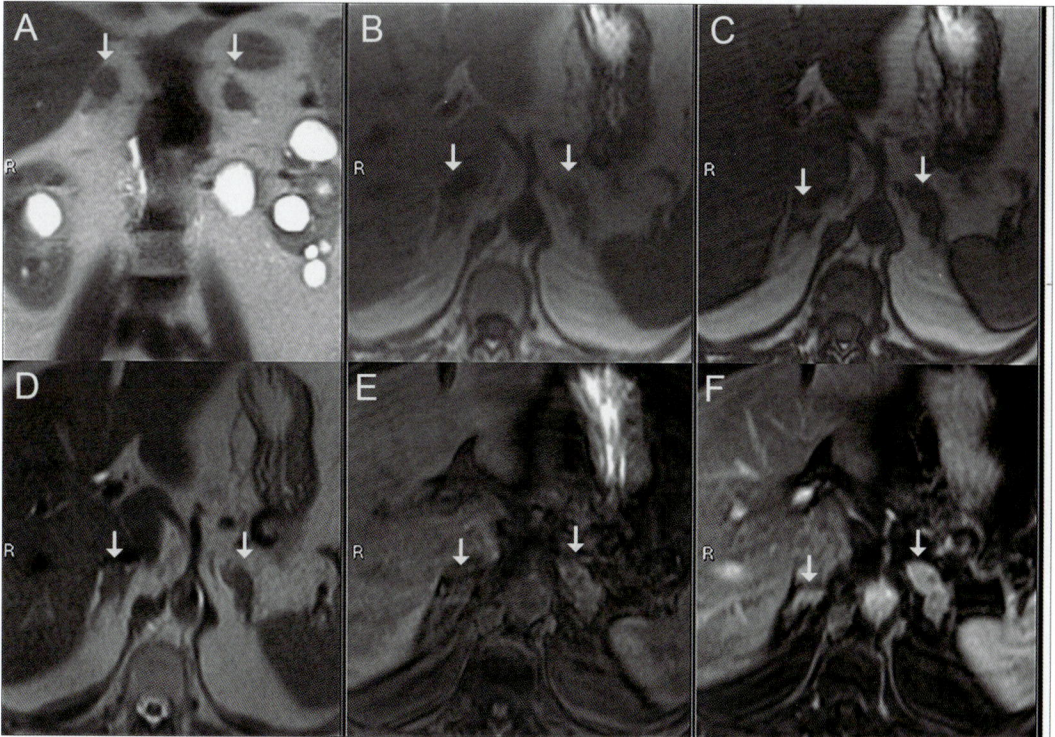

A. Coronal T2-weighted single-shot FSE/TSE. **B**. Axial in-phase and (**C**) opposed-phase T1-weighted gradient echo. **D**. Axial T2-weighted single-shot FSE/TSE. **E**. Pre- and (**F**) post-contrast-enhanced T1-weighted gradient echo with fat saturation.

Case 10 Bilateral Adrenal Hyperplasia

Findings

▶ Bilateral nodular adrenal enlargement (*arrows*) without distorting the adreniform shape

▶ Small bilateral adrenal lesions (<2 cm). Cysts in both kidneys.

▶ The signal intensity is similar on both sides, following that of normal adrenal glands on all sequences.

▶ The lesions decrease slightly in signal intensity on the opposed-phase gradient-echo image (**C**) compared with the in-phase image (**B**).

Differential diagnosis

▶ Bilateral adrenal adenomas

▶ Metastatic disease

▶ Bilateral pheochromocytomas (associated with von Hippel-Lindau syndrome)

Teaching points

▶ The distinction between bilateral adrenal adenomas and bilateral adrenal hyperplasia is not critical clinically so long as the patient undergoes an endocrine evaluation to determine adrenal endocrine hyperfunction. Hyperplasia is favored in this case since the enlarged adrenal glands maintain their normal shape.

▶ These lesions show a mild decrease in signal intensity on opposed-phase images compared with in-phase images. This is evidence of sufficient lipid within these lesions for them to represent adrenal cortical tissue, allowing the exclusion of metastatic disease. To confirm the presence of intracellular lipid, an adrenal-to-spleen signal intensity index could be calculated, as necessary.

▶ Metastatic disease is a possible diagnosis to consider. The apparent lipid content within these masses is evidence of functioning adrenal tissue, however, and excludes metastatic disease. Metastatic disease generally does not contain fat and the normal shape of the adrenal glands is distorted.

▶ Bilateral pheochromocytomas are a diagnostic possibility, except the adrenal glands are usually distorted by these masses. There is no history of hypertension or associated findings of von Hippel-Lindau syndrome in this case.

Management

▶ A cross-sectional imaging study is recommended to be performed at 3 months to 1 year to confirm stability of the adrenal lesions.

▶ Endocrinologic evaluation should include tests to exclude pheochromocytoma and subclinical Cushing syndrome. Exclusion of pheochromocytoma can be done on clinical grounds (is there hypertension, with bouts of diaphoresis, headaches, and palpitations?) or biochemically (serum resting catecholamine levels, 24-hour urine collection to assay for catecholamine metabolites). Exclusion of subclinical Cushing syndrome is performed using a dexamethasone suppression test.

Further reading

1. Doppman JL, Miller DL, Dwyer AJ, et al. Macronodular adrenal hyperplasia in Cushing disease. Radiology 1988;166:347–352.
2. Premkumar A, Chow CK, Choyke PL, Doppman JL. Stress-induced adrenal hyperplasia simulating metastatic disease: CT and MR findings. AJR Am J Roentgenol 1992;159:675–676.
3. Bassignani MJ. Adrenal and retroperitoneal MR. In: Brant WE, de Lange EE (eds), Essentials of Body MR Imaging. New York: Oxford University Press, 2012.

History

▶ 45-year-old obese woman presents with right upper quadrant pain. Abdominal ultrasound examination was reported to be normal.

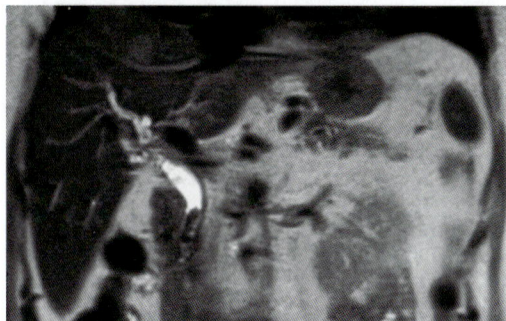

A

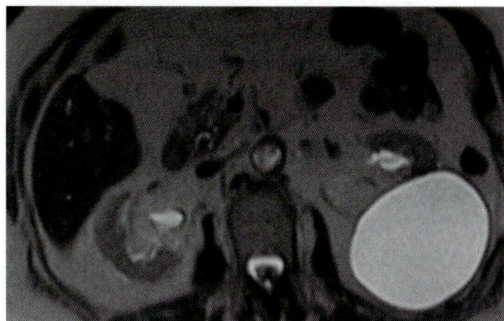

B

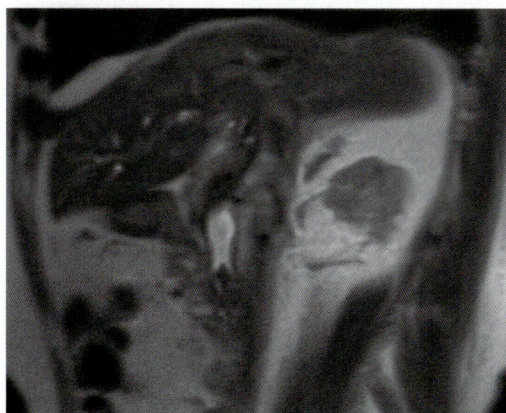

C

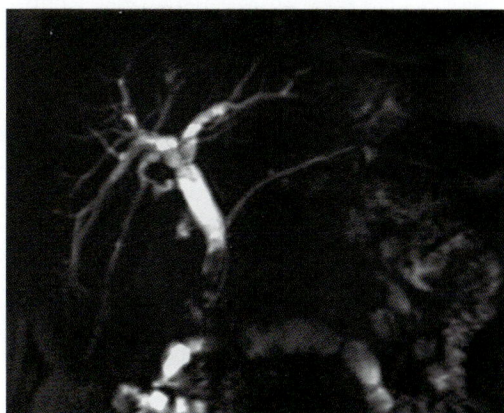

D

A. Coronal, (**B**) axial, and (**C**) sagittal T2-weighted single-shot FSE/TSE. **D**. T2-weighted MRCP (thick-slab single-shot FSE/TSE with fat suppression).

Case 11 Choledocholithiasis

Findings
- ▶ Signal voids caused by gallstones are present within the distal common bile duct.
- ▶ The biliary tree is mildly dilated.
- ▶ A rim or crescent of high-signal-intensity biliary fluid helps to identify the stones in the distal common bile duct (the "ring" or "crescent" sign) (**B**).
- ▶ A large benign left renal cyst is evident in **B**.

Differential diagnosis
- ▶ Cholangiocarcinoma
- ▶ Ampullary carcinoma
- ▶ Sphincteric contraction
- ▶ Air bubbles

Teaching points
- ▶ Whereas ultrasound has a sensitivity for detecting choledocholithiasis of only 21% to 63%, MR cholangiography has sensitivity of 89% to 100%, with specificity of 83% to 100%. MR can demonstrate ductal stones as small as 2 mm in size even in the absence of ductal dilatation, though its sensitivity for detecting tiny stones is lower and requires thin-section imaging.
- ▶ On T2-weighted images biliary ductal stones appear as signal voids, often with an angulated or geometric shape and a lamellated appearance.
- ▶ Stones layer dependently and are typically outlined anteriorly by a crescent of high-signal-intensity bile on axial T2-weighted images (the "crescent sign").
- ▶ Biliary segments with multiple impacted stones and with little to no surrounding bile fluid may be mistaken for a ductal stricture.
- ▶ Pneumobilia also produces a signal void on all MR sequences and may mimic stones in the duct. However, in contrast to stones, the signal voids from air bubbles are in a non-dependent position. Susceptibility artifact such as blooming on gradient-echo images is also evidence of ductal air rather than stones.
- ▶ Periductal edema and inflammation caused by irritation of the duct wall by impacted stones may be seen as wall thickening, stranding in the periductal fat, and mural enhancement.

Management
- ▶ Stones smaller than 3 mm may pass without intervention.
- ▶ Stones in the range of 3 to 10 mm generally require intervention with endoscopic retrograde cholangiography (ERCP) and balloon sweep of the common bile duct.

Further reading
1. Bortoff GA, Chen MYM, Ott DJ, et al. Gallbladder stones: imaging and intervention RadioGraphics 2000;20:751–766.
2. Olazagasti J. Biliary system MR imaging. In: Brant WE, de Lange EE (Eds), Essentials of Body MRI. New York: Oxford University Press, 2012.
3. Yeh BM, Liu PS, Soto JA, et al. MR imaging and CT of the biliary tract RadioGraphics 2009;29:1669–1688.

History

▶ 54-year-old women with history of rectosigmoid colectomy with primary anastomosis for colon carcinoma. Routine follow-up examination.

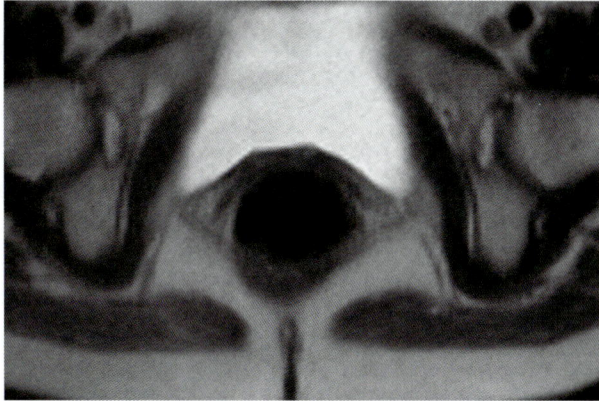

A

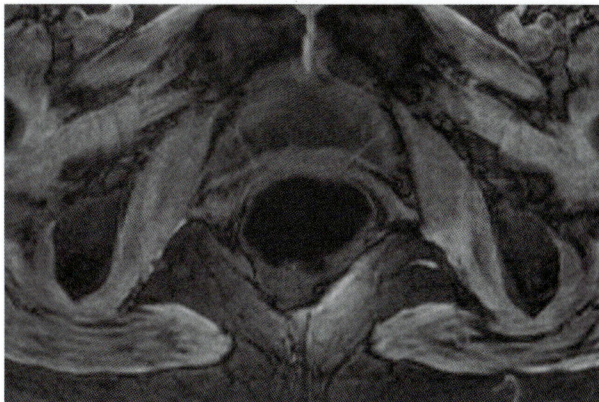

B

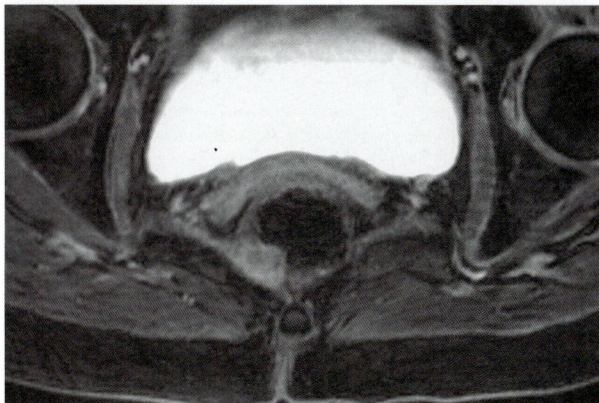

C

A. Axial T2-weighted single-shot FSE/TSE, **B**. Axial pre-contrast-enhanced and (**C**) post-gadolinium contrast-enhanced T1-weighted gradient echo with fat saturation.

Case 12   Recurrent Adenocarcinoma of the Colon

Findings

▶ Nodular wall thickening at the anastomosis shows enhancement following gadolinium contrast material administration. Biopsy of nodule revealed adenocarcinoma.

Differential diagnosis

▶ Postsurgical granulation tissue/scarring—post-radiation fibrosis

Teaching points

▶ Colorectal carcinoma recurs in approximately one third of patients following surgical resection. Half of the recurrences are detected within 1 year of resection and 70% to 80% are detected within 2 years. Approximately 3% to 5% of patients develop a second primary colon cancer at a different location.

▶ Recurrence is most common locally at the colonic anastomosis (60% of recurrences). Distant metastases occur in 26% and local recurrence plus distant metastases occur in 14%.

▶ Recurrent colon cancers display moderately high signal intensity on T2-weighted images and relatively low signal intensity on T1-weighted images. Moderate enhancement post-gadolinium contrast material administration is typical.

▶ Post-radiation fibrosis may show increased signal intensity on T2-weighted images for up to 1 year, and may show contrast enhancement for 1.5 to 2 years following treatment. After 1 year post-radiation fibrosis shows low signal intensity on both T1- and T2-weighted images. However, postsurgical granulation tissue may demonstrate high signal intensity for up to 3 years following surgery. Differentiation is made by shape, changes over time, and clinical factors. Recurrent tumor is usually nodular in shape, while fibrosis and granulation tissue is typically linear, plaque-like and shows stranding. Fibrosis contracts over time while recurrent tumor grows. Diffusion-weighted images (not shown) may be helpful for differentiating between tumor and scar tissue. Recurrence of pain and elevation of carcinoembryonic antigen (CEA) levels suggest tumor recurrence.

Management

▶ Colonoscopic or image-guided biopsy is needed for pathologic confirmation.

Further reading

1. Brant WE, Lambert DL. Gastrointestinal tract, peritoneal cavity, and spleen MR imaging. In: Brant WE, de Lange EE (eds), Essentials of Body MRI. New York: Oxford University Press, 2012.
2. de Lange EE, Fechner RE, Wanebo HJ. Suspected recurrent rectosigmoid carcinoma after abdomino-perineal resection: MR imaging and histopathologic correlation. Radiology 1989;170;323–328.
3. Sugimura K, Carrington BM, Quivey JM, Hricak H. Postirradiation changes in the pelvis: assessment with MR imaging. Radiology 1990;175:805–813.

History

▶ 33-year-old woman with twin pregnancy at 14 weeks' gestation presents with worsening right lower quadrant pain. Ultrasound examination was equivocal.

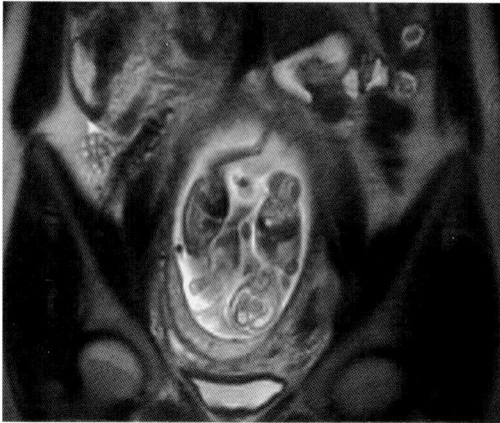

A

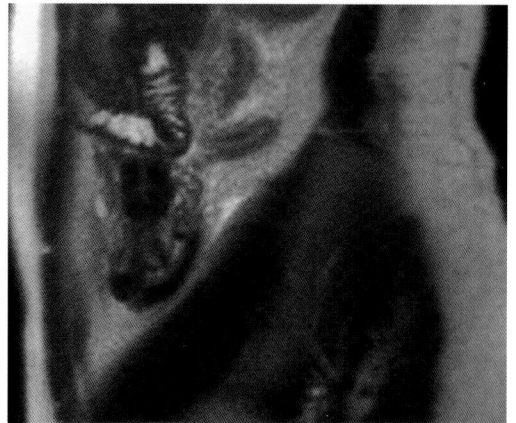

B

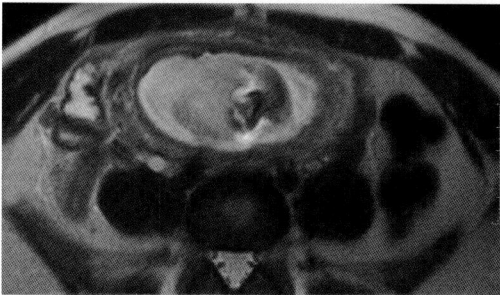

C

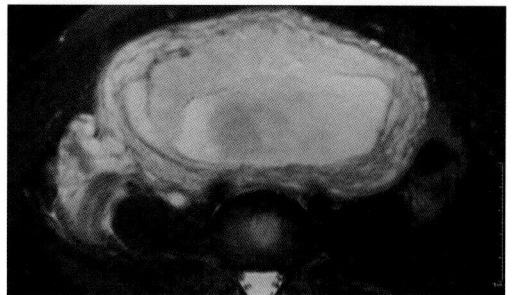

D

A. Coronal, (**B**) sagittal, and (**C**) axial T2-weighted single-shot FSE/TSE. **D**. Axial T2-weighted FSE/TSE with fat saturation.

Case 13 Acute Appendicitis in Pregnancy

Findings

▶ T2-weighted images (**A**, **B**, **C**) show a dilated (8 mm in diameter), thick-walled (3 mm), fluid-filled appendix.

▶ The T2-weighted image with fat saturation (**D**) shows periappendiceal high signal intensity indicative of inflammation and edema.

▶ Note the relatively high position of the appendix in the right mid-abdomen (**A**). The appendix is displaced by the enlarged uterus containing the twin pregnancy.

▶ The diagnosis was confirmed at surgery.

Differential diagnosis

▶ Terminal ileitis
▶ Diverticulitis
▶ Colitis

Teaching points

▶ Ultrasound is generally considered the imaging method of choice for assessing the appendix in a pregnant patient with abdominal pain. However, ultrasound is limited by dependence on a skilled operator. Further, the appendix is considerably more difficult to identify in the pregnant patient than when there is no pregnancy, and the examination may be equivocal. A non–contrast-enhanced MR study then becomes the imaging method of choice. Gadolinium contrast agent is not approved for use in pregnancy.

▶ A normal appendix can be visualized with MR in 85% of pregnant patients. In the second and third trimester the gravid uterus displaces the appendix superiorly into the right mid-abdomen or sometimes even into the right upper quadrant. The normal appendix measures less than 6 mm in diameter with wall thickness less than 2 mm and commonly contains air or orally administered contrast material. On T2-weighted images the wall of the appendix displays low signal intensity whereas the mucosa/submucosa shows high signal intensity. On T1-weighted images the normal appendix is uniformly low in signal intensity.

▶ In acute appendicitis the appendix is filled with fluid and exceeds 7 mm in diameter. The wall thickness commonly exceeds 2 mm. Periappendiceal inflammation appears on T2-weighted images as a high-signal-intensity band surrounding the appendix. On MR the appendix is best visualized on single-shot FSE/TSE images. Periappendiceal edema is best visualized on fat-suppressed T2-weighted images. Rupture of the appendix often results in an abscess cavity shown as a fluid collection confined by a well-defined wall. Acute appendicitis may be confined to the tip of the appendix, and hence it is important that the entire appendix be assessed for diagnosing the condition.

Management

▶ Appendectomy

Further reading

1. Basaran A, Basaran M. Diagnosis of acute appendicitis during pregnancy: a systematic review. Obstet Gynecol Surv 2009;64:481–488.
2. Heverhagan JT., Klose KJ. MR imaging for acute lower abdominal and pelvic pain. RadioGraphics 2009;29:1781–1796.
3. Pedrosa I, Zeikus EA, Levine D, Rofsky NM. MR imaging of acute right lower quadrant pain in pregnant and nonpregnant patients. RadioGraphics 2007;27:721–753.

History

▶ 55-year-old man with history of pancreatitis presents with increasing epigastric pain.

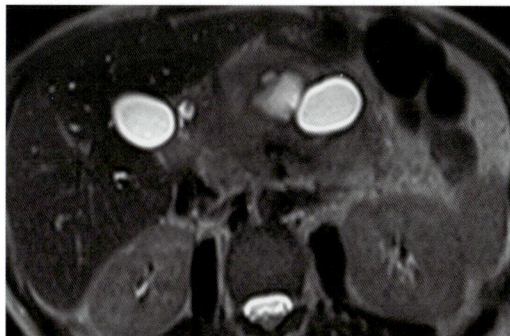

A

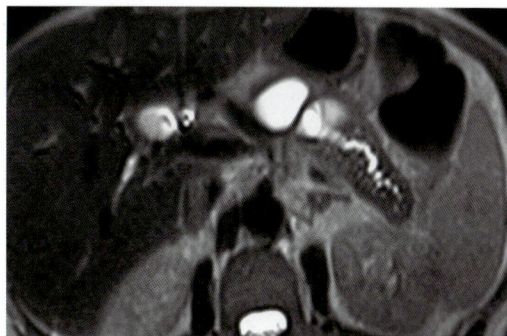

B

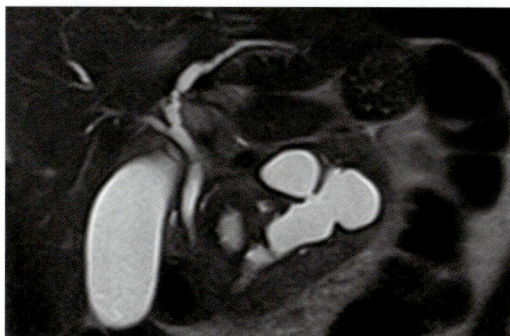

C

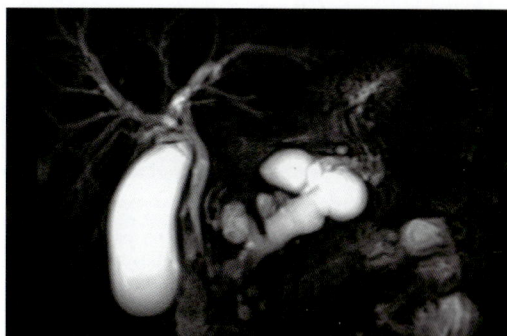

D

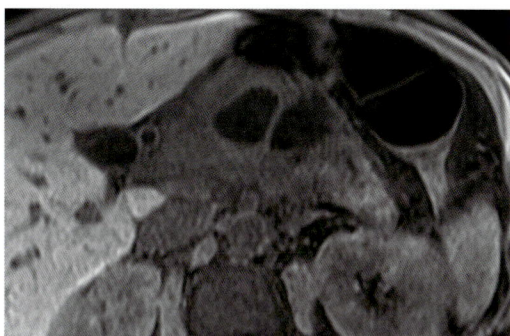

E

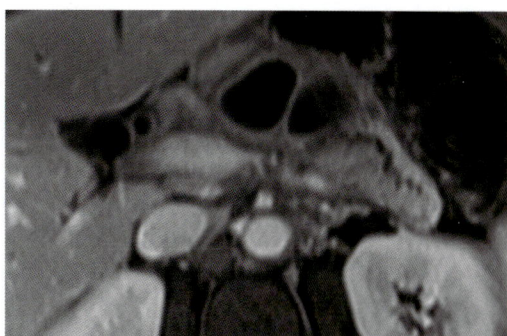

F

A, B. Axial T2-weighted single-shot FSE/TSE at different levels. **C**. Coronal T2-weighted single-shot FSE. **D**. Thick-slab MRCP using single-shot FSE/TSE. **E**. Axial pre-contrast and (**F**) post-gadolinium contrast-enhanced gradient echo with fat saturation.

Case 14 Acute-On-Chronic Severe Pancreatitis

Findings

- ▶ Enlarged pancreatic head with increased signal intensity on T2-weighted images
- ▶ Decreased parenchymal signal on T1-weighted fat-suppressed images
- ▶ Poor, delayed enhancement of the pancreatic head and body corresponding to the edematous tissue
- ▶ Marked dilatation of the main and side-branch pancreatic ducts

Differential diagnosis

- ▶ Intraductal papillary mucinous neoplasm (IPMN)—main duct type
- ▶ Pancreatic adenocarcinoma with pancreatic ductal obstruction
- ▶ Pseudocyst

Teaching points

- ▶ Findings of early chronic pancreatitis include low-signal-intensity pancreatic parenchyma on T1-weighted fat-suppressed images, delayed and diminished parenchymal enhancement following intravenous gadolinium contrast material administration, and dilatation of the side branches of the pancreatic duct.
- ▶ Findings seen in longstanding chronic pancreatitis include pancreatic atrophy, masslike focal enlargement of the pancreatic parenchyma, and beaded dilatation of the pancreatic duct with areas of stricture.
- ▶ The degree of decreased or delayed enhancement helps to differentiate involved fibrotic parenchyma from viable parenchyma.
- ▶ The extent of main pancreatic duct dilatation and the number of dilated side branches predict the degree of severity of chronic pancreatitis.

Management

- ▶ Supportive medical management
- ▶ Placement of a pancreatic duct stent
- ▶ Pancreatic transplant

Further reading

1. Balci NC, Bieneman BK, Bilgin M, Akduman, et al. Magnetic resonance imaging in pancreatitis. Top Magn Reson Imaging 2009;20:25–30.
2. Miller FH, Keppke AL, Wadhwa A, et al. MRI of pancreatitis and its complications: part 2, chronic pancreatitis. AJR Am J Roentgenol 2004;183:1645–1652.
3. Sandrasegaran K, Lin C, Akisik FM, Tann M. State-of-the-art pancreatic MRI. AJR Am J Roentgenol 2010;195:42–53.

History

▶ 48-year-old man with abnormal liver function tests.

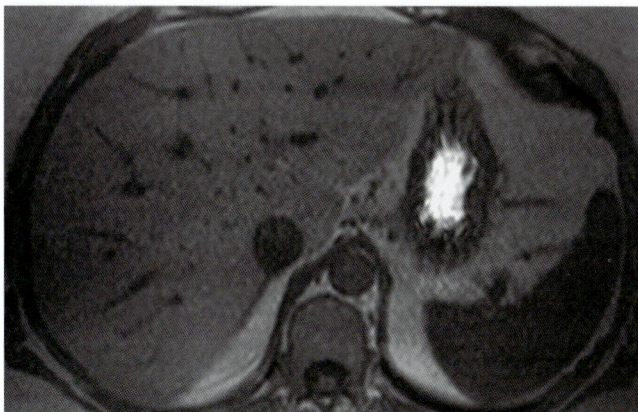

A

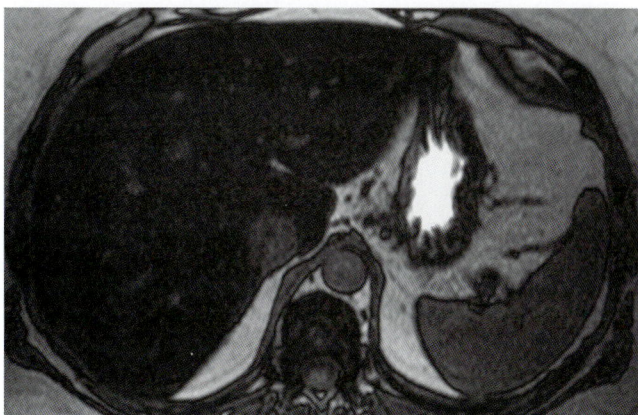

B

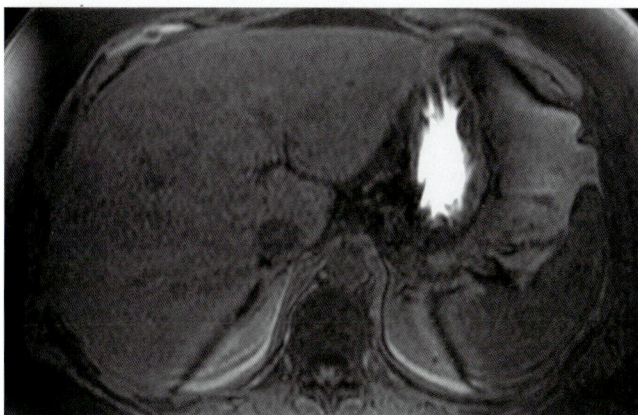

C

A. Axial in-phase and (**B**) opposed-phase T1-weighted gradient echo. **C**. Axial unenhanced T1-weighted gradient echo with fat saturation.

Case 15   Hepatic Steatosis (Diffuse Fatty Liver)

Findings

▶ The liver parenchyma shows a marked decrease in signal intensity on the phase-opposed image (B) compared with the in-phase gradient-echo image (A). This finding is highly indicative of fatty liver.

▶ The fat-suppressed image (C) shows only little signal loss of the liver parenchyma.

Differential diagnosis

Hemochromatosis

Teaching points

▶ Hepatic steatosis, the accumulation of fat within hepatocytes, is the most common cause of chronic liver disease in both children and adults in the United States.

▶ Fatty liver has numerous causes including excessive alcohol use, chemotherapy and numerous medications and liver toxins, malnutrition, total parenteral nutrition, glycogen storage disease, severe weight loss, hepatitis C, and human immunodeficiency virus infection.

▶ Non-alcoholic steatohepatitis (NASH) is one of the most common causes of hepatic steatosis, involving up to 20% of patients with fatty liver and up to 3% of Americans overall. Obesity, commonly associated with diabetes, is the major risk factor for NASH. NASH progresses to cirrhosis in 3% to 10% of cases and to liver failure in 2% to 3% of cases.

▶ Chemical shift (in-phase/opposed-phase gradient-echo) imaging takes advantage of the fact that the hydrogen nuclei in water-containing tissue precess faster than those in fat. The difference in precessional frequency between the protons in water and fat causes periodic variation in signal when a voxel contains a mixture of water and fat. When an echo time (TE) is chosen at which the fat and water signals within the same voxel are in phase the signals are summed, and when the TE is chosen at which the fat and water signals are out of phase the signals cancel. An organ or lesion that shows decrease in signal on out-of-phase images compared to in-phase images is composed of a mixture of water and fat. Absence of signal loss on the out-of-phase image indicates that the organ or lesion contains only water or only fat. In this example, there is almost complete loss of signal on the out-of-phase image, indicating that the signals for water and fat are about equal.

Further reading

1. Cassidy FH, Yokoo T, Aganovic L, et al. Fatty liver disease: MR imaging techniques for the detection and quantification of liver steatosis. RadioGraphics 2009;29:231–260.
2. de Lange EE, Mugler JP III. Basic MR physics. In: Brant WE, de Lange EE. Essentials of Body MR Imaging. New York: Oxford University Press, 2012.
3. Lall CG, Aisen AM, Bansal N, Sandrasegaran K. Nonalcoholic fatty liver disease. AJR Am J Roentgenol 2008;190:993–1002.

History

▶ 65-year-woman who developed gross hematuria.

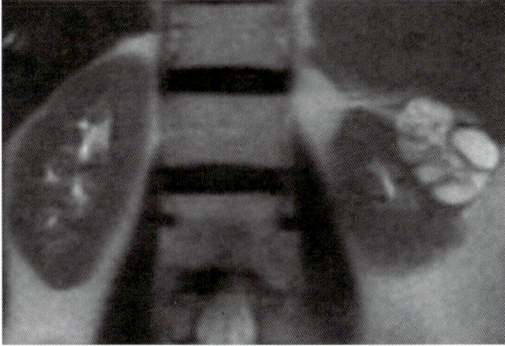

A

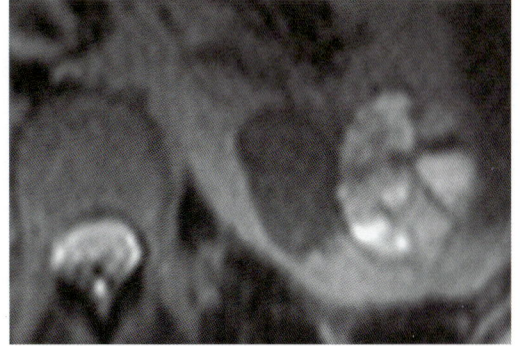

B

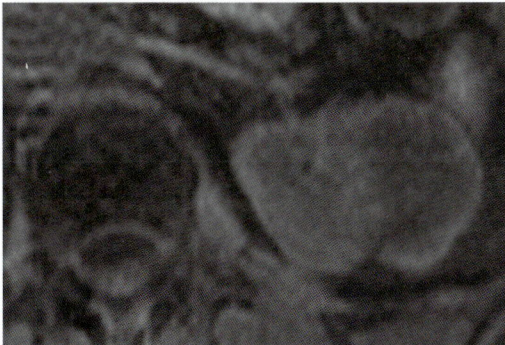

C

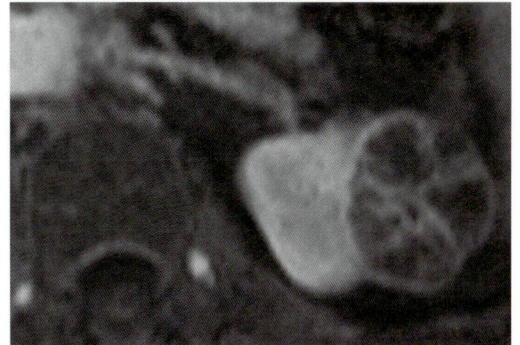

D

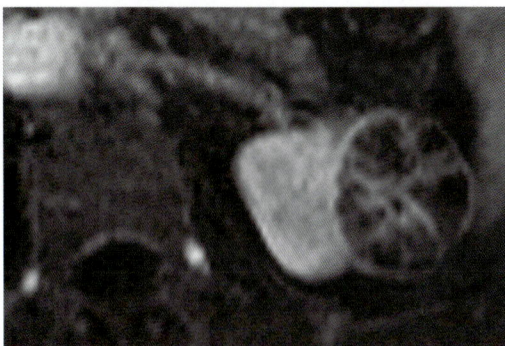

E

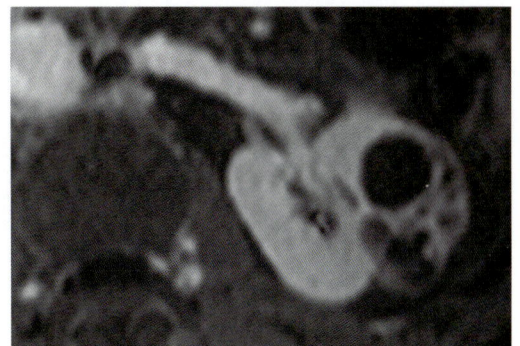

F

A. Coronal and (**B**) axial T2-weighted single-shot FSE/TSE. **C**. Axial pre- and (**D**) post- gadolinium contrast-enhanced (nephrographic phase) T1-weighted gradient echo with fat saturation, and (**E**) subtraction image of **D. F**. Pyelographic-phase subtraction image from a level slightly caudad to **E**.

Case 16   Multiloculated Cystic Mass, Bosniak Classification III

Findings

- ▶ A multiloculated cystic mass arises from the upper mid-pole of the left kidney.
- ▶ The septations within the mass are of variable thickness.
- ▶ The wall, septa, and solid components of the mass show distinct contrast enhancement.

Differential diagnosis

- ▶ Multilocular cystic nephroma
- ▶ Multilocular cystic renal cell carcinoma
- ▶ Multilocular benign cyst

Teaching points

- ▶ The Bosniak classification of renal cysts, first published in 1986, is widely used by urologists and radiologists to classify renal cysts as: benign simple cyst (Bosniak I), definitely benign complicated cyst (II), indeterminate benign or malignant multilocular cyst (III), and definitely malignant cystic mass (IV). While initially applied to CT, the criteria for classification have been extended to MR imaging.
- ▶ The complex cystic renal mass (Bosniak category III) is the most problematic as these lesions may be either benign or malignant. The class III cystic mass is characterized by grossly thickened wall or septa, which show distinct contrast enhancement. Etiologies that may fall into this category include chronic abscess, chronically infected renal cyst, hemorrhagic cyst, benign complex multiloculated cyst, benign localized renal cystic disease, multilocular cystic nephroma, and the multiloculated cystic form of renal cell carcinoma. The malignant tumor is characterized by clear cell carcinoma lining the walls and septa of the cystic mass.
- ▶ Prior imaging, evolution of findings, or stability over time may assist in characterizing the class III cystic mass as likely benign. Biopsy is usually not helpful, as a biopsy showing benign tissue does not exclude malignancy in these lesions.

Management

- ▶ Surgical removal is generally recommended for Bosniak class III cystic lesions. Imaging follow-up is an alternative in patients who are not considered to be safe surgical candidates.

Further reading

1. Bosniak MA. The current radiological approach to renal cysts. Radiology 1986;158:1–10.
2. Freire M, Remer EM. Clinical and radiologic features of cystic renal masses. AJR Am J Roentgenol 2009;192:1367–1372.
3. Hartman DS, Choyke PL, Hartman MS. A practical approach to the cystic renal mass. RadioGraphics 2004;24:S101–S115.
4. Israel GM, Bosniak MA. Pitfalls in renal mass evaluation and how to avoid them. RadioGraphics 2008;28:1325–1338.

History

▶ 39-year-old man with longstanding type 2 diabetes presents with abdominal pain, and was incidentally found to have elevated troponin cardiac enzymes, and inferior Q waves and lateral repolarization abnormalities on electrocardiography.

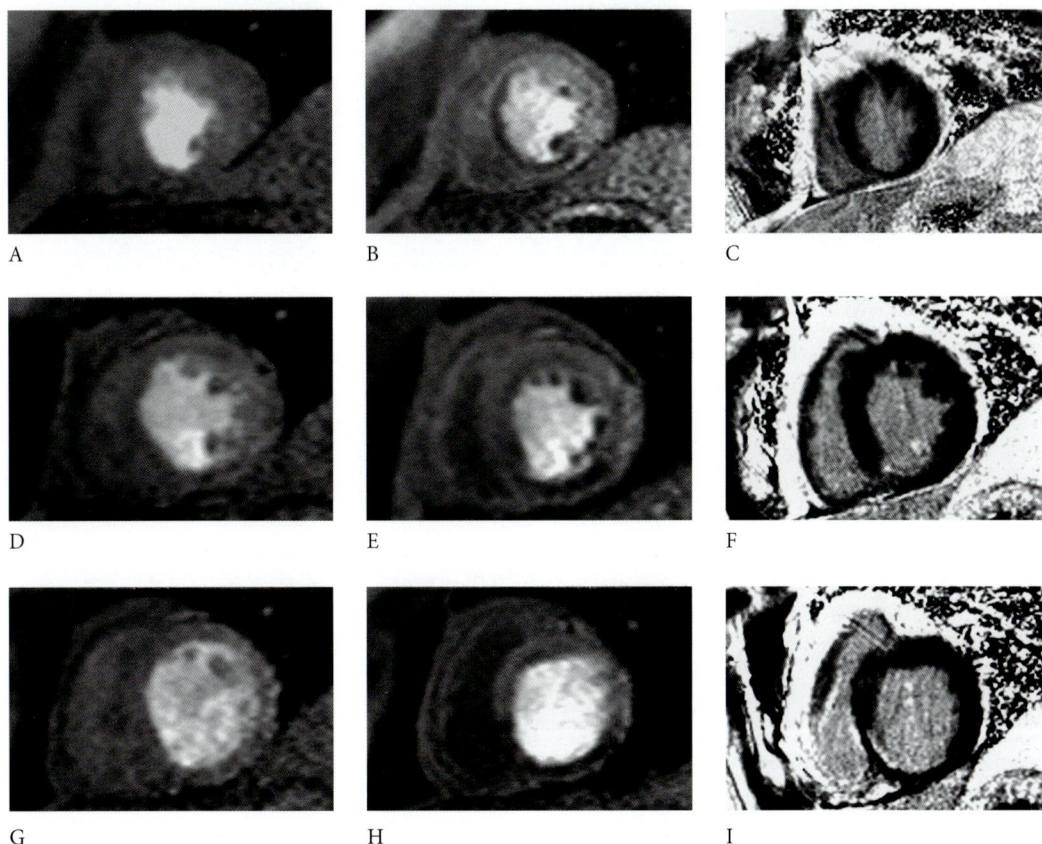

Short-axis views of the left ventricle (apex, midportion, and base) during rest (left column) and adenosine stress (middle column) perfusion imaging using gradient echo with segmented echo-planar readout and late gadolinium-enhanced (LGE) phase-sensitive inversion recovery (PSIR) gradient echo (right column). **A**. Apical at rest and (**B**) with stress. **C**. Apical LGE. **D**. Mid at rest and (**E**) with stress. **F**. Mid LGE. **G**. Base at rest and (**H**) with stress. **I**. Base LGE.

Case 17 Chronic Myocardial Infarction in the RCA Territory with Stress-Induced Myocardial Ischemia in the LAD and LCx Territory

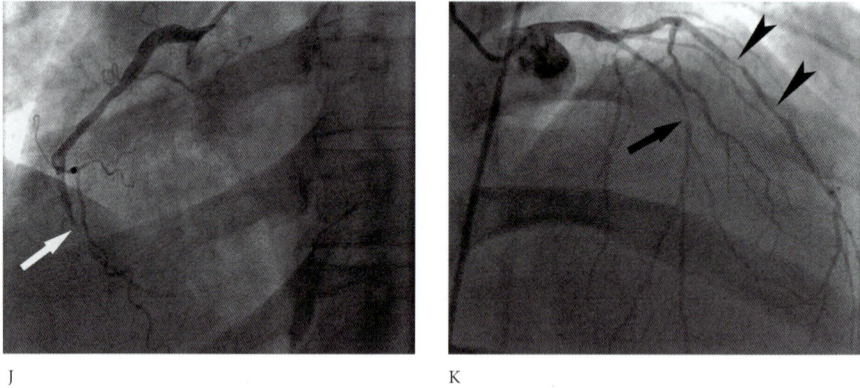

J

K

Findings

▶ Dense perfusion defects on stress imaging in the inferior wall (**E, H**) correlating with subendocardial infarction in the same location, demonstrated on late gadolinium enhancement (LGE) imaging (**F, I**)

▶ Stress-induced ischemia without infarction in the apical septum (**B**) and septum, anterior, and lateral wall of the mid-ventricle (**E**)

▶ Right coronary angiogram (J) Angiogram shows occluded (*arrow*) mid-right coronary artery (RCA). Left Main coronary angiogram (K) shows and high-grade tandem stenoses in the left anterior coronary artery (LAD) (*arrowheads*) and obtuse marginal artery (*arrow*), a branch of the left circumflex artery (LCx).

Teaching points

▶ Subendocardial late gadolinium enhancement isolated to a coronary vascular territory is specific for myocardial infarction. Adenosine stress imaging demonstrates reduced perfusion.

▶ Chronic myocardial infarctions demonstrate late enhancement and thinning of the myocardium.

▶ Using adenosine, stress-induced ischemia appears as subendocardial hypoperfusion not seen at rest.

▶ Subendocardial low signal intensity on both rest and stress images is indicative of artifact.

▶ Myocardium is considered viable if the territory has subendocardial enhancement that involves less than 50% of the wall thickness.

Management

▶ Intervention during a myocardial infarction is aimed at rapid restoration of coronary blood flow. This is performed using thrombolytic agents or mechanical devices, such as stents and/or angioplasty.

▶ Coronary artery bypass grafting is used to revascularize multiple coronary artery territories. Cardiac MR imaging can be used to determine which coronary territories have viable myocardium appropriate for revascularization.

Further reading

1. Norton PT. Cardiac MR imaging. In: Brant WE, de Lange EE (eds), Essentials of Body MR Imaging. New York: Oxford University Press, 2012.
2. Reeder SB, Du YP, Lima JA, Bluemke DA. Advanced cardiac MR imaging of ischemic heart disease. RadioGraphics 2001;21:1047–1074.

▶ 54-year-old woman with history of endometrial carcinoma. MR imaging is performed for a lesion seen on CT in the posterior aspect of the left liver lobe (segment 2) suspicious for metastasis.

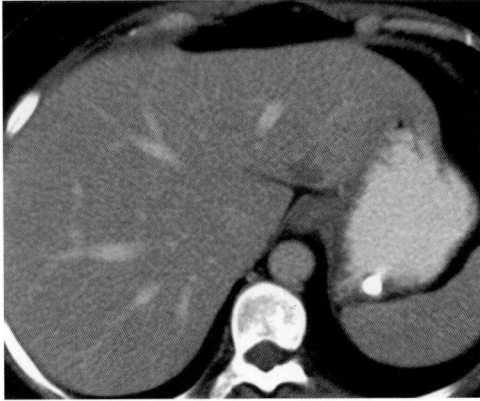

A

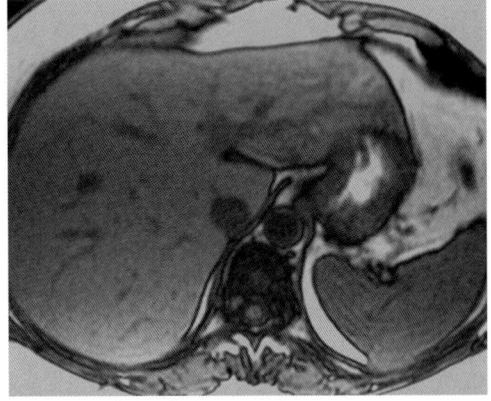

B

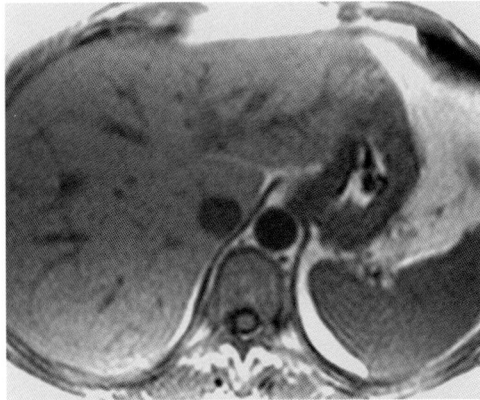

C

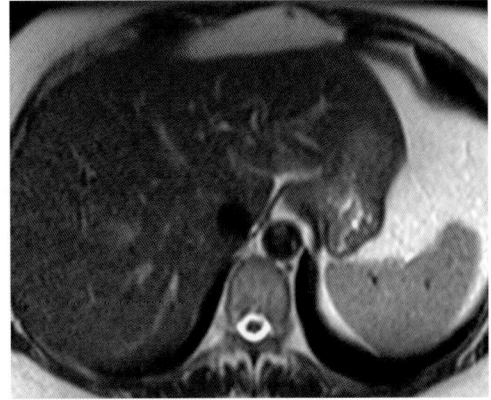

D

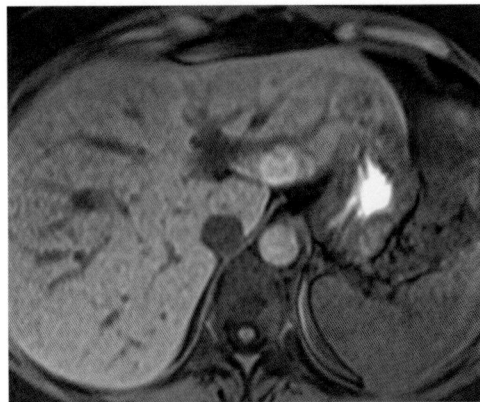

E

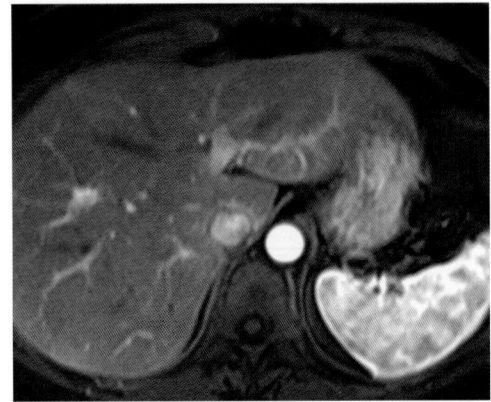

F

A. Axial CT. **B**. Axial opposed-phase and (**C**) in-phase T1-weighted gradient echo. **D**. Axial T2-weighted single-shot FSE/TSE.
E. Pre-contrast-enhanced and (**F**) arterial-phase post-gadolinium contrast-enhanced T1-weighted gradient echo with fat saturation.

Case 18 Flow Artifact

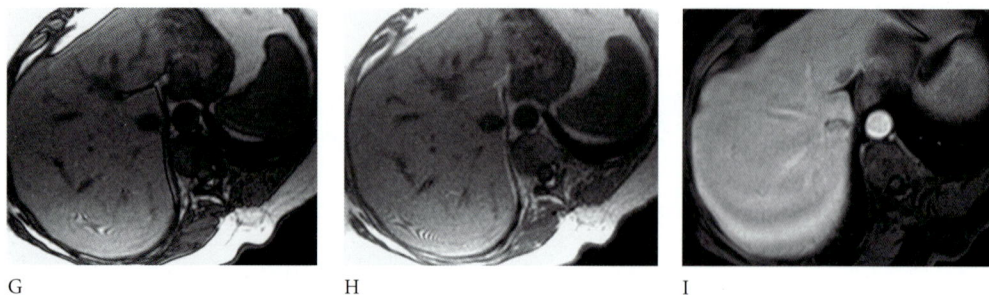

G

H

I

Findings

▶ On the opposed-phase (**B**) image there is a focal area of decreased signal at the posterior margin of segment 2 compared to the in-phase (**C**) image suggestive of fatty infiltration; however, assessment is hampered by flow artifact from the aorta obscuring the area.

▶ The lesion displays slightly increased signal intensity on the T2-weighted image (**D**).

▶ Pre- and post-gadolinium contrast-enhanced images (**E, F**) are of limited value because of flow artifact from the aorta obscuring the area.

▶ Flow artifact from the aorta over the area of interest makes it difficult to definitively determine whether there is a real lesion or focal fatty infiltration.

Teaching points

▶ Flow artifact from vessels is primarily seen in the phase-encoding direction and resembles the shape of the vessel, in this case the aorta.

▶ Flow artifacts from vessels can be suppressed by adding presaturation pulses.

▶ In this case a spatial presaturation RF pulse was placed cranial to the most superior slice of the image set of the gradient-echo sequence to suppress the signal from blood flowing in the craniocaudal direction, as in the aorta. However, despite the presaturation pulse flow artifacts from the aorta were not completely suppressed, obscuring the area of interest in the liver.

▶ In the T2-weighted single-shot FSE/TSE image (**B**) there are no flow artifacts associated with the blood flowing in the aorta and because the blood that flows into the slice section does not experience the 90° excitation RF pulse that initiates the echo train and hence provides no signal contribution.

Management

▶ Increase the thickness of the presaturation pulse to better suppress signal from inflowing blood

▶ Obtain images with the patient partially turned on the right side as shown (**G,** opposed-phase; **H,** in-phase; **I,** late-phase contrast-enhanced gradient-echo) so that pulsation artifacts from the aorta do not obscure the liver. The diagnosis of focal fatty infiltration can now be definitely made.

Further reading

1. de Lange EE, Mugler JP. MR Acquisition Techniques & Practical Considerations for Abdominal Imaging. In: Brant WE, de Lange EE (eds), Essentials of Body MR Imaging. New York: Oxford University Press, 2012.

History

▶ Incidental finding at MR imaging performed to evaluate biliary colic

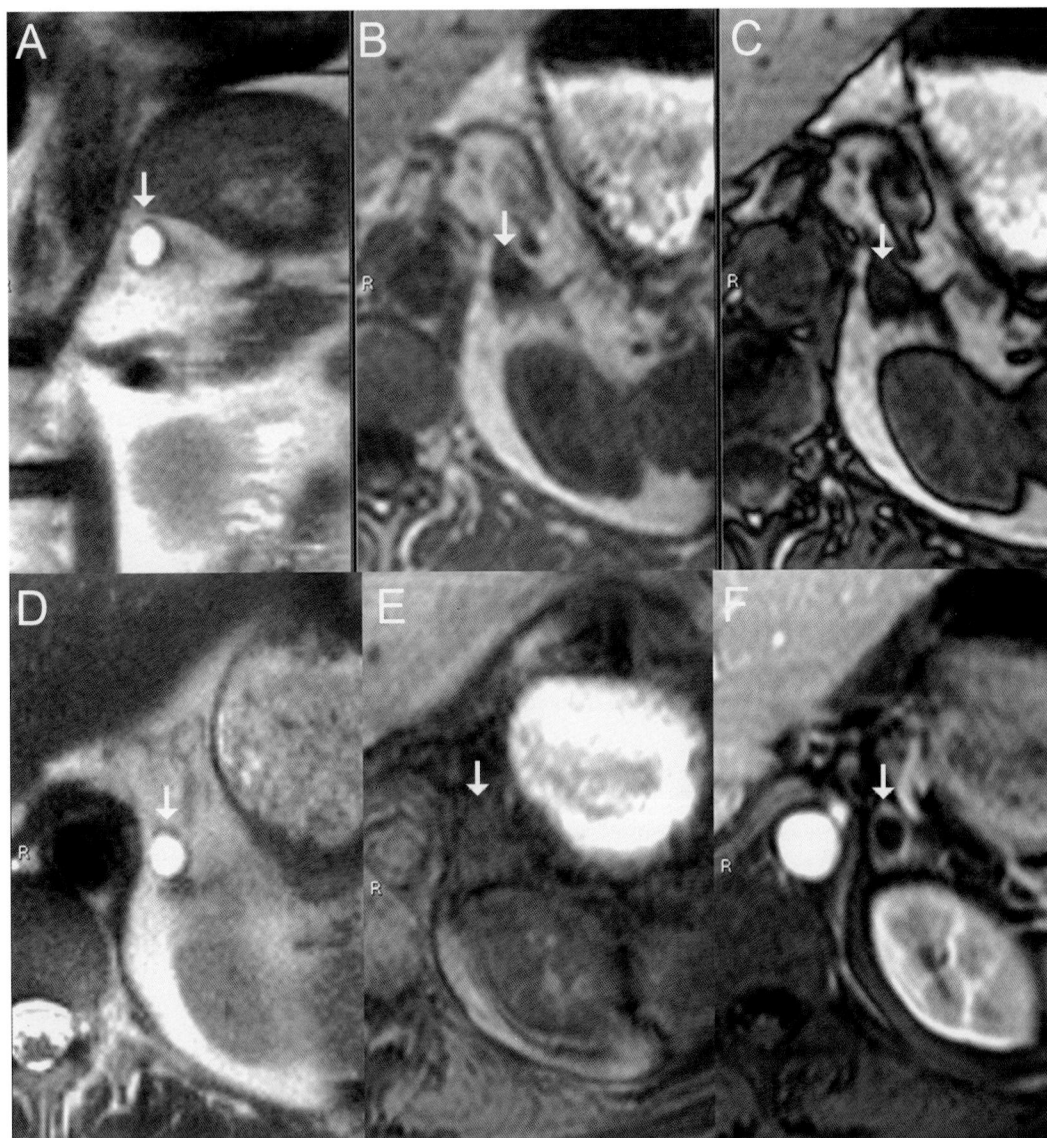

A. Coronal T2-weighted single-shot FSE/TSE. (**B**) Axial in-phase and (**C**) opposed-phase T1-weighted gradient echo. **D**. Axial T2-weighted single-shot FSE/TSE. **E**. Pre- and (**F**) post-gadolinium contrast-enhanced axial T1-weighted gradient echo with fat saturation.

Case 19 Benign Simple Adrenal Cyst

Findings

- A small well-defined round left adrenal mass (*arrows*) follows the signal intensity of simple fluid on all sequences and does not enhance.
- High-signal-intensity lesion on T2-weighted images (**A** and **D**)
- Low-signal-intensity lesion on T1-weighted images (**B** and **C**)
- No signal-intensity loss on opposed-phase (**C**) compared with in-phase image (**B**)
- The limbs of the adrenal gland surrounding the lesion enhance following gadolinium-based contrast material administration (**F**), but no enhancement is present inside the lesion.

Differential diagnosis

- Adrenal hematoma
- Adrenal pseudocyst
- Cystic pheochromocytoma
- Cystic primary adrenal carcinoma

Teaching points

- This lesion contains simple fluid and is well defined with no internal enhancing elements, which is indicative of a simple adrenal cyst.
- Adrenal hematomas demonstrate signal characteristics of hemorrhage and evolve to resolution over time.
- Adrenal pseudocysts are more complex than simple adrenal cysts, showing calcification, hemorrhage, or complex fluid, and occasionally enhancing elements.
- There are case reports of cystic pheochromocytomas and cystic adrenal cortical carcinomas, but in these the solid components were not detectable on imaging.

Management

- Simple adrenal cysts can be followed over time with imaging to confirm stability.
- Pheochromocytoma can be excluded biochemically.
- Adrenal cysts can be surgically removed if symptomatic.

Further reading

1. Erickson LA, Lloyd RV, Hartman R, Thompson G. Cystic adrenal neoplasms. Cancer 2004;101:1537–1544.
2. Ishigami K, Stolpen AH, Sato Y, et al. Adrenal adenoma with organizing hematoma: diagnostic dilemma at MRI. Magn Reson Imaging 2004;22:1157–1159.
3. Lal TG, Kaulback KR, Bombonati A, et al. Surgical management of adrenal cysts. Am Surg 2003;69:812–814.
4. Nigawara T, Sakihara S, Kageyama K, et al. Endothelial cyst of the adrenal gland associated with adrenocortical adenoma: preoperative images simulate carcinoma. Internal Medicine 2009;48:235–240.

History

▶ 53-year-old man with weight loss of 16 kg over 7 months

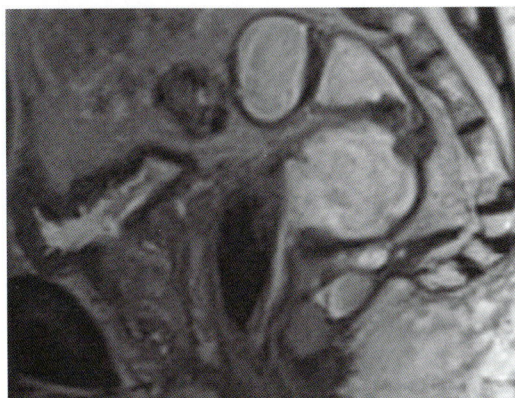

A

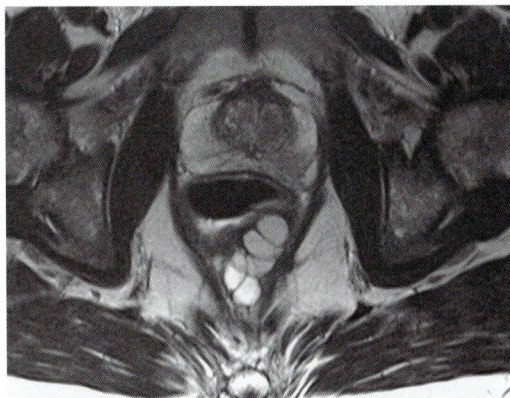

B

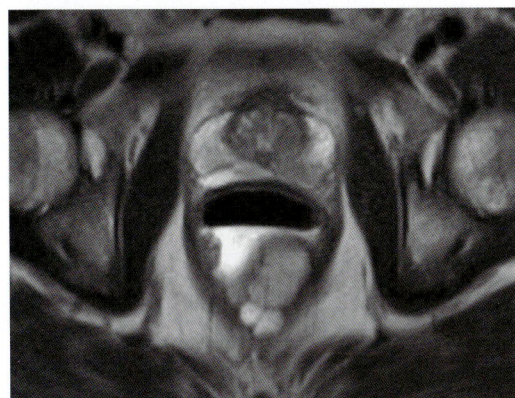

C

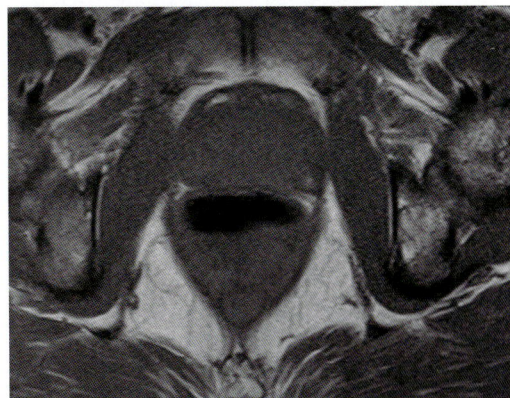

D

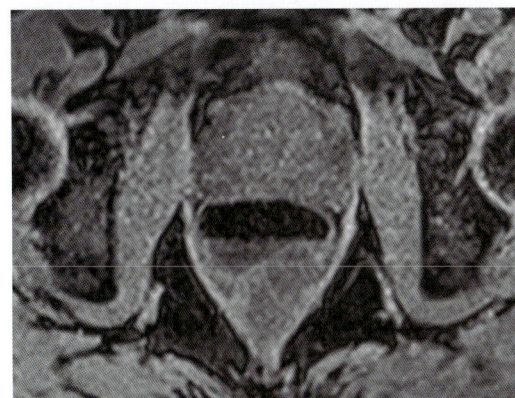

E

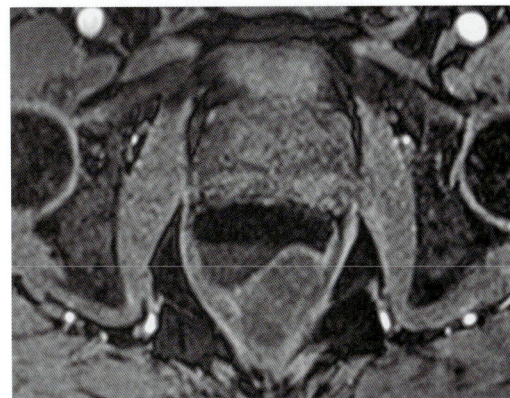

F

A. Sagittal and (**B, C**) axial T2-weighted FSE/TSE at different levels. **D**. Axial T1-weighted spin echo. **E**. Pre- and (**F**) post-contrast-enhanced T1-weighted gradient echo with fat saturation.

Case 20 Tailgut Cyst, also called a Retrorectal Cystic Hamartoma

Findings

- Well-defined multiloculated cystic lesion seen posterior to the rectum but not infiltrating the surrounding structures
- Low-signal-intensity component inferiorly in image **A** represents proteinaceous material or hemorrhage.
- No enhancing wall, septum, or soft tissue nodule
- Note that the sacrum and coccyx are normal.

Differential diagnosis

Multilocular Cyst
- Tailgut cyst
- Cystic lymphangioma

Unilocular Cyst
- Epidermoid cyst
- Dermoid cyst
- Rectal duplication cyst
- Anterior meningocele (associated with bony defect)

Teaching points

- Tailgut cyst or retrorectal cystic hamartoma is a rare congenital lesion. The remnants of the primitive gut that fail to regress are believed to form tailgut cysts. More common in women, tailgut cysts are asymptomatic but may be found in patients with constipation or abdominal pain.
- MRI is the recommended imaging modality in evaluating tailgut cysts for diagnosis and determination of resectability.

Management

- Complete surgical excision is the treatment of choice because of the risk of malignant transformation.
- Biopsy should not be attempted because of the risk of rupture and subsequent spread of dysplastic cells in the pelvis.

Further reading

1. Hjermstad BM, Helwig EB. Tailgut cysts. Report of 53 cases. Am J Clin Pathol 1988;89:139–147.
2. Yang DM, Park CH, Jin W, et al. Tailgut cyst: MRI evaluation. AJR Am J Roentgenol 2005;184:1519–1523.

History

▶ 52-year-old woman with abnormal liver function tests

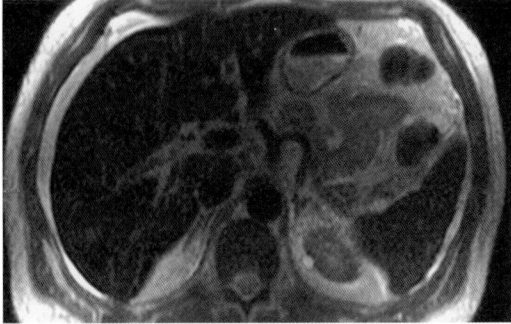

A

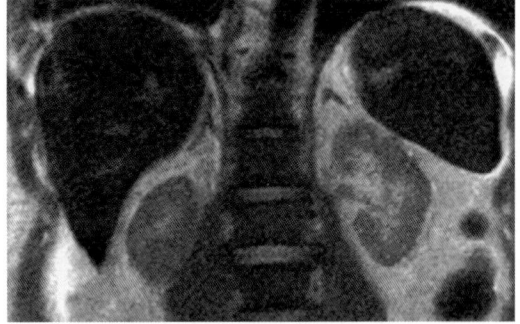

B

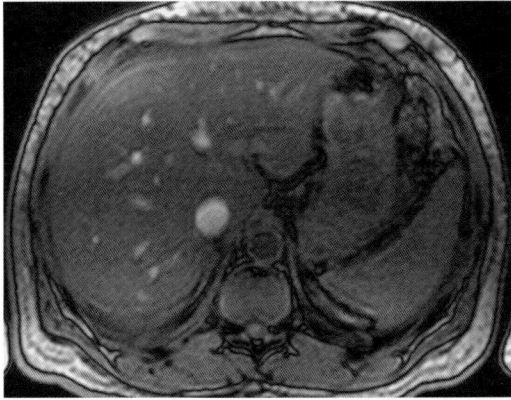

C

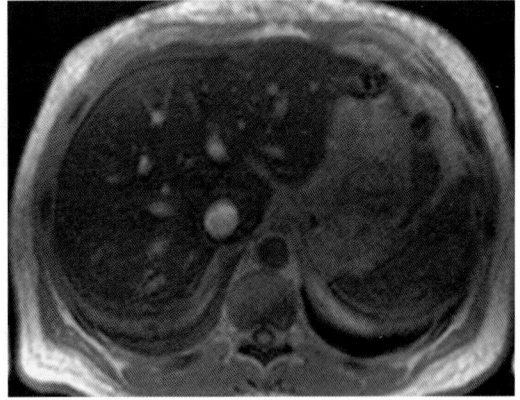

D

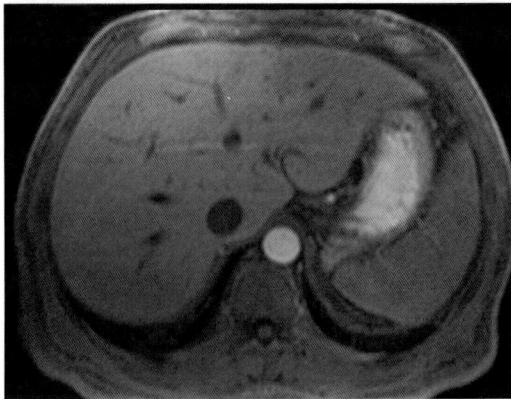

E

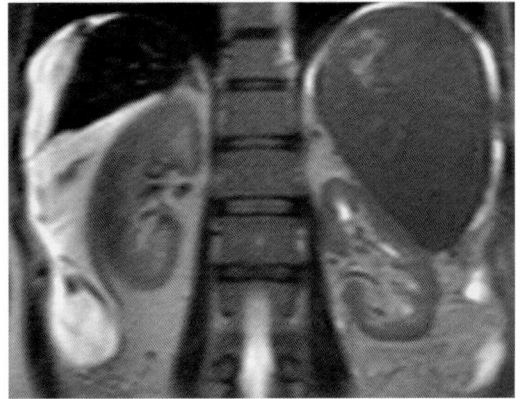

F

A. Axial and (**B**) coronal T2-weighted single-shot FSE/TSE. **C**. Axial phase-opposed (TE 2.4 ms) and (**D**) in-phase (TE 4.8 ms) T1-weighted gradient echo. **E**. Axial arterial-phase T1-weighted gradient echo with fat saturation. **F**. Coronal T2-weighted single-shot FSE/TSE image obtained in a different patient than figures **A–E**.

Case 21 Hemochromatosis (reticuloendothelial pattern), hemochromatosis-gene negative, secondary hemochromatosis

Findings

► T2-weighted images (**A, B**) show low signal intensity in liver, spleen, and bone marrow.
► On gradient-echo images (**D, C**) signal loss is greatest on the image obtained with the longest TE.
► T1-weighted image with fat saturation (**E**) shows no abnormalities.
► Findings represent a reticuloendothelial pattern of excessive iron deposition.
► T2-weighted image of a comparison patient (**F**) with the parenchymal pattern of iron deposition shows low liver signal, and normal spleen and bone signal.

Teaching points

► Primary hemochromatosis is an autosomal recessive disorder that promotes an increase in iron absorption from the gut.
► Secondary hemochromatosis refers to nongenetic causes of excess iron accumulation such as multiple blood transfusions, excessive iron ingestion or parenteral administration, and excess iron absorption. Hemosiderosis refers to excess deposition of hemosiderin and is usually related to hemolytic disorders.
► The accumulated iron shortens T1, T2, and especially T2* relaxation times, resulting in a signal loss that is proportional to the iron deposition. Dual-echo gradient-echo images show a decrease in signal intensity on long-TE images compared to short TE-images. For most 1.5T scanners the opposed-phase image is obtained with short TE and the in-phase image with long TE. On these scanners the aforementioned effect is opposite to that seen with hepatosteatosis, in which case the liver signal is higher on the long-TE (in-phase) image compared to the short-TE (opposed-phase) image.
► The *parenchymal distribution pattern* is caused by excessive iron absorption. Excess iron is present in the liver, pancreas, and thyroid, sparing the spleen and bone marrow. This pattern of iron deposition is the most toxic.
► The *reticuloendothelial deposition pattern* is caused by multiple blood transfusions with iron deposition in the reticuloendothelial system of the liver, spleen, and bone marrow. This pattern is not associated with tissue damage.

Management

► Reticuloendothelial hemochromatosis is generally not treated. Treatment options for parenchymal hematomatosis include periodic phlebotomy and use of chelating agents.

Further reading

1. Queiroz-Andrade M, Blasbalg R, Ortega CD, et al. MR imaging findings of iron overload. RadioGraphics 2009;29:1575–1589.
2. Westphalen ACA, Qayyum A, Yeh BM, et al. Liver fat: effect of hepatic iron deposition on evaluation with opposed-phase MR imaging. Radiology 2007;242:450–456.

History

▶ 56-year-old woman with mass in the liver reported on outside CT

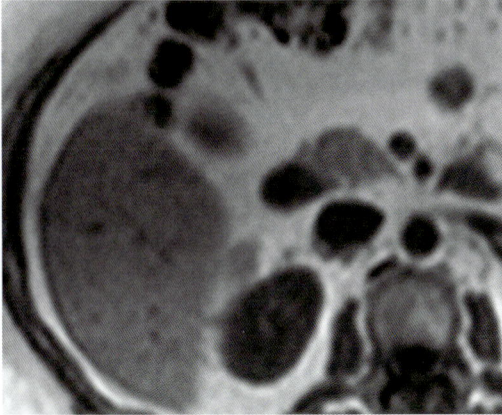

A

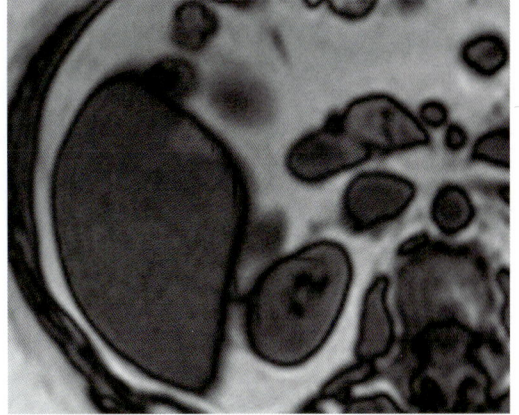

B

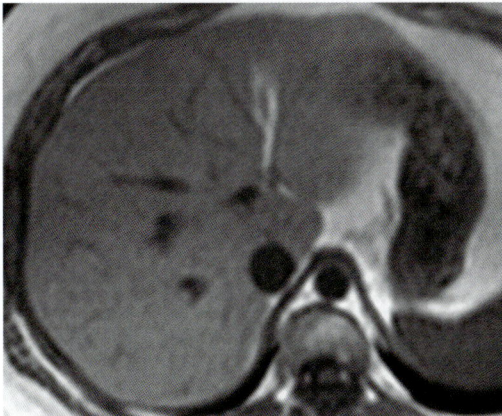

C

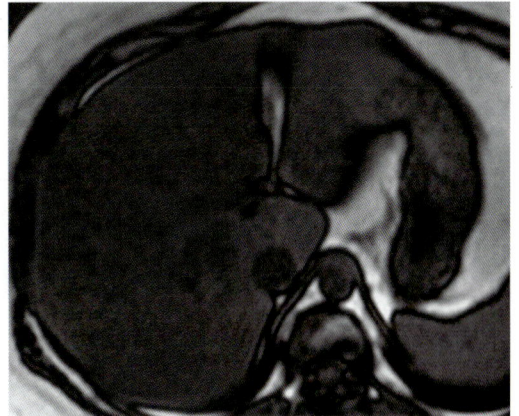

D

A, C. Axial in-phase and (**B, D**) opposed-phase T1-weighted gradient echo.

Case 22 Diffuse Hepatic Steatosis with Focal Fatty Sparing

Findings

▶ Opposed-phase (chemical shift) images show diffuse heterogeneous loss of signal intensity compared to in-phase images indicating hepatic steatosis.

▶ On the out-of-phase images focal sparing of fatty infiltration results in higher signal intensity than that of the remaining liver as seen in the caudate lobe and as a small triangular area at the gallbladder fossa margin of segment 5.

Differential diagnosis

▶ Metastatic disease

▶ Primary hepatic tumor

Teaching points

▶ Chemical-shift MR imaging has become the noninvasive imaging method of choice to detect the presence or absence of fat within the liver parenchyma or within liver nodules. The signal-intensity loss within a liver lesion on opposed-phase images indicates the presence of fat within the lesion. Conversely, the absence of signal loss on out-of-phase images indicates the absence of fat within the lesion. In the case that is shown the absence of signal loss indicates normal liver parenchyma that is spared from the fatty infiltration affecting the remainder of the liver.

▶ Focal fatty sparing occurs most commonly in the areas of the liver that are also most commonly affected by focal fatty infiltration. These include the areas of segments 4 and 5 near the gallbladder fossa, and the liver tissue adjacent to the porta hepatis and subcapsular regions. Focal fatty sparing, like focal fatty infiltration, is believed to be secondary to altered arterial or portal venous blood flow. In the region of the gallbladder fossa, the altered blood flow may be the result of changes in systemic venous drainage.

▶ Focal fatty sparing may also occur around liver lesions, especially metastases. This is because compression of the peritumoral liver parenchyma by the growing tumor alters the portal venous blood flow, which in turn can lead to the deposition of fat.

Management

▶ Recognition of the characteristic features of focal fatty sparing in the setting of diffuse hepatic steatosis will avoid diagnostic errors and unnecessary invasive procedures.

Further reading

1. Chung J-J, Kim M-J, Kim JH, et al. Fat sparing of surrounding liver metastasis in patients with fatty liver: MR imaging with histopathologic correlation. AJR Am J Roentgenol 2003;180:1347–1350.
2. Tom WW, Yeh BM, Cheng JC, et al. Hepatic pseudotumor due to nodular fatty sparing: the diagnostic role of opposed-phase MRI. AJR Am J Roentgenol 2004;183;721–724.

Case 23

History

▶ 63-year-old woman with a history of deep venous thrombosis in the lower extremities

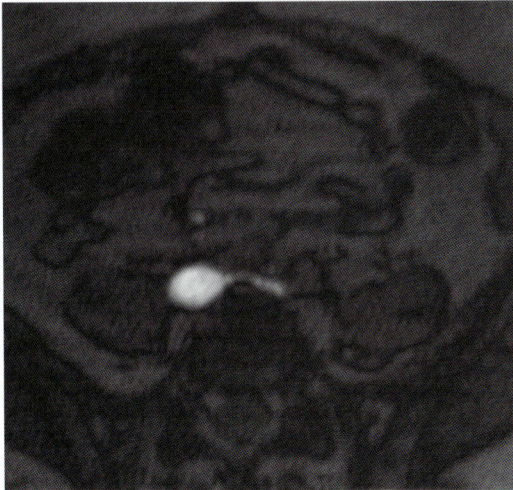

A

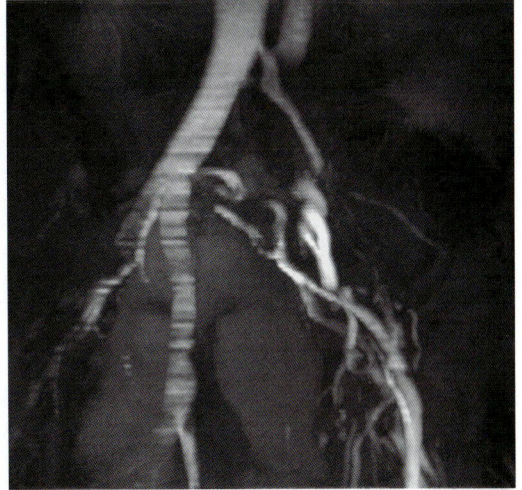

B

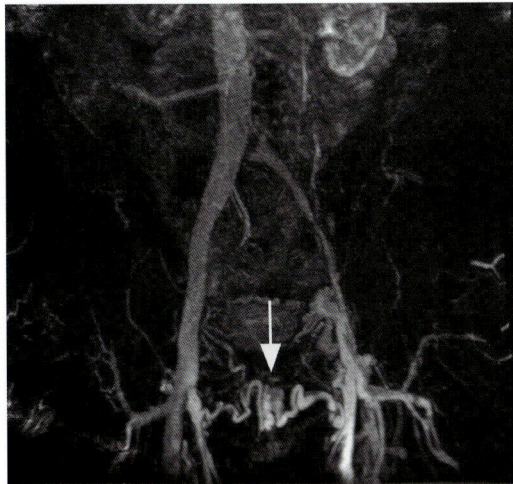

C

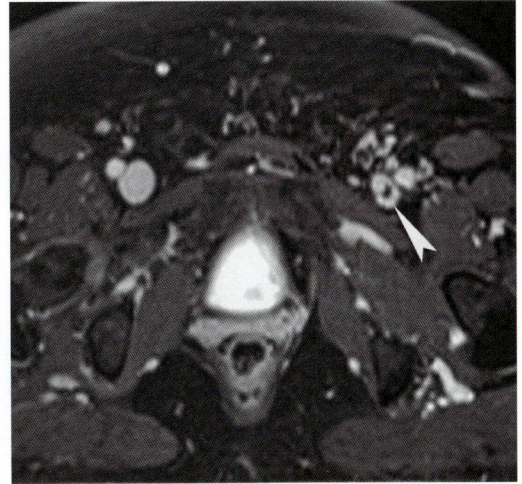

D

A. Axial 2D time-of-flight gradient echo (arterial flow suppressed with presaturation pulse). **B**. Coronal right anterior oblique maximum intensity projection (MIP) image generated from a 2D time-of-flight gradient-echo sequence obtained in axial orientation with presaturation pulse suppressing arterial flow. **C**. Coronal MIP image from gadolinium contrast-enhanced MR venogram. **D**. Gadolinium contrast-enhanced gradient echo with fat suppression.

Case 23 May-Thürner Syndrome

Findings

▶ The left common iliac vein is compressed by the overlying right common iliac artery (**A**).

▶ Thrombosis of the left iliac vein with extensive venous collateralization (**B**)

▶ Superficial collateral veins extend over the pubic symphysis (*arrow* in **C**).

▶ Synechiae in the left common femoral vein (*arrowhead* in **D**)

Differential diagnosis

▶ External compression of the iliac vein by mass, nodal tissue, or fibrosis

Teaching points

▶ The main anatomic component of the syndrome described by May and Thürner is compression of the left common iliac vein by the overlying right common iliac artery and the underlying fifth lumbar vertebral body. This appearance may also be present in asymptomatic patients.

▶ In the setting of venous compression, the presence of collateral veins in the absence of thrombosis is supportive of the diagnosis.

▶ MR time-of-flight sequences allow for the selective saturation of the signals from the arteries or veins in order to interrogate these systems individually.

▶ Compression of the vein results in stasis of blood as well as direct injury of the endothelium with development of chronic fibrous webs. Both factors precipitate deep venous thrombosis.

▶ The majority of cases of May-Thürner syndrome involve young and middle-aged women.

▶ Endovascular therapies including angioplasty and stenting have been shown to improve quality of life with patency rates that are comparable to or better than conventional surgical therapies.

▶ When left untreated, patients have a high risk of developing post-thrombotic syndrome. Post-thrombotic syndrome refers to a spectrum of manifestations including telangiectasias, varicosities, edema, pain, ulceration, and ischemia resulting from venous incompetence occurring as a complication of deep venous thrombosis.

Management

Thrombolysis followed by angioplasty and stenting

Further reading

1. Norton P, Hagspiel K. Vascular MR imaging. In: Brant WE, de Lange EE (eds), Essentials of Body MRI. New York: Oxford University Press, 2012.
2. Titus JM, Moise MA, Bena J, et al. Iliofemoral stenting for venous occlusive disease. J Vasc Surg 2011;53:706–712.
3. Wolpert LM, Rahmani O, Stein B, et al. Magnetic resonance venography in the diagnosis and management of May-Thurner Syndrome. Vasc Endovascular Surg 2002;36:51–57.

History

▶ 86-year-old man with suspected gallstone pancreatitis and cholangitis, unable to complete outside Endoscopic Retrograde Cholangiopancreatography (ERCP) due to difficult anatomy

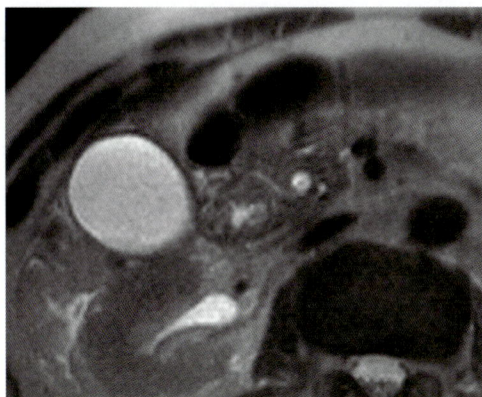

A

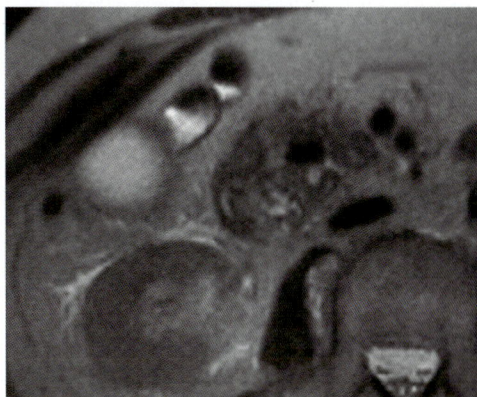

B

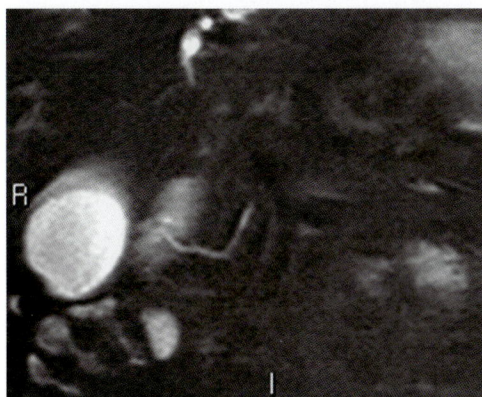

C

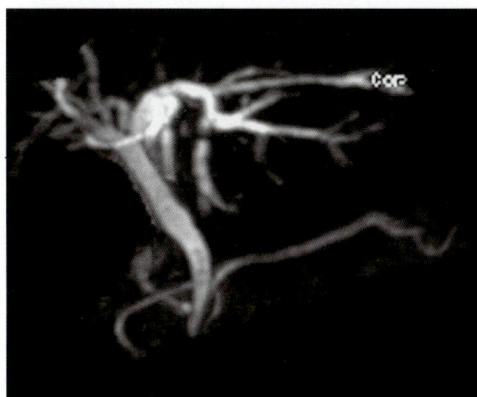

D

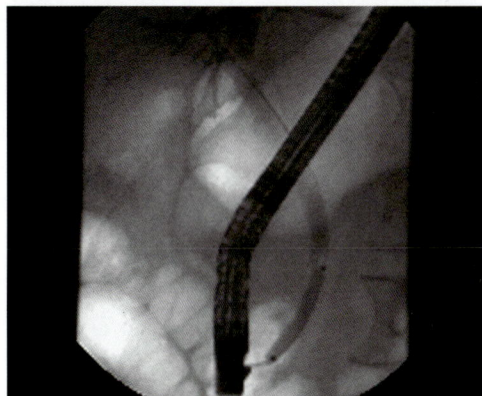

E

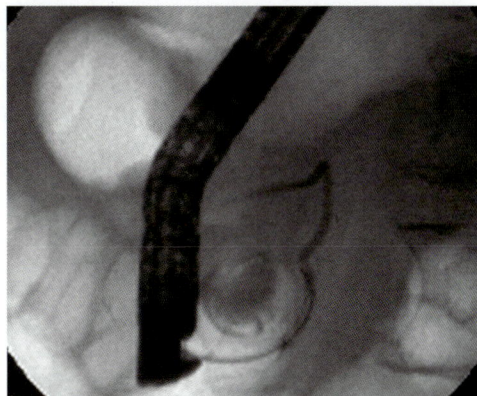

F

A, B. Axial T2-weighted single-shot FSE/TSE at different levels. **C**. Coronal T2-weighted single-shot FSE/TSE. **D**. Maximum intensity projection MRCP generated from 3D FSE/TSE. **E**. ERCP showing common bile duct and (**F**) pancreatic duct.

Case 24 Annular Pancreas

Findings

▸ Accessory annular ducts are noted coursing anterior and posterior to the duodenum (**A**), with the continuation of the posterior annular duct coursing within annular pancreatic tissue (**B**). Signal void in **B** is a duodenal diverticulum.

▸ Coronal image shows anterior annular duct connection to the main pancreatic duct (**C**).

▸ MRCP (**D**) shows the main pancreatic duct with connection to the anterior annular duct and the posterior annular duct with connection to the common bile duct. Signal voids in the distal common bile duct are air bubbles introduced during prior ERCP.

▸ ERCP shows cannulation of the common bile duct (**E**) and of the posterior annular duct (**F**). The pool of contrast material in F is within the duodenal diverticulum.

Differential diagnosis

▸ None

Teaching points

▸ Annular pancreas is a relatively rare congenital anomaly in which one of the ventral buds of the pancreas fails to regress, or the right ventral bud does not rotate normally behind the duodenum, resulting in a ring of pancreatic tissue around the duodenum.

▸ It is estimated to occur in 1:12,000 to 15,000 live births.

▸ The ring of tissue surrounding the descending duodenum can be either complete (25%) or partial (75%).

▸ It can be associated with other congenital anomalies, including esophageal atresia, imperforate anus, congenital heart disease, midgut malrotation, and Down syndrome.

▸ In approximately half of symptomatic cases it will manifest in the neonate with gastrointestinal tract obstruction, possibly associated with pancreatitis. In symptomatic adults it may manifest with symptoms of peptic ulcer disease, duodenal obstruction, or pancreatitis. In general, there is duodenal obstruction in 10% of cases.

Management

▸ Surgical correction can be required when there is duodenal obstruction. Duodenoduodenostomy is performed in neonates, whereas duodenojejunostomy or gastrojejunostomy is recommended in adults because the duodenum has limited mobility.

Further reading

1. Mortelé KJ, Rocha TC, Streeter JL, Taylor AJ. Multimodality imaging of pancreatic and biliary congenital anomalies. RadioGraphics 2006;26:715–731.
2. Sandrasegaran K, Patel A, Fogel EL, et al. Annular pancreas in adults. AJR Am J Roentgenol 2009;193:455–460.
3. Tadokoro H, Takase M, Nobukawa B. Development and congenital anomalies of the pancreas. Anatomy Research International, vol. 2011, Article ID 351217, 7 pages, 2011. doi:10.1155/2011/351217

History

▶ 46-year-old man with a family history of renal disease presents with renal failure.

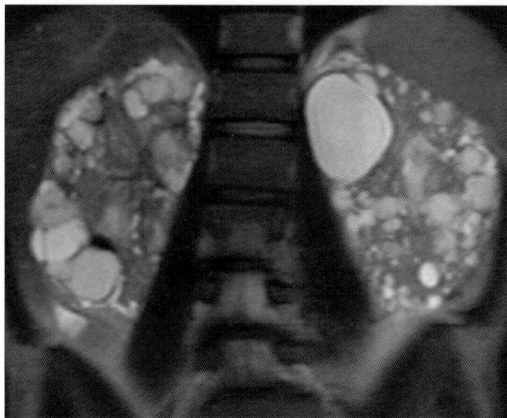

A

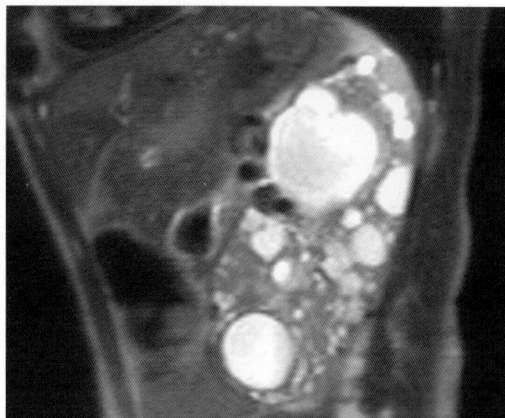

B

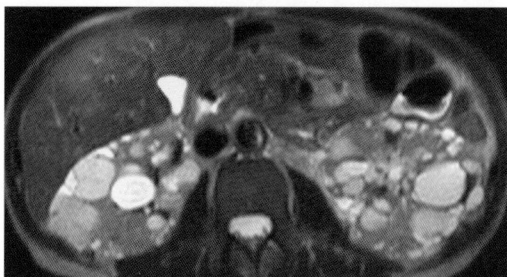

C

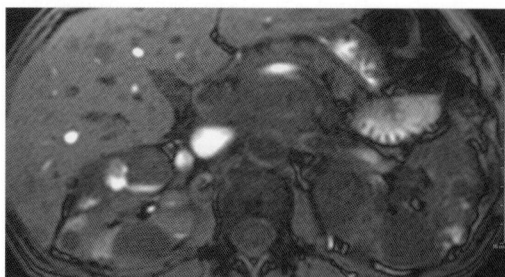

D

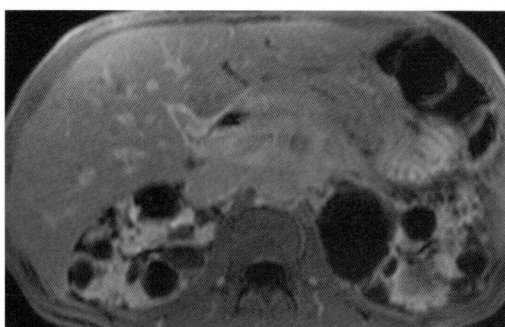

E

A. Coronal, (**B**) sagittal, and (**C**) axial T2-weighted single-shot FSE/TSE. **D**. Axial opposed-phase T1-weighted gradient echo. **E**. Axial post-gadolinium contrast-enhanced T1-weighted gradient echo with fat saturation.

Case 25 Autosomal Dominant Polycystic Kidney Disease (ADPCKD)

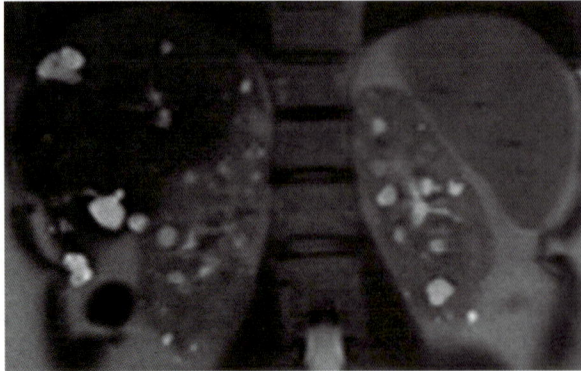

F

Findings

- ► Bilateral very large kidneys with innumerable cysts of varying size largely replacing the renal parenchyma
- ► The cysts show variable signal intensity and fluid–fluid levels indicating the presence of blood products from prior hemorrhage and varying protein content of the cyst fluid.
- ► A few small cysts are seen in the liver.
- ► Coronal single-shot T2-weighted FSE/TSE image(**F**) from another patient with similar disease at an earlier stage shows more cysts in the liver.

Differential diagnosis

- ► Multiple simple renal cysts
- ► Tuberous sclerosis, von Hippel-Lindau disease

Teaching points

- ► ADPCKD, also called adult polycystic disease, affects about 1 in 1,000 people in the general population and is the third most common cause of end-stage renal disease.
- ► The cysts may be seen in utero and in childhood, though they are usually small and do not affect the renal function. The cysts enlarge progressively over time. Most patients have cysts apparent at imaging by age 30. About 45% of patients develop end-stage renal failure by age 60.
- ► The renal cysts are commonly complicated by hemorrhage or infection, or rarely by cyst rupture. In most patients imaging demonstrates extrarenal cysts in the liver, pancreas, seminal vesicles, and spleen. Associated abnormalities include intracranial aneurysms, aortic aneurysms, abdominal wall hernias, aortic and mitral valve disease, and colon diverticula.
- ► MR allows assessment of the kidney and cyst volumes, which serve as indicators of disease progression or response to treatment.

Management

- ► Treatment involves control of blood pressure and metabolic conditions associated with renal failure, as well as prevention and treatment of urinary tract infections.

Further reading

1. Hilpert PL, Friedman AC, Radecki PD, et al. MRI of hemorrhagic renal cysts in polycystic kidney disease. AJR Am J Roentgenol 1986;146:1167–1172.
2. Katabathina VS, Kota G, Dasyam AK, et al. Adult renal cystic disease: a genetic, biological, and developmental primer. RadioGraphics 2010;30:1509–1523.

History

▸ 54-year-old woman with a history of neurofibromatosis type 1 presents with a history of weight loss, vague abdominal pain, diarrhea, nausea, and vomiting.

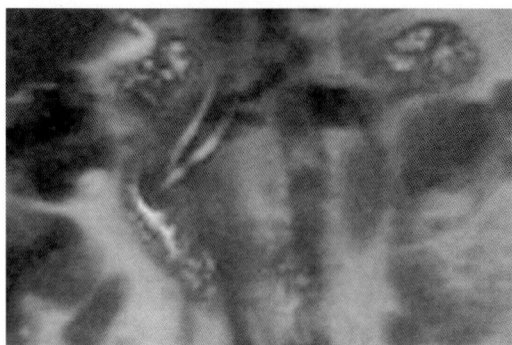
A

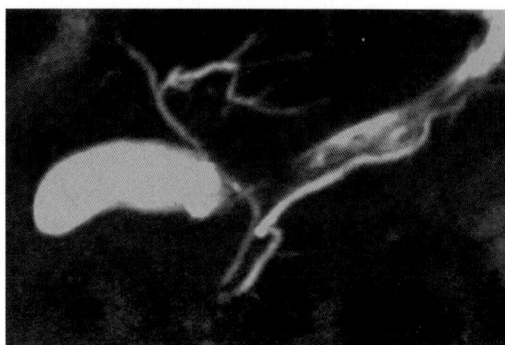
B

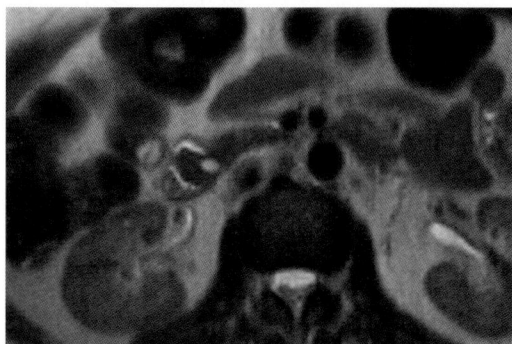
C

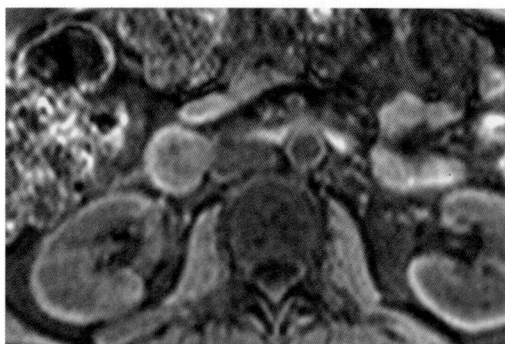
D

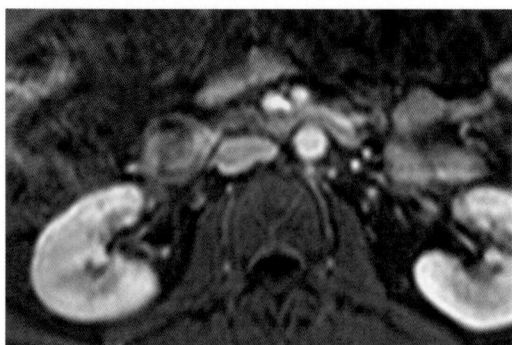
E

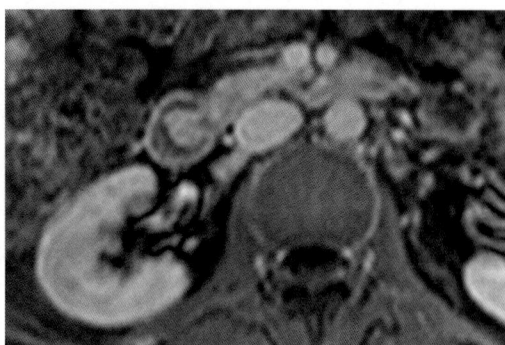
F

A. Coronal T2-weighted single-shot FSE/TSE. **B**. Thick-slab T2-weighted single-shot FSE/TSE MRCP image. **C**. Axial T2-weighted single-shot FSE/TSE. **D**. Pre-contrast-enhanced and (**E**, **F**) delayed gadolinium contrast-enhanced T1-weighted gradient echo with fat saturation

Case 26 Carcinoid Tumor of the Duodenum

Findings

- A well-defined lobulated polypoid mass projects into the lumen of the descending duodenum at the level of the ampulla.
- Though the common bile duct and pancreatic duct course through the mass they are not dilated.
- The mass displays relatively low signal intensity on both T1- and T2-weighted images.
- The mass shows early and persistent contrast enhancement.

Differential diagnosis

- Duodenal/pancreatic/biliary ductal adenocarcinoma
- Gastrointestinal stromal tumor
- Metastatic disease

Teaching points

- Carcinoid tumor is the second most common primary small bowel malignancy after adenocarcinoma.
- Carcinoid tumors occur sporadically and are also associated with multiple endocrine neoplasia, type 1 and neurofibromatosis, type 1.
- Primary carcinoid tumors and their metastases often demonstrate avid early arterial enhancement. The more common adenoma/adenocarcinoma shows minimal early enhancement.
- Carcinoid tumors can express a variety of neuropeptides, leading to characteristic symptoms and syndromes. However, the classic carcinoid syndrome occurs in less than 10% of patients.
- While the distal ileum is the most common site for gastrointestinal carcinoid tumors, they can arise anywhere along the gastrointestinal tract from the neuroendocrine cells populating the mucosa and submucosa.
- Avoid satisfaction of search when the lesion is found, as synchronous disease occurs in 29% to 41% of patients, and 29% to 53% of patients will have a second primary malignancy, most often in the gastrointestinal tract.

Management

- The diagnosis can be confirmed with endoscopic biopsy. In this case the lesion was confined to the muscularis propria of the duodenum.
- Nuclear scans with MIBG or octreotide can be helpful in evaluating the extent of disease or in cases where the primary lesion is not found at endoscopy.
- Surgical resection is the mainstay of treatment. Nonresectable lesions can be treated with surgical debulking and symptomatic palliation using octreotide.

Further reading

1. Horton KH, Kamel I, Hofmann L, Fishman EK. Carcinoid tumors of the small bowel: a multitechnique imaging approach. AJR Am J Roentgenol 2004;182:559–567.
2. Levy AD, Sobin LH. From the archives of the AFIP: gastrointestinal carcinoids imaging features with clinicopathologic comparison. RadioGraphics 2007;27:237–257.

History

▶ 45-year-old man complains of abdominal pain.

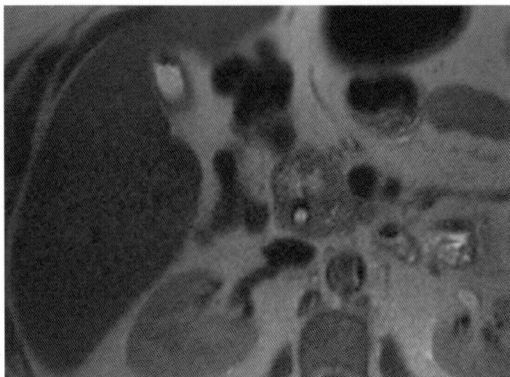

A

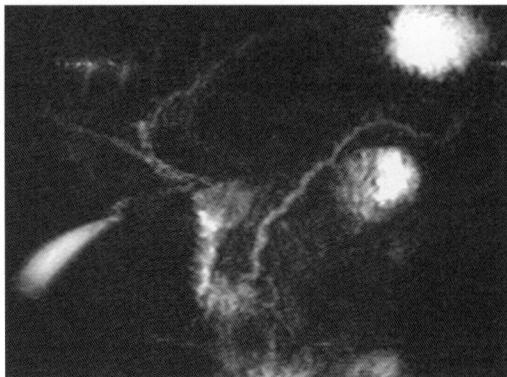

B

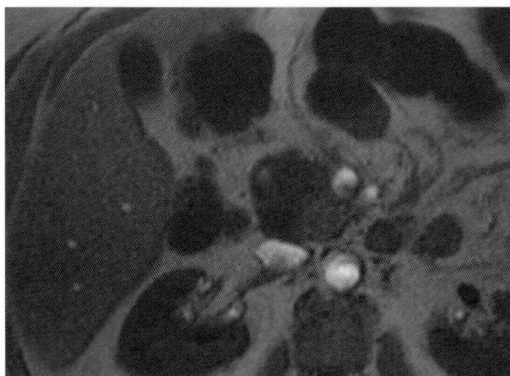

C

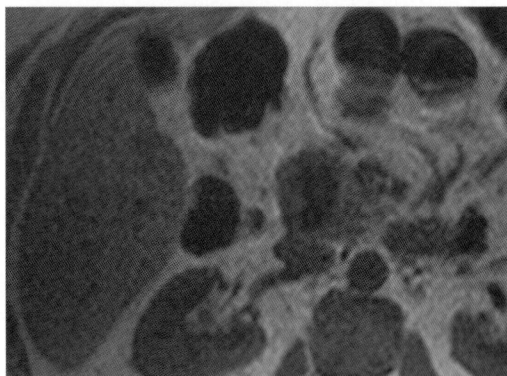

D

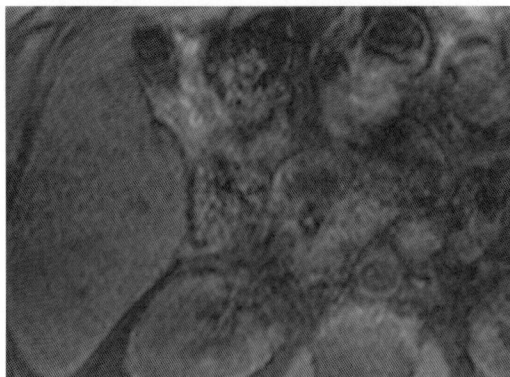

E

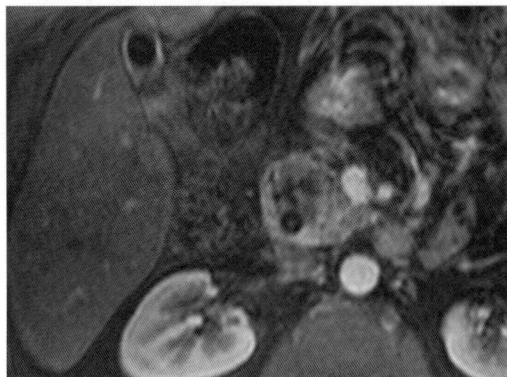

F

A. Axial T2-weighted single-shot FSE/TSE. **B**. MRCP using thick-slab single-shot FSE/TSE with fat saturation. **C**. Axial magnetization-prepared T1-weighted gradient echo (MPGRE). **D**. Axial T1-weighted gradient echo. **E**. Axial pre-contrast-enhanced and (**F**) post-gadolinium contrast-enhanced T1-weighted gradient echo with fat saturation.

Case 27 Pancreas Adenocarcinoma—Potentially Resectable

Findings

▶ Heterogeneous tumor mass in the pancreatic head without evidence of vascular involvement. A distinct border of normal-appearing pancreatic tissue separates the enhancing tumor from the superior mesenteric vein.

▶ The magnetization-prepared gradient-echo (MPGRE) sequence typically shows the tumor well with marked low signal intensity, and although differentiation with surrounding edema is difficult, the technique can be particularly helpful for detecting small tumors also in cases with no abnormalities on diffusion-weighted images (not shown).

▶ A wall stent is in place in the common bile duct. Note there is only little artifact from the stent.

▶ Surgical findings were a well-differentiated mucinous non-cystic adenocarcinoma, stage T3, N0, M0, extension beyond the pancreas without vascular involvement. At 5 years of follow-up this patient has no evidence of recurrent or metastatic disease.

Differential diagnosis

▶ Neuroendocrine tumor
▶ Chronic pancreatitis

Teaching points

▶ Pancreatic adenocarcinoma has an overall 5-year survival rate of only 4%. Surgical resection offers the only chance for longevity with this disease, with a 5-year survival rate of 35% for surgically resectable disease.

▶ Tumors classified by MR as surgically resectable show no evidence of involvement of the celiac axis or superior mesenteric artery (stage T3 or lower) and no evidence of metastatic disease (stage N0 and M0).

▶ Tumors classified by MR as being borderline surgically resectable include T4 (N0, M0) lesions with:
  - Less than 50% (<180°) tumor abutment of the celiac axis or superior mesenteric artery
  - Short segment abutment or encasement of the common hepatic artery
  - Segmental venous occlusion that allows venous reconstruction (adequate segment of superior mesenteric vein below and portal vein above the area of tumor involvement)

Management

▶ Whipple or modified Whipple procedure is generally the surgery of choice.

Further reading

1. American Joint Committee on Cancer. AJCC Cancer Staging Manual, 7th ed. New York: Springer, 2010.
2. Sahani DV, Shah ZK, Catalano OA, et al. Radiology of pancreatic carcinoma: current status of imaging. J Gastroent Hepatol 2008;23:23–33.
3. Sarti M. Pancreas MR imaging. In: Brant WE, de Lange EE (eds), Essentials of Body MRI. New York: Oxford University Press, 2012.
4. Varadhachary GR, Kim YH, Baki NC, et al. Borderline resectable pancreatic cancers: definitions, management, and role of preoperative therapy. Ann Surg Oncol 2006;13:1035–1046.

History

▶ 48-year-old man presents with headaches that are increasing in frequency, anxiety attacks, and intermittent hypertension. A CT scan performed for chest pain revealed a right adrenal mass.

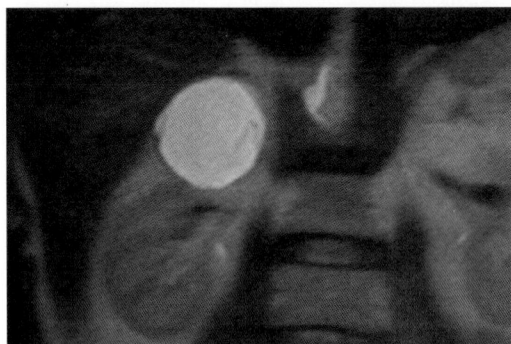

A

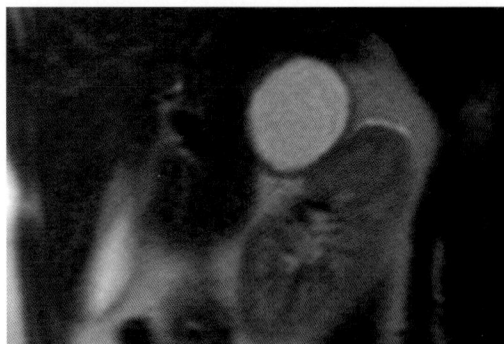

B

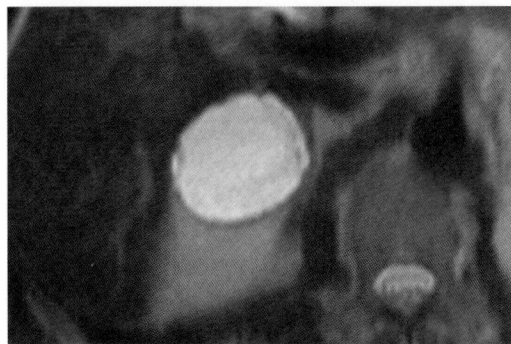

C

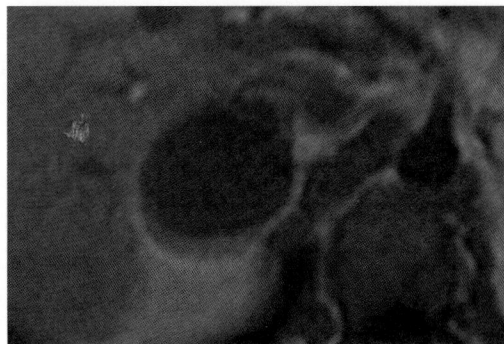

D

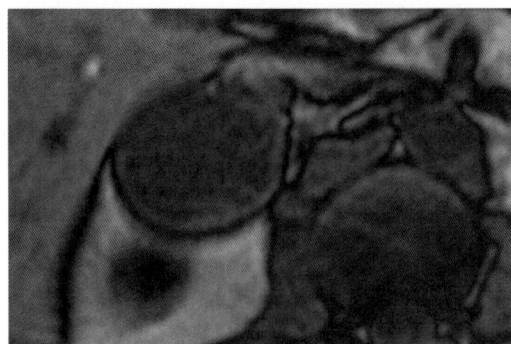

E

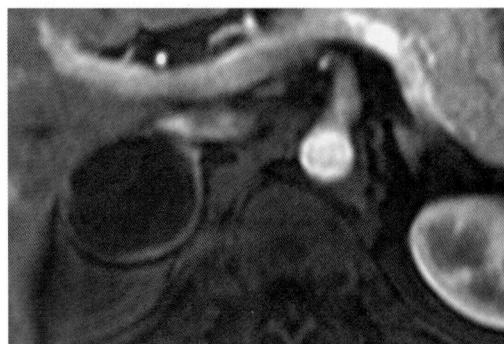

F

A. Coronal, (**B**) sagittal, and (**C**) axial T2-weighted single-shot FSE/TSE. (**D**) Axial in-phase and (**E**) opposed-phase T1-weighted gradient echo. (**F**) Gadolinium contrast-enhanced T1-weighted gradient echo with fat saturation.

Case 28 Cystic Pheochromocytoma

Findings

▶ Multiplanar MR imaging confirms a 5-cm right adrenal mass that is clearly separate from the right kidney and liver.
▶ The mass has cystic characteristics with an irregular and slightly nodular wall as well as a few thin septations. Internal contents displays low signal intensity on T1-weighted and high signal intensity on T2-weighted images, indicating simple fluid.
▶ In-phase/opposed-phase gradient-echo and fat-suppressed sequences show no evidence of microscopic or macroscopic (adipose) internal fat content.
▶ The wall of the lesion enhances while its contents does not.
▶ Adrenalectomy revealed a cystic pheochromocytoma containing gelatinous material.

Differential diagnosis

▶ Simple adrenal cysts (endothelialized cysts) contain simple fluid, have thin walls and no solid tissue components and do not enhance.
▶ Adrenal pseudocysts result from an episode of adrenal hemorrhage. They are more complicated in appearance than simple cysts, with thicker walls, septations, and internal contents reflecting blood products and thrombus. Calcification in the wall is common but often not appreciated on MR.
▶ Cystic lymphangiomas appear as thin-walled cysts and demonstrate low signal intensity on T1-weighted and high signal intensity on T2-weighted images. They do not enhance.
▶ Cystic metastases have irregular soft tissue components and wall nodularity and contain hemorrhagic and necrotic fluid.

Teaching points

▶ Pheochromocytoma is a rare cause of hypertension, accounting for less than 0.5% of cases with hypertension. Most small pheochromocytomas are solid lesions.
▶ While necrosis and hemorrhage are common in large pheochromocytomas, cystic degeneration is rare. Most reported cystic pheochromocytomas have septations. The wall of the lesion may contain only a few cells identifiable as pheochromocytoma.
▶ Radioscintigraphy using iodine-131 metaiodobenzylguanidine (I-131 MIBG) is effective in localizing the primary tumor. However, its use may be problematic in cystic lesions because the radionuclide is taken up only by the solid components of the tumor and the resulting faint radioactivity may be overlooked, as it was in this case (MIBG study not shown).
▶ Because solid tissue is sparse in cystic pheochromocytoma, the avid enhancement characteristic of most pheochromocytomas is usually not evident.

Management

▶ Surgical resection is indicated.

Further reading

1. Blake MA, Kalra MK, Maher MM, et al. Pheochromocytoma: an imaging chameleon. RadioGraphics 2004;24:S87–S99.
2. Lee TH, Slywotzky CM, Lavelle MT, Garcia RA. Cystic pheochromocytoma. RadioGraphics 2002;22:935–940.

History

▶ 72-year-old man with weight loss and increasing abdominal pain

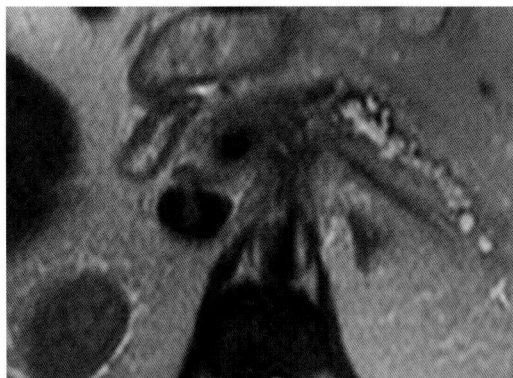

A

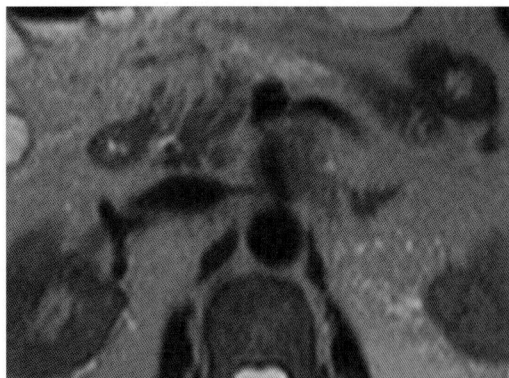

B

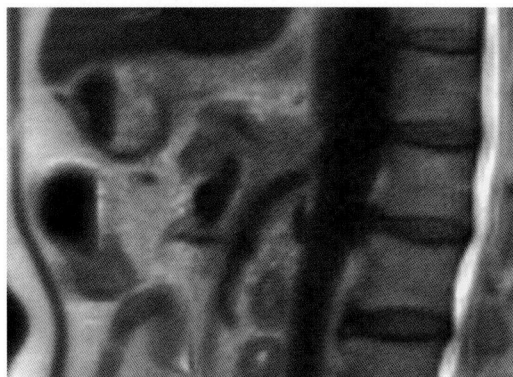

C

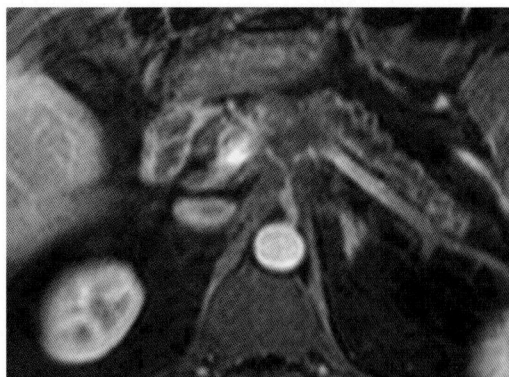

D

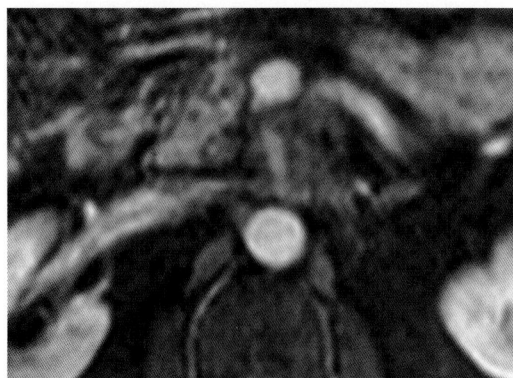

E

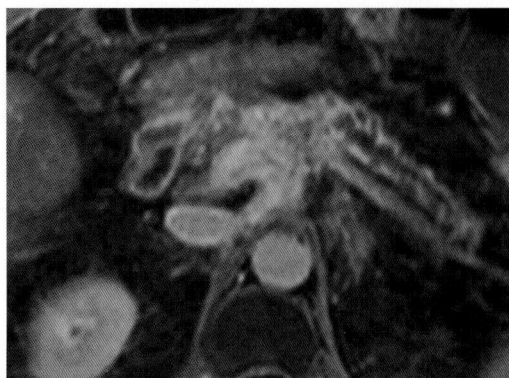

F

(**A, B**) Axial T2-weighted single-shot FSE/TSE (**B** at lower level than **A**). **C**. Sagittal T2-weighted single-shot FSE/TSE. (**D, E**) Axial post-gadolinium contrast-enhanced T1-weighted gradient echo with fat saturation (**E** at same level as **B**). **F**. Axial delayed-phase contrast-enhanced gradient echo with fat saturation (**F** at same level as **D**).

Case 29 Non-surgically-resectable ductal adenocarcinoma of the pancreas (tumor stage T4)

Findings

► Pancreatic tumor extends beyond the pancreas to completely encase the celiac axis (**A**, **C**, **D**, **F**) and superior mesenteric artery (**B**, **C**, **E**).
► The pancreatic duct proximal to the tumor is diffusely dilated and the pancreatic parenchyma is diffusely atrophic (**A**, **D**, **F**).

Differential diagnosis

► Chronic pancreatitis

Teaching points

► Current criteria for unresectability of pancreatic adenocarcinoma include extrapancreatic spread of tumor with invasion of major blood vessels. This is defined on MR as continuity of the tumor to vessel of greater than 50%. The major vessels whose involvement defines unresectability include the celiac axis and superior mesenteric artery (tumor stage T4). Massive involvement of the common hepatic artery, portal vein, and superior mesenteric vein with or without thrombosis also precludes surgical resection.
► Distant metastases, involvement of the liver, regional lymph nodes, or omentum (stage N1 or M1) are contraindications to surgical resection.
► With the use of modern surgical techniques, limited venous involvement without thrombosis does not preclude surgical resection.
► The sensitivity of MR and helical CT for determination of tumor resectability are the same, reported at 81% to 82%.
► Pancreatic ductal adenocarcinoma is variable in signal intensity on T2-weighted images depending primarily on the desmoplastic response associated with the tumor. Tumors usually display relatively low signal intensity on T1-weighted images. Dynamic post-gadolinium contrast-enhanced sequences generally show less tumor enhancement than normal parenchyma on early-phase images with progressively increased enhancement on delayed-phase images.

Management

► For non-surgically-resectable pancreatic cancer, chemotherapy and radiation therapy, alone or combined, offer palliation.

Further reading

1. American Joint Committee on Cancer. AJCC Cancer Staging Manual, 7th ed. New York: Springer, 2010.
2. Sahani DV, Shah ZK, Catalano OA, et al. Radiology of pancreatic carcinoma: current status of imaging. J Gastroent Hepatol 2008;23:23–33.
3. Sarti M. Pancreas MR imaging. In: Brant WE, de Lange EE (eds), Essentials of Body MRI. New York: Oxford University Press, 2012.
4. Varadhachary GR, Kim YH, Baki NC, et al. Borderline resectable pancreatic cancers: definitions, management, and role of preoperative therapy. Ann Surg Oncol 2006;13:1035–1046.

History

▶ 48-year-old man with incidentally noted liver lesion

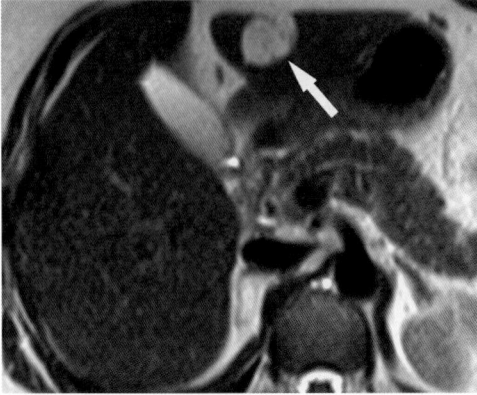

A

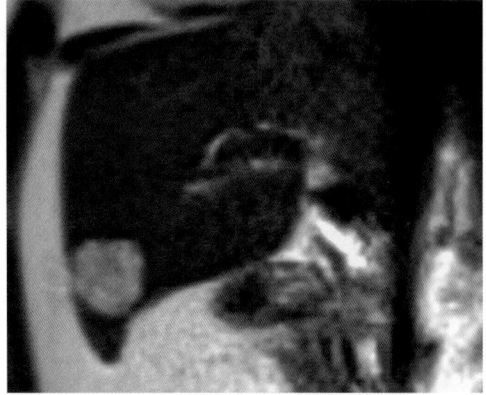

B

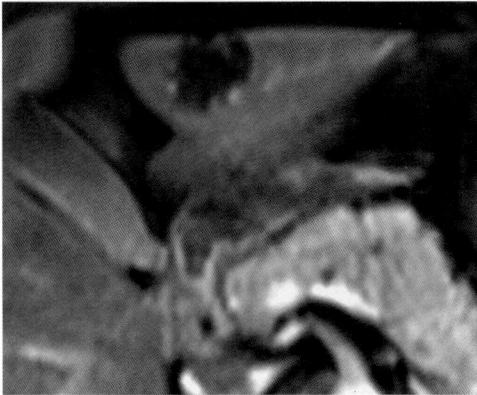

C

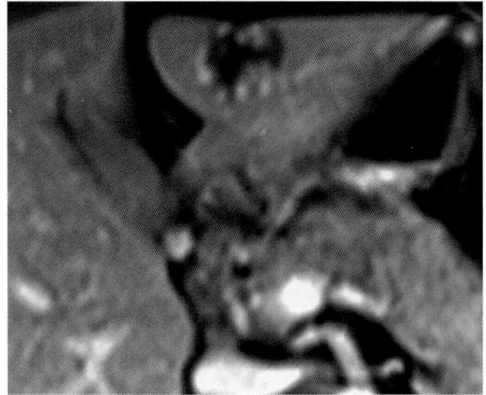

D

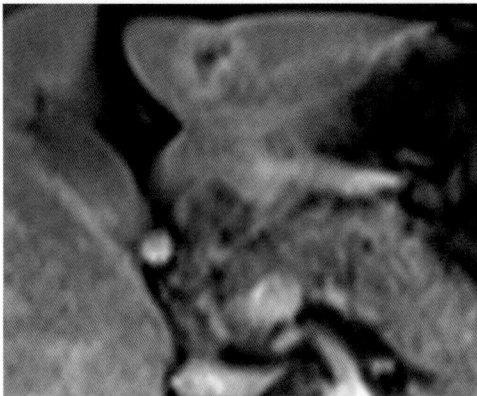

E

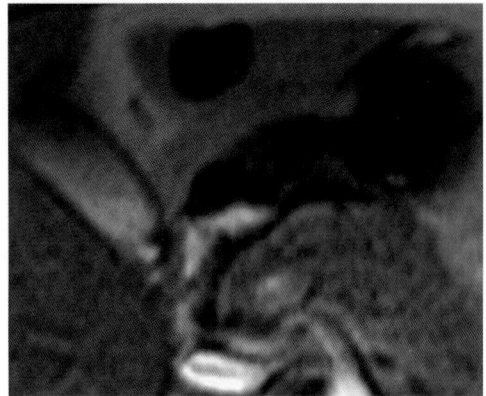

F

A. Axial and (**B**) sagittal T2-weighted single-shot FSE/TSE. **C**. Arterial phase, (**D**) hepatic venous phase, and (**E**) 10-minute delayed-phase contrast-enhanced axial T1-weighted gradient echo with fat saturation. **F**. Unenhanced axial T1-weighted magnetization-prepared gradient echo.

Case 30 Hepatic Cavernous Hemangioma, Classic MRI Findings

Findings

▶ A well-marginated, mildly lobulated mass (*arrow*) in the left hepatic lobe. The mass is hypointense on T1-weighted images and demonstrates discontinuous peripheral nodular enhancement on early contrast-enhanced images. Enhancement progresses from the periphery to the center of the lesion on later phases.

▶ The lesion is hyperintense on T2-weighted images, but not as high in signal intensity as cerebrospinal fluid.

▶ Delayed post-contrast-enhanced images reveal a central scar that remains low in signal intensity.

▶ The lesion demonstrates extremely low signal intensity on T1-weighted MPGRE images.

Differential diagnosis

▶ Hepatocellular carcinoma (HCC): small (i.e., "capillary") hemangiomas often enhance homogeneously and may mimic small HCC.

▶ Hypervascular metastasis

▶ Peripheral cholangiocarcinoma shows increased enhancement on delayed contrast-enhanced images but is less well circumscribed than hemangioma and displays lower signal intensity on T2-weighted images.

▶ Hepatic angiosarcoma is usually multifocal, and exhibits local and vascular invasion

Teaching points

▶ Hepatic cavernous hemangioma is a benign tumor consisting of endothelium-lined vascular spaces of various sizes, which are separated by fibrous septa. No bile ducts or hepatocytes are present.

▶ The increased volume of distribution within the vascular channels and fibrous tissue both contribute to the progressive centripetal enhancement—a virtually pathognomonic feature.

▶ Hyperintensity on T2-weighted images is due to slow-flowing blood; however, this may be countered by fibrous tissue within the lesion or thrombosis, which may cause hypointensity.

▶ For example, a giant hemangioma (i.e., >10 cm) can be quite heterogeneous in signal and demonstrate a central hypointense cleft on T2-weighted as well as on post-contrast-enhanced T1-weighted images.

Management

▶ If classic imaging features are present, no further follow-up is needed.

Further reading

1. Elsayes KM, Menias CO, Dillman JR, et al. Vascular malformation and hemangiomatosis syndromes: spectrum of imaging manifestations. AJR Am J Roentgenol 2008;190:1291–1299.
2. Tung GA, Vaccaro JP, Cronan JJ, Rogg JM. Cavernous hemangioma of the liver: pathologic correlation with high-field MR imaging. AJR Am J Roentgenol 1994;162:1113–1117.

History

▸ A 52-year-old man developed chronic right flank pain and an abscess two years after a laparoscopic cholecystectomy for gallstones. Several attempts with percutaneous catheter drainage were unsuccessful at resolving the abscess.

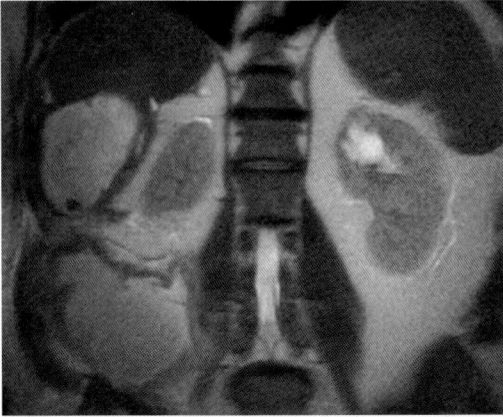

A

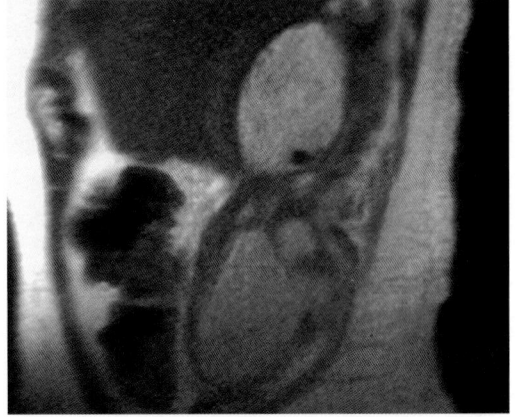

B

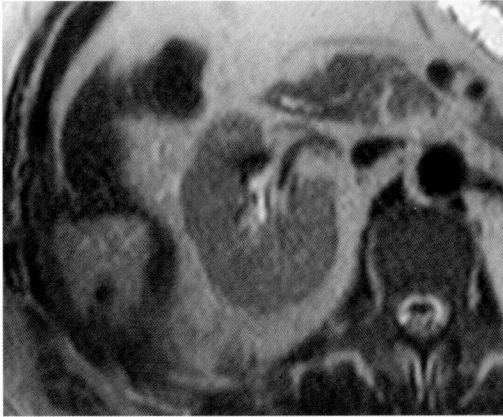

C

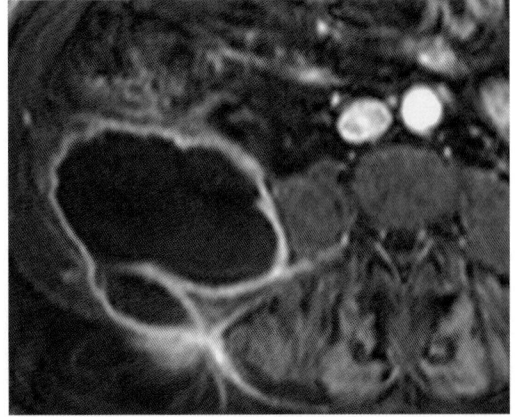

D

A. Coronal, (**B**) sagittal, and (**C**) axial T2-weighted single-shot FSE/TSE. **D**. Axial contrast-enhanced T1-weighted gradient echo with fat saturation.

Case 31 Gallstone-Induced Chronic Abdominal Abscess with Gallstone Granuloma—Spilled Gallstone

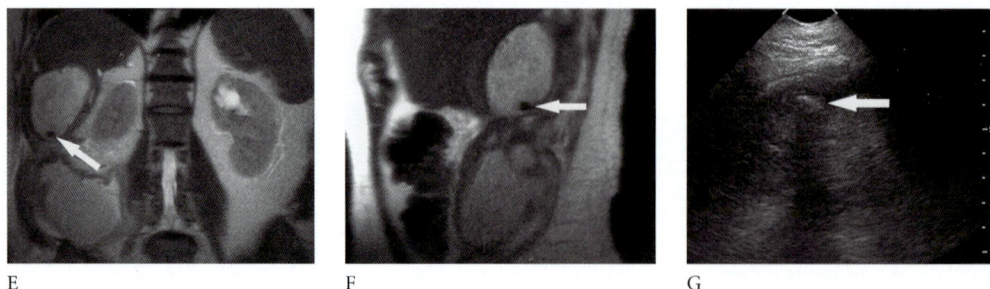

E

F

G

Findings

▶ A subhepatic mixed-consistency fluid collection contains a non-enhancing round 6 mm low-signal-intensity lesion (*arrows*) (**E, F**). Inferiorly, a right flank collection extends into the quadratus muscle and communicates with the subhepatic collection.

▶ Ultrasound (**G**) of the abscess performed after the MRI demonstrates an echogenic lesion (*arrow*) with acoustic shadowing consistent with a spilled gallstone adherent to surrounding tissue.

▶ At surgery a 1-cm gallstone with surrounded granulomatous tissue was removed from the abscess cavity. Cultures of the thick abscess fluid grew *E. coli* and *Klebsiella*.

Differential diagnosis

▶ Diverticulitis with abscess

▶ Postoperative hematoma or biloma serving as a nidus for recurrent infection

Teaching points

▶ Spillage of gallstones into the peritoneal cavity is a relatively common occurrence during laparoscopic cholecystectomy. Most spilled gallstones remain clinically silent.

▶ Potential complications of a spilled gallstone include intra-abdominal abscess formation, gallstone granuloma, percutaneous peritoneal sinus-tract formation, and erosion of the gallstone into the gastrointestinal tract with risk of cholelithoptysis (coughing up gallstones).

▶ The spilled gallstones may rarely serve as a nidus for a chronic foreign body–type intraperitoneal or abdominal wall granulomatous reaction. The inflammatory reaction can cause the gallstone to erode into the abdominal wall. Dropped gallstones must be suspected even if not visible on imaging.

▶ The inflammatory response can result in abdominal and pelvic adhesions, mimicking endometriosis.

Management

▶ Surgical resection of the gallstone and granulomatous tissue

Further reading

1. Schäfer M, Suter C, Klaiber C, et al. Spilled gallstones after laparoscopic cholecystectomy. A relevant problem? A retrospective analysis of 10,174 laparoscopic cholecystectomies. Surg Endosc 1998;12:305–309.
2. Tham CH, Ng BK. Gallstone granuloma: a rare complication of laparoscopic cholecystectomy. Singapore Med J 2001;42:174–175.

History

▶ 64-year-old man with biopsy-proven prostate carcinoma for staging

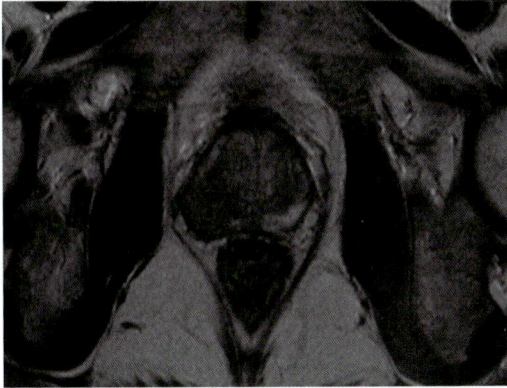

A

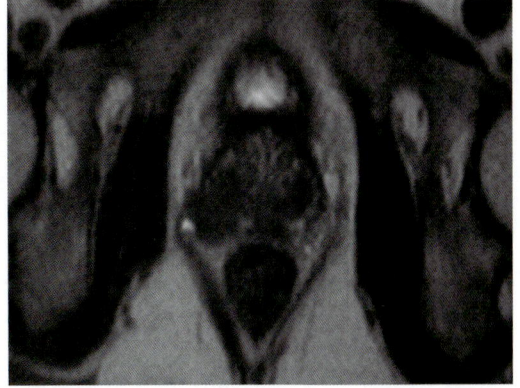

B

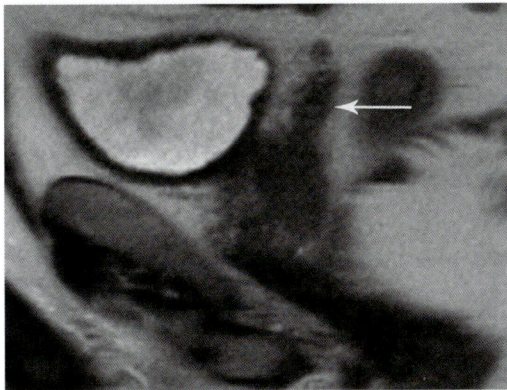

C

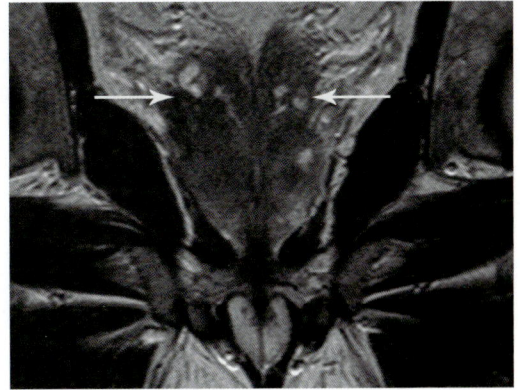

D

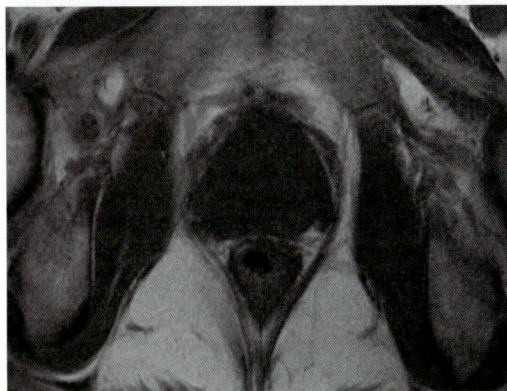

E

A. Axial T2-weighted FSE/TSE and (**B**) T2-weighted single-shot FSE/TSE. **C**. Sagittal T2-weighted single-shot FSE/TSE (*arrow*, seminal vesicle). **D**. Coronal T2-weighted FSE/TSE (*arrows*, seminal vesicles). **E**. Axial T1-weighted spin echo.

Case 32 Stage T3 Prostate Carcinoma

Findings

► In **A** and **B**, low-signal-intensity tumor (right posterior/lateral aspect of the prostate) replaces the high-signal-intensity peripheral-zone parenchyma and bulges posterolaterally on the right consistent with extracapsular spread. The tumor crosses the midline and invades the peripheral zone on the left anteriorly, abutting the central gland.
► In **C** and **D**, the tumor invades both seminal vesicles, replacing and encasing the high-signal-intensity tubules with low-signal-intensity tumor.
► T1-weighted images do not allow differentiation of tumor from normal prostate parenchyma. Differentiation is well done with diffusion-weighted images (not shown)

Differential diagnosis

► Besides cancer, other causes of low signal intensity in the peripheral zone include scarring, parenchymal atrophy, hemorrhage, prostatitis, cryosurgery, and hormonal therapy.

Teaching points

► Local staging with MR is used to differentiate stage T1 or T2 disease, confined to the prostate, from T3 disease with extracapsular spread of tumor with involvement of the neurovascular bundles or seminal vesicles.
► The neurovascular bundles are seen at the 5-o'clock and 7-o'clock positions on axial images of the prostate gland. The tumor shown here involved the neurovascular bundle on the right.
► Approximately 70% of cancers arise in the peripheral zone of the prostate gland.
► On T2-weighted images the peripheral zone is homogeneous with high signal intensity, while cancer displays low signal intensity replacing the peripheral zone tissue.
► The central gland is often affected by benign prostatic hypertrophy appearing as nodules showing variable, usually intermediate, signal intensity.
► Criteria for extracapsular spread of tumor include irregular focal bulge of the prostate contour, obliteration of the angle between the rectum and prostate, and encasement of the neurovascular bundles.
► Seminal vesicle involvement on T2-weighted images is evidenced by focal low signal intensity replacing the high-signal-intensity fluid and obliterating the tubular structures.
► T1-weighted images provide limited assessment of the prostate parenchyma but are useful for evaluating the contour of the prostate, and for detection of post-biopsy hemorrhage and involvement of the neurovascular bundles.

Management

► Treatment remains controversial, with options including prostatectomy, cryo- or radiofrequency ablation, brachytherapy in case of organ-confined disease, and hormone and/or radiation therapy for extracapsular disease.

Further reading

1. Bonekamp D, Jacobs MA, El-Khouli R, et al. Advancements in MR imaging of the prostate: from diagnosis to interventions. RadioGraphics 2011;31:677–703.
2. Hricak H, Choyke PL, Eberhardt SC, et al. Imaging prostate cancer: a multidisciplinary perspective. Radiology 2007;243:28–53.

History

▶ 58-year-old man referred for evaluation of liver lesion

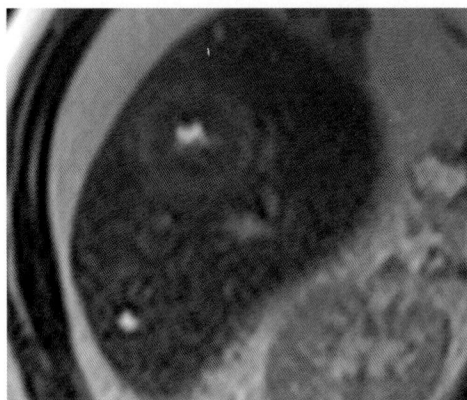
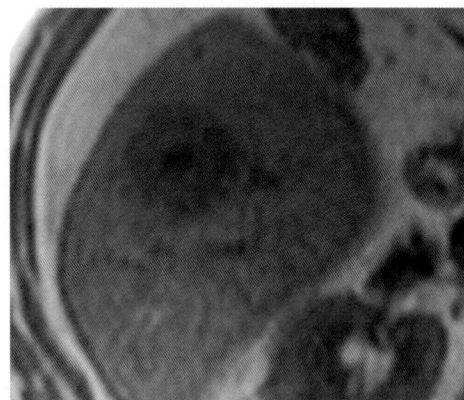

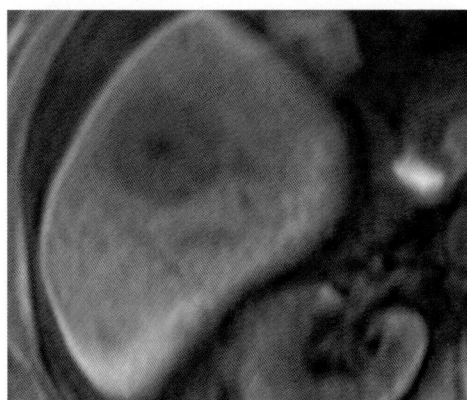
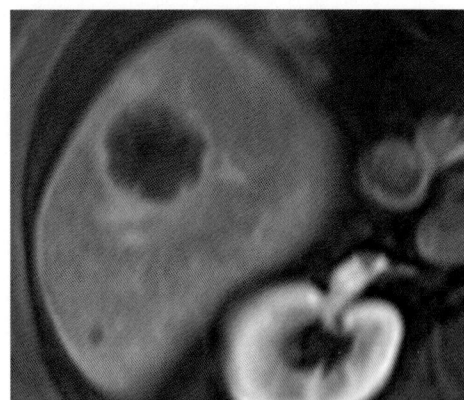

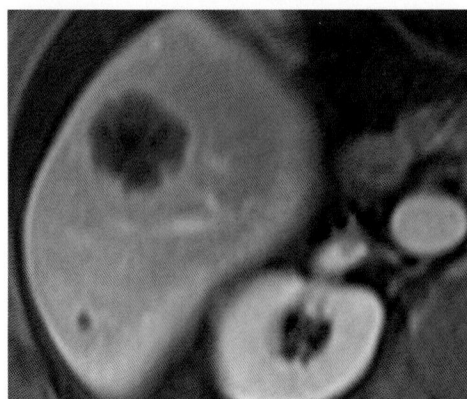
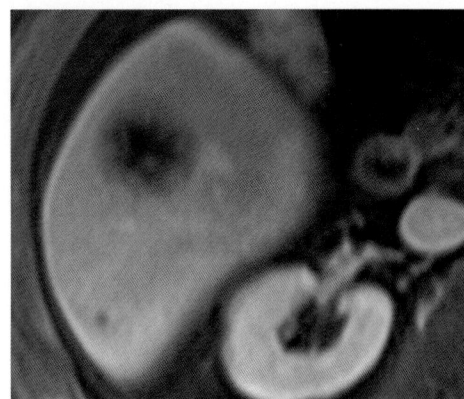

A. Axial T2-weighted single-shot FSE/TSE. **B**. Axial T1-weighted gradient echo. **C**. Pre-contrast-enhanced and (**D**) arterial phase, (**E**) portal venous phase, and (**F**) delayed enhancement phase of dynamically obtained contrast-enhanced axial T1-weighted gradient echo with fat saturation.

Case 33 Metastasis to the Liver. Primary Lesion: Colon Carcinoma.

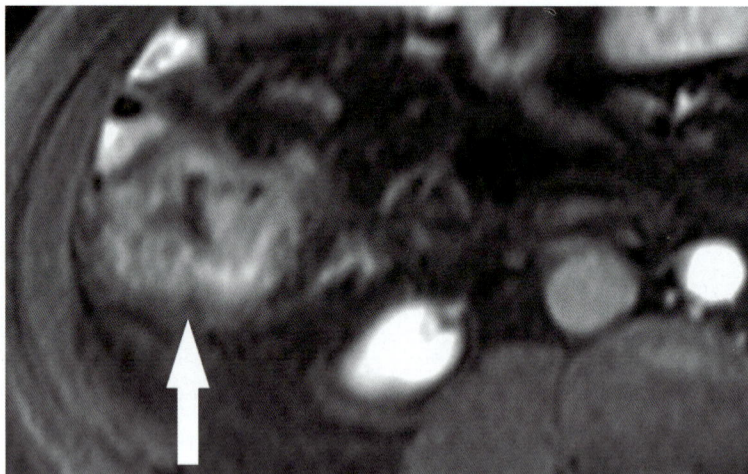

G

Findings

► Mildly hyperintense round lesion in the liver on T2-weighted images with central high-signal-intensity focus representing area of necrosis.
► On dynamic post-contrast-enhanced images, the liver lesion has early ring-like peripheral enhancement and late continuous interstitial enhancement.
► A tiny simple liver cyst showing high signal intensity on T2-weighted image and no contrast enhancement is also noted posterior to the larger lesion.
► A mass (*arrow*) is seen in the right colon in contrast-enhanced image **G** obtained at a level inferior to the liver.

Differential diagnosis

► Hemangioma
► Primary hepatic neoplasm

Teaching points

► Interstitial continuous peripheral enhancement that fills in the lesion differentiates this metastatic lesion from hemangiomas, which characteristically have discontinuous peripheral nodular enhancement with progressive fill-in.
► Ring-like enhancement has been shown to be predictive of metastasis.
► When metastatic liver disease is suspected, all images of the MRI study must be carefully inspected for evidence of a primary lesion elsewhere.

Further reading

1. Goshima S, Kanematsu M, Watanabe H, et al. Hepatic hemangioma and metastasis: differentiation with gadoxetate disodium–enhanced 3-T MRI. AJR Am J Roentgenol 2010;195:941–946.
2. Motosugi U, Ishikawa T, Onohara K, et al. Distinguishing hepatic metastases from hemangiomas using gadoxetic acid-enhanced magnetic resonance imaging. Invest Radiol 2011;46:359–365.

History

▶ 45-year-old woman with right upper quadrant pain

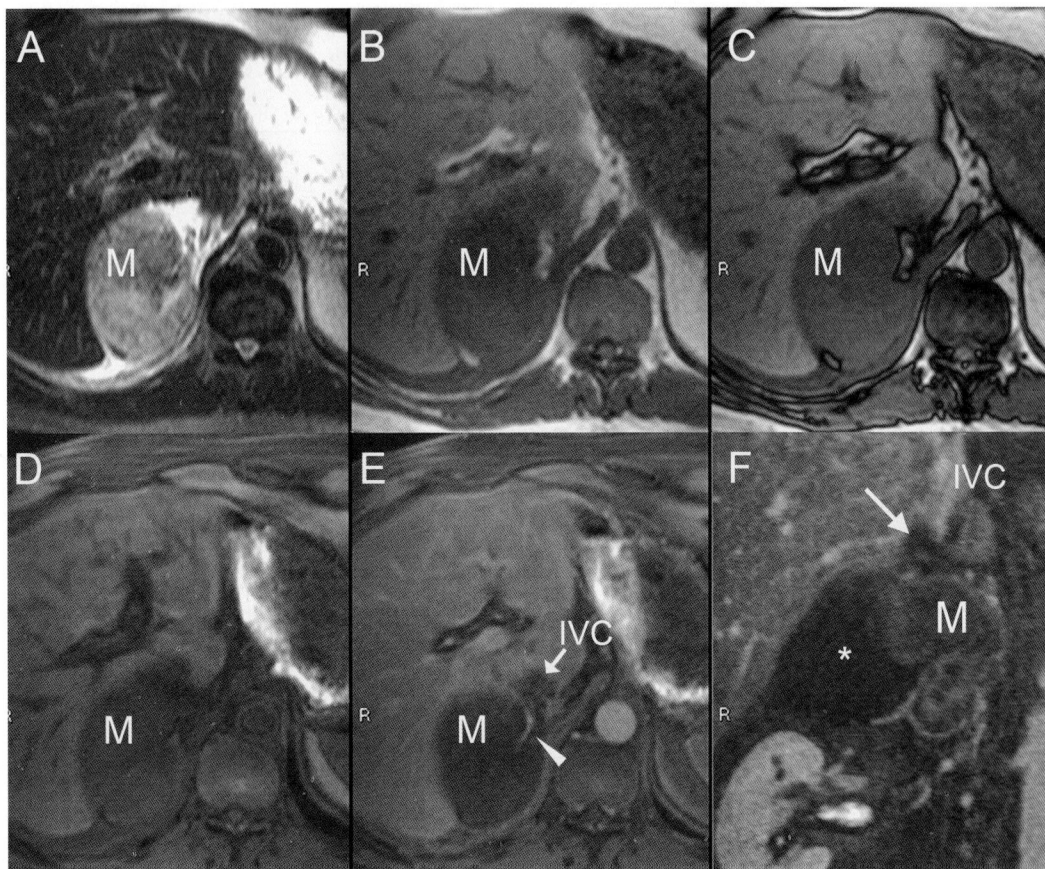

A. Axial T2-weighted single-shot FSE/TSE. **B**. Axial in-phase and (**C**) opposed-phase T1-weighted gradient echo. **D**. Pre- and (**E**) post-contrast-enhanced axial T1-weighted gradient echo with fat saturation. **F**. Coronal post-contrast-enhanced T1-weighted gradient echo with fat saturation. *M*, mass. *IVC*, inferior vena cava. *Asterisk* indicates the non-enhancing portion of the right adrenal mass.

Case 34 Adrenal Cortical Carcinoma

Findings

▶ 6-cm right adrenal lesion (*M*) with mass effect on the adjacent liver with tumor growth into the inferior vena cava (*IVC*)

▶ The mass displays high signal intensity on T2-weighted images (**A**).

▶ There is no loss of signal intensity on opposed-phase image (**C**) compared with in-phase (**B**) gradient-echo image.

▶ Most of the mass shows minimal enhancement following intravenous gadolinium contrast material administration (**E**), but there is tumor vascularity (*arrow* in **E**) growing into the inferior vena cava.

Differential diagnosis

▶ Metastatic disease

▶ Pheochromocytoma (malignant)

▶ Retroperitoneal sarcoma

▶ Non-Hodgkin's lymphoma

Teaching points

▶ The biological behavior of this tumor is aggressive, with evidence of vascular invasion by enhancing tumor. This is characteristic of primary adrenal carcinoma. Also, most primary adrenal carcinomas are quite large at diagnosis, as is seen with this case.

▶ A metastatic deposit in the adrenal gland from another primary tumor, such as lung, can become quite large, but no history of a primary extra-adrenal malignancy is given. Metastatic disease would rarely invade the IVC.

▶ Malignant pheochromocytoma is a possible consideration, but there is no history of hypertension.

▶ Retroperitoneal sarcoma and non-Hodgkin's lymphoma are also entities that cannot be excluded.

Management

▶ Both primary adrenal carcinoma and retroperitoneal sarcoma will undergo resection for diagnosis and staging of the tumor.

▶ If lymphoma is highly likely, percutaneous image-guided fine-needle aspiration biopsy can be performed for cytologic analysis and flow cytometry. Lymphoma is treated with chemotherapy and not by surgery.

Further reading

1. Allolio B, Fassnacht M. Clinical review: adrenocortical carcinoma: clinical update. J Clin Endocrinol Metab 2006;91:2027–2037.
2. Hueman MT, Herman JM, Ahuja N. Management of retroperitoneal sarcomas. Surg Clin North Am 2008;88:583–597.
3. Lau SK, Weiss LM. Adrenocortical neoplasms. Pathology Case Reviews 2005;219–227.
4. Lee FT, Jr, Thornbury JR, Grist TM, Kelcz F. MR imaging of adrenal lymphoma. Abdom Imaging 1993;18:95–96.
5. Zhang LJ, Yang GF, Shen W, Qi J. Imaging of primary adrenal lymphoma: case report and literature review. Acta Radiol 2006;47:993–997.

History:

▶ 20-year-old man presents with chest pain, shortness of breath, and tachycardia

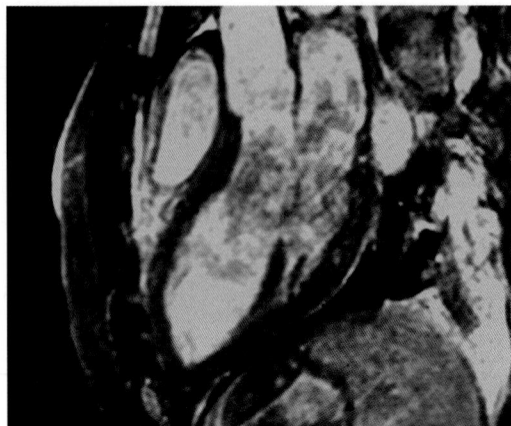

A

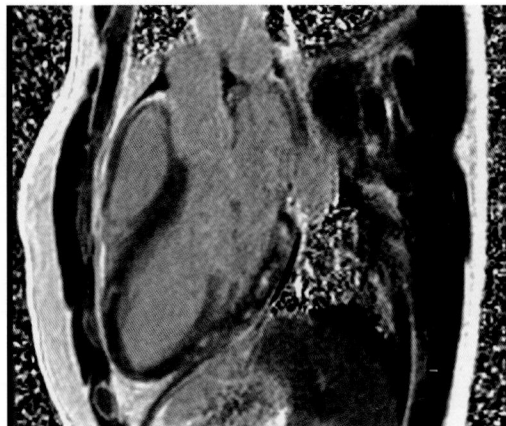

B

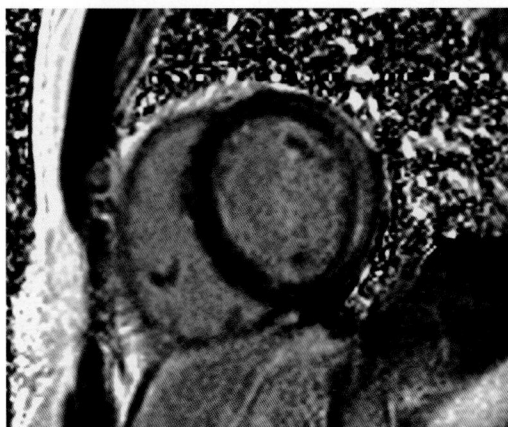

C

A. Three-chamber long-axis T2-weighted balanced steady-state free precession (SSFP). **B**. Three-chamber long-axis late gadolinium enhancement (LGE) phase-sensitive inversion recovery (PSIR). **C**. Short-axis LGE PSIR.

Case 35 Myocarditis

Findings

▶ Increased signal on T2-weighted image in the basal inferolateral wall (**A**) represents edema from inflammation.
▶ Patchy mid-wall late gadolinium enhancement (LGE) in the mid- and basal inferolateral wall (**B**) corresponding with the area of edema
▶ Extensive mid-wall LGE in the lateral wall (**C**)

Differential diagnosis

▶ Sarcoidosis
▶ Chagas disease

Teaching points

▶ Myocarditis is characterized by inflammatory infiltration of the myocardium with degeneration of adjacent myocytes.
▶ Most common etiologies are viral and are the result of Coxsackie B, adenovirus, parvovirus, Ebstein-Barr virus, and echovirus.
▶ Myocarditis may be clinically silent or present with symptoms such as chest pain, fatigue, decreased exercise intolerance, or fulminant heart failure
▶ Often leads to elevation of cardiac enzyme levels and erythrocyte sedimentation rate
▶ Cardiac MRI is most useful in discriminating between myocarditis and cardiac ischemia.
▶ Functional imaging typically demonstrates diffuse left ventricular hypokinesis.
▶ T2-weighted images may reveal increased signal intensity within the wall of the left ventricle secondary to inflammation.
▶ Delayed gadolinium contrast enhancement involving the subepicardial or mid-wall regions is the most specific finding for myocarditis, but may not always be present.
▶ Diagnosis of myocarditis with MRI is based on the clinical history and the presence of subepicardial or mid-wall LGE or edema.
▶ The most common location of LGE is the inferolateral wall of the left ventricle.

Management

▶ Management depends on the severity of presentation, but usually consists of avoidance of exercise, monitoring with electrocardiograms, treatment of congestive heart failure, and administration of antiarrhythmic agents in patients who develop resultant arrhythmias.
▶ A third of patients will recover completely with return of normal left ventricular function; another third will have some residual cardiac dysfunction; the rest will develop a dilated cardiomyopathy.

Further reading

1. Cummings KW, Bhalla S, Javidan-Nejad C, et al. A pattern-based approach to assessment of delayed enhancement in nonischemic cardiomyopathy at MR imaging. RadioGraphics 2009;29: 89–103.
2. Goitein O, Matetzky S, Beinart R, et al. Acute myocarditis: noninvasive evaluation with cardiac MRI and transthoracic echocardiography. AJR Am J Roentgenol 2009;192:254–258.
3. Laissy JP, Hyafil F, Feldman LJ, et al. Differentiating acute myocardial infarction from myocarditis: Diagnostic value of early- and delayed-perfusion cardiac MR imaging. Radiology 2005;237:75–82.

History

▶ 54-year old woman with uncontrolled hypertension

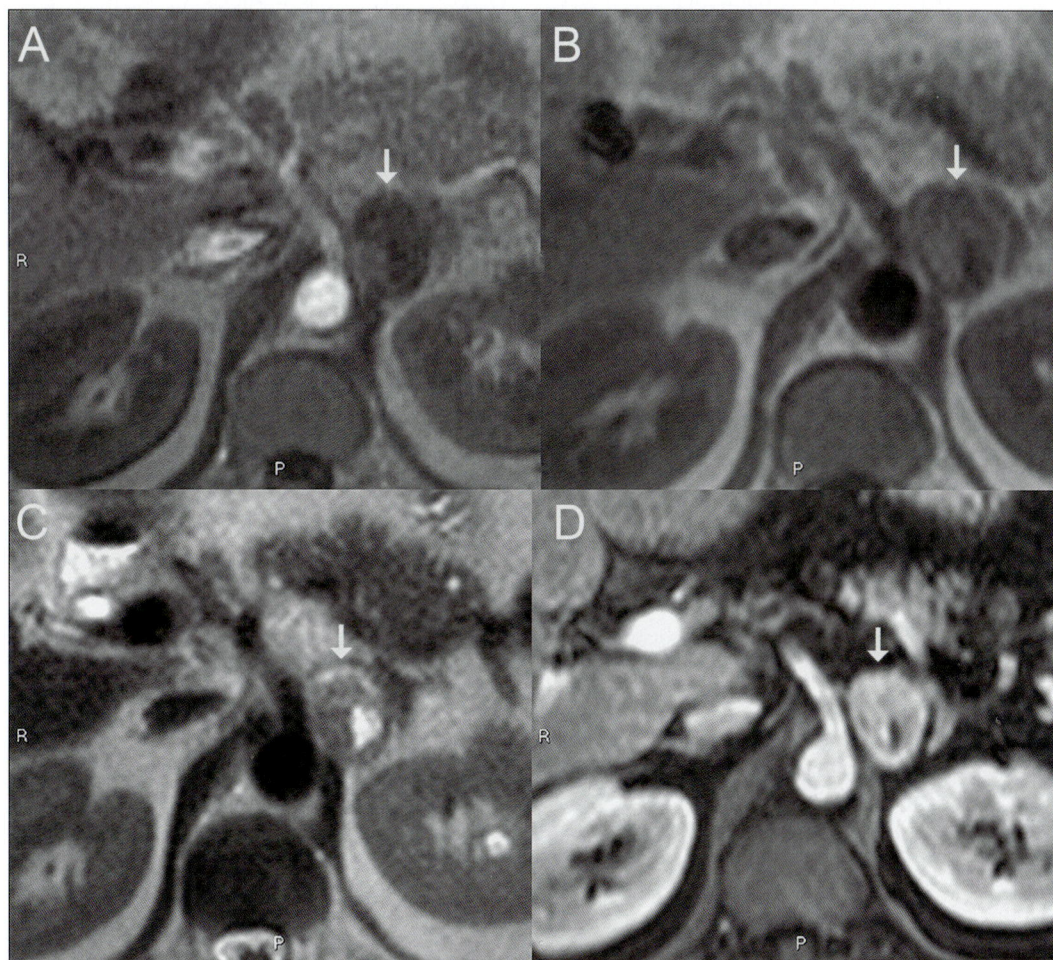

A and **B**. Axial magnetization-prepared T1-weighted gradient echo. **B**. Axial T1-weighted gradient echo. **C**. Axial T2-weighted single-shot FSE/TSE. **D**. Axial gadolinium-contrast-enhanced T1-weighted gradient echo with fat saturation.

Case 36   Pheochromocytoma Left Adrenal Gland

Findings

- ▶ Solid left adrenal mass (*arrows*) with an area of cystic degeneration
- ▶ The lesion does not contain macroscopic fat (adipose tissue) on T1-weighted gradient-echo images (**A** and **B**).
- ▶ Cystic area follows signal of simple fluid on all sequences.
- ▶ The mass enhances avidly following gadolinium contrast-material enhancement (**D**).

Differential diagnosis

- ▶ Lipid-poor adrenal adenoma
- ▶ Adrenal metastasis
- ▶ Primary adrenal cortical carcinoma
- ▶ Rare lesions (ganglioneuroma, lymphoma)

Teaching points

- ▶ This lesion could represent any of the lesions in the differential diagnosis.
- ▶ Pheochromocytoma is an imaging "chameleon" as its features can be quite variable.
- ▶ In the setting of uncontrolled hypertension, pheochromocytoma becomes the most likely diagnosis.
- ▶ Pheochromocytoma characteristically shows marked early enhancement following intravenous gadolinium contrast material administration.
- ▶ Hemorrhage, necrosis, and cystic degeneration are common findings in pheochromocytoma.
- ▶ Primary adrenal cortical carcinoma is usually larger than 6 cm at diagnosis, making this entity less likely.

Management

- ▶ Radioscintigraphy with I-131 metaiodobenzylguanidine (MIBG) study could be obtained to confirm the nature of the adrenal lesion and search for secondary foci of pheochromocytoma prior to surgery.
- ▶ The patient must undergo "adrenergic blockage" with alpha- and beta-blockers prior to any biopsy or surgical manipulation of the adrenal mass to control blood pressure and prevent hypertensive crisis.

Further reading

1. Blake MA, Kalra MK, Maher MM, et al. Pheochromocytoma: an imaging chameleon. RadioGraphics 2004;24:S87–S99.
2. Elsayes KM, Narra VR, Leyendecker JR, et al. MRI of adrenal and extraadrenal pheochromocytoma. AJR Am J Roentgenol 2005;184:860–867.
3. Lee TH, Slywotzky CM, Lavelle MT, Garcia RA. Cystic pheochromocytoma. RadioGraphics 2002;22:935–940.
4. Tischler AS. Pheochromocytoma and extra-adrenal paraganglioma: updates. Arch Pathol Lab Med 2008;132:1272–1284.

▶ Identify normal anatomy of the biliary system.

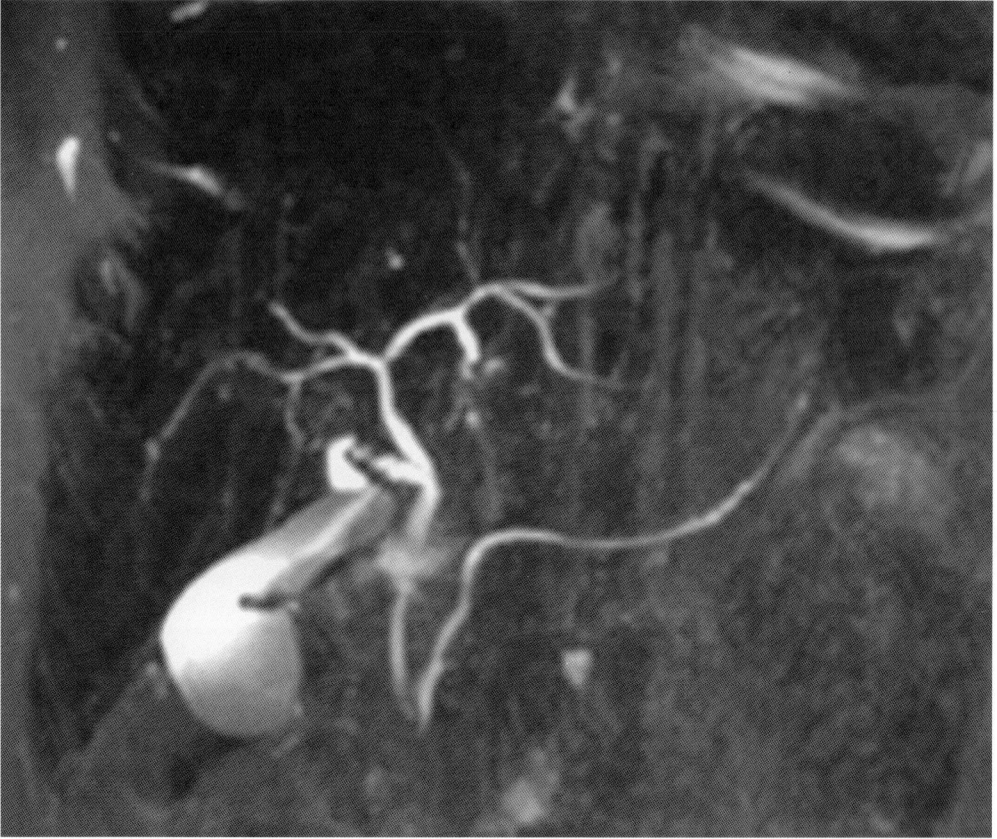

A. Maximum intensity projection MRCP image generated from respiratory gated 3D FSE/TSE with fat saturation.

Case 37 Normal Anatomy of the Biliary System

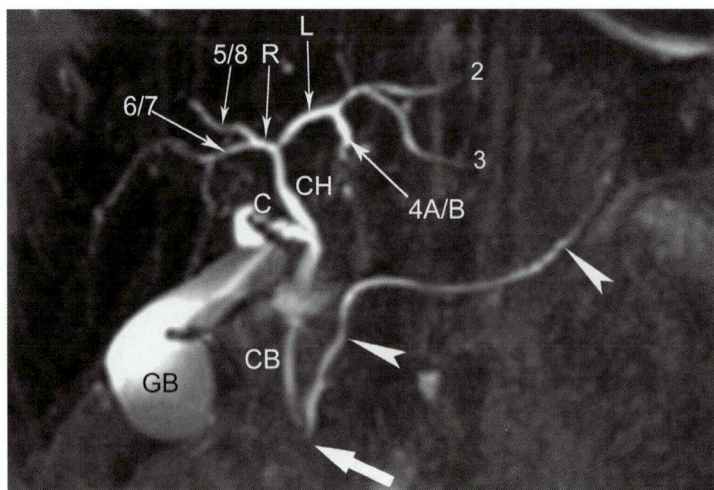

Findings

Normal biliary tree anatomy

► The main right hepatic duct (*R*) is formed by the junction of the right posterior hepatic duct (*6/7*) draining segments 6 and 7 and the right anterior hepatic duct (*5/8*) draining segments 5 and 8.
► The left hepatic duct (*L*) is formed by the ducts draining segments *2*, *3*, and *4A/B*.
► The duct of the caudate lobe joins either *L* or *R*. The duct of the caudate lobe is small and not seen in this example.
► The common hepatic duct (*CH*) is formed by the junction of main left (*L*) and main right (*R*) *hepatic duct.*
► The cystic duct (*C*) draining the gallbladder (*GB*) joins the *CH* to form the common bile duct (*CB*).
► The main pancreatic duct (*arrowheads*) joins the *CB* at the sphincter of Oddi (*fat arrow*).

Teaching points

► The classic configuration of the biliary tree is present in only 50% to 60% of the population.
► Common variants:
  ▪ The right posterior hepatic duct (6/7) drains into the left hepatic duct (L) usually within a few centimeters from the confluence of the right and left hepatic ducts (13% to 19% of the population).
  ▪ The trifurcation pattern (11% of the population), with a common confluence of the right anterior, right posterior, and left hepatic duct
  ▪ These two variants are important findings when considering potential living donors for right hepatic lobe transplantation—11% of the population.

Further reading

1. Mortele KJ, Rocha TC, Streeter JL, Taylor AJ. Multimodality imaging of pancreatic and biliary congenital anomalies. RadioGraphics 2006;26:715–731.
2. Mortele KJ, Ros PR. Anatomic variants of the biliary tree: MR cholangiographic findings and clinical applications. AJR Am J Roentgenol 2001;177:389–394.

History

▶ 59-year-old man, with history of orthotopic liver transplantation for primary sclerosing cholangitis 10 years ago, presents with fevers and chills.

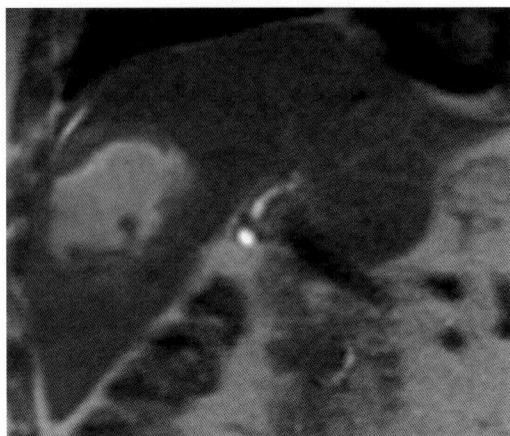

A

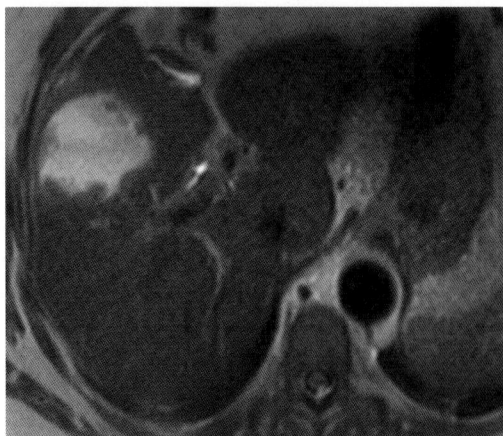

B

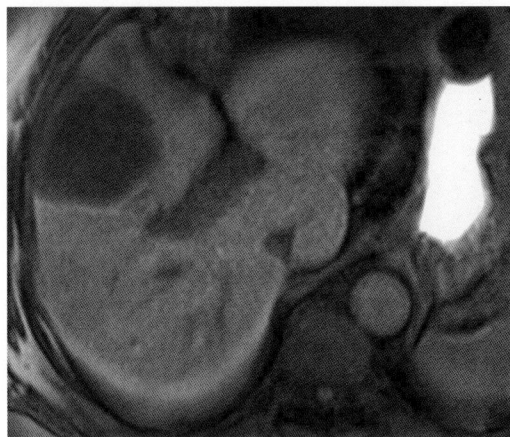

C

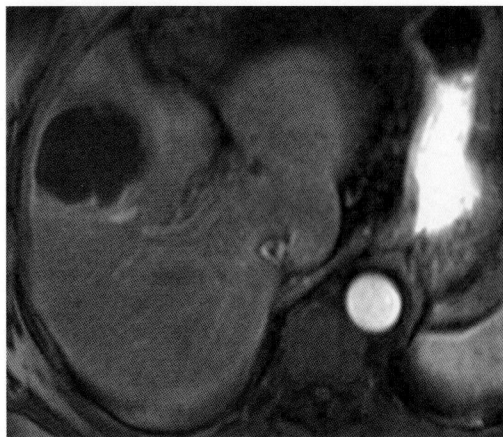

D

A. Coronal and (**B**) axial T2-weighted single-shot FSE/TSE. **C**. Axial pre- and (**D**) post-contrast-enhanced T1-weighted gradient echo with fat saturation.

Case 38 Pyogenic Liver Abscess

Findings

▶ Unilocular cystic lesion in the right lobe of the liver with irregular enhancing wall
▶ The inflammatory edema shows as increased signal intensity in the adjacent parenchyma in images **A** and **B**.
▶ Culture of aspirate showed *Enterococcus faecalis*.

Differential diagnosis

▶ Necrotic tumor (metastasis, hepatocellular carcinoma, cholangiocarcinoma)
▶ Cavernous hemangioma
▶ Hematoma/biloma

Teaching points

▶ Liver abscesses can be classified as pyogenic, amebic, or fungal. Pyogenic hepatic abscesses are the most common.
▶ Infections following solid-organ transplants are a major cause of morbidity and mortality. Mortality is higher in transplanted than nontransplanted patients.
▶ Hepatic abscess is a rare complication after liver transplantation. Etiology of liver abscess after orthotopic liver transplantation is complex. The predisposing factors reported frequently include hepatic artery thrombosis or stenosis, cholangitis, and biliary interventional therapy.

Management

▶ Prolonged antibiotic therapy, percutaneous drainage, and even retransplantation may be required to improve the outcome in these patients.

Further reading

1. Mortele KJ, Ros PR. Cystic focal liver lesions in adult: Differential CT and MRI imaging features. RadioGraphics 2001;21:895–910.
2. Tachopoulou OA, Vogt DP, Henderson JM, et al. Hepatic abscess after liver transplantation: 1990–2000. Transplantation 2003;75:79–83.
3. Vachha B, Sun MRM, Siewert B, Eisenberg RL. Cystic lesions of the liver. AJR Am J Roentgenol 2011;196:W355–W366.

History

▶ 21-year-old man with jaundice and abdominal pain

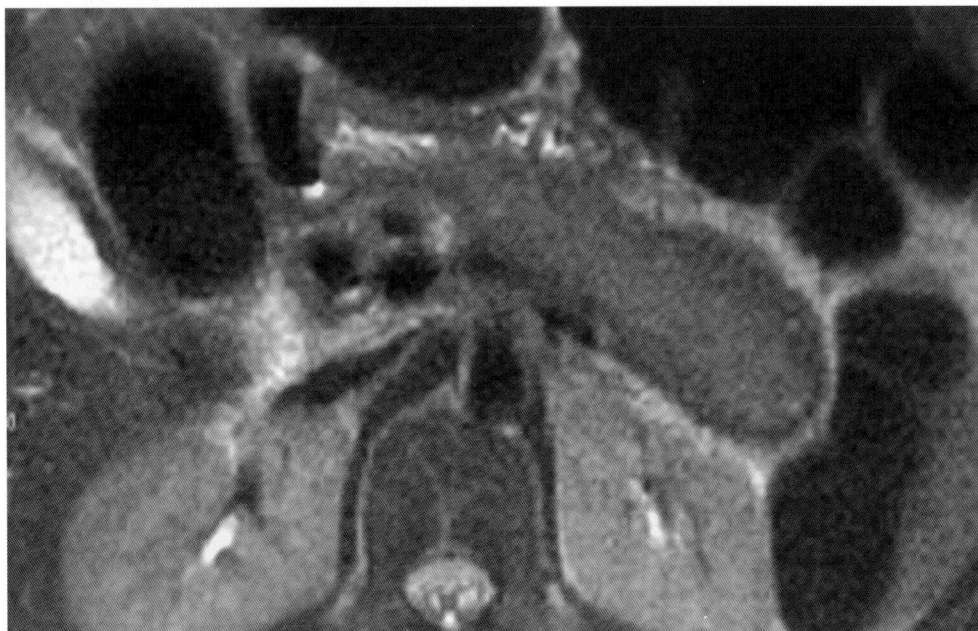

A

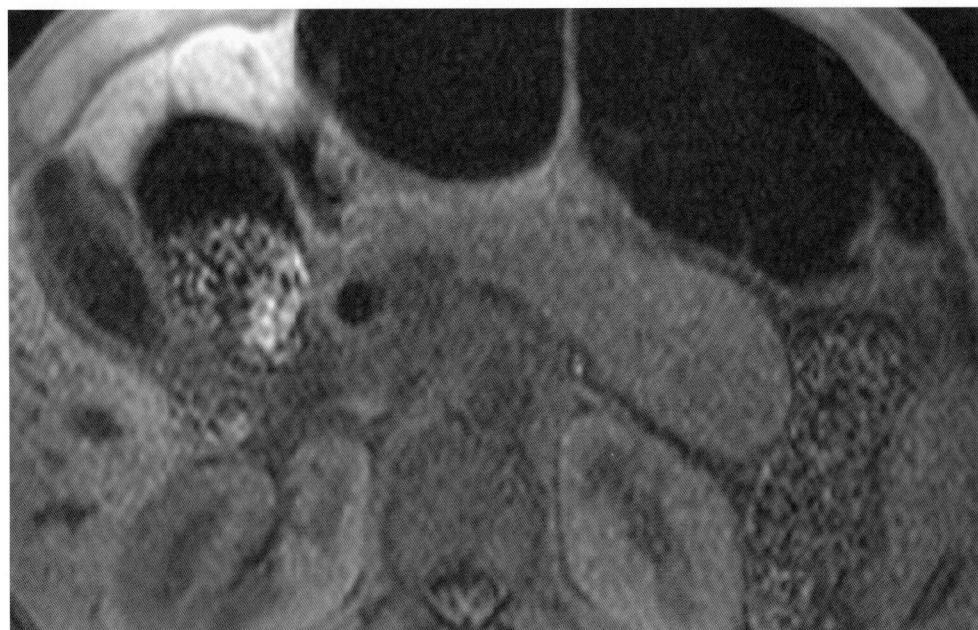

B

A. Axial T2-weighted single-shot FSE/TSE. **B**. Unenhanced axial T1-weighted gradient echo with fat saturation.

Case 39 Autoimmune Pancreatitis

Findings

- ► Diffuse enlargement of the pancreatic parenchyma
- ► Pancreas displays slightly increased signal intensity compared to liver on T2-weighted images and slightly decreased signal intensity on T1-weighted images.
- ► Note a capsule-like hypointense rim surrounding the pancreas.

Differential diagnosis

- ► Chronic pancreatitis
- ► Pancreatic ductal carcinoma

Teaching points

- ► Autoimmune form of chronic pancreatitis that responds well to steroid therapy
- ► Diffuse enlargement of pancreatic parenchyma with a halo of decreased signal intensity on T2-weighted images is a characteristic finding of autoimmune pancreatitis. The halo is thought to be related to peripancreatic inflammation.
- ► The pancreas becomes sausage-like, with loss of fatty lobulation and minimal peripancreatic stranding.
- ► Jaundice, weight loss, and diabetes are the most common clinical findings.
- ► Diffuse or segmental narrowing of the main pancreatic duct can be seen as well as strictures of the common bile duct and intrahepatic ducts resembling primary sclerosing cholangitis.

Management

- ► Slowly progresses to end-stage pancreatic disease unless treated
- ► Usually responds well to steroid therapy with normalization of all clinical and imaging abnormalities

Further reading

1. Kamisawa T, Chen PY, Tu Y, et al. MRCP and MRI findings in 9 patients with autoimmune pancreatitis. World J Gastroenterol 2006;12: 2919–2922.

History

▶ 42-year-old man presents with weight loss. No known primary malignancy.

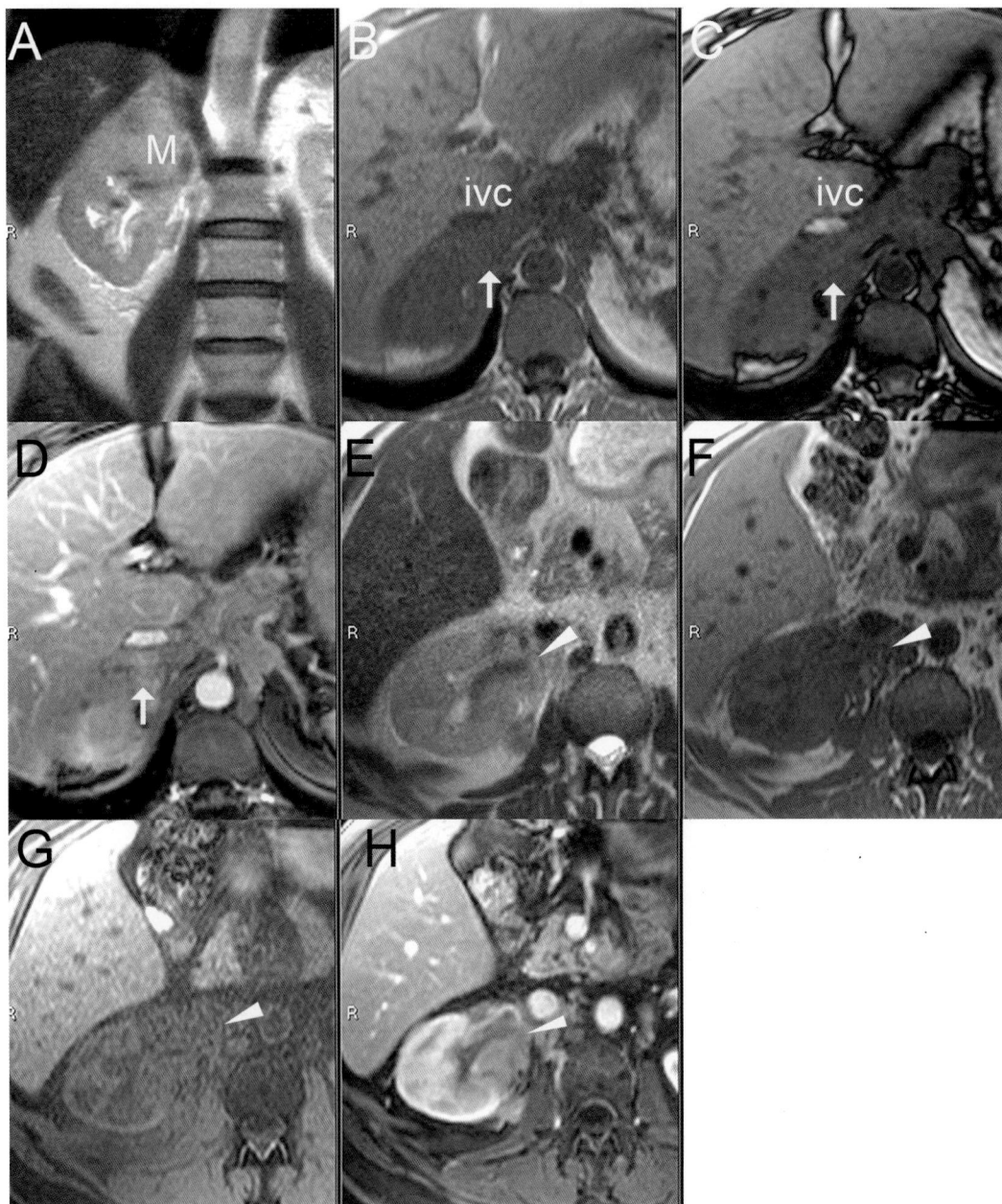

A. Coronal T2-weighted single-shot FSE/TSE of the left adrenal gland as well as (**B**) axial in-phase and (**C**) opposed-phase T1-weighted gradient echo and (**D**) axial contrast-enhanced T1-weighted gradient echo with fat saturation. **E**. Axial T2-weighted single-shot FSE/TSE obtained through the level of the right renal hilum as well as (**F**) axial T1-weighted gradient echo, (**G**) axial pre-contrast-enhanced, and (**H**) post-contrast-enhanced T1-weighted gradient echo with fat saturation. *Arrow* points to right adrenal fossa. *Arrowhead* points to renal hilum. *M* = mass. *ivc* = inferior vena cava.

Case 40 Adrenal Lymphoma

Findings

- ▶ A large mass engulfs the right adrenal gland and infiltrates the right renal hilum.
- ▶ The mass is not invading the inferior vena cava (**B**, **C**, and **D**).
- ▶ The infiltrating mass causes little mass effect but rather travels along fascial planes.
- ▶ The mass is relatively homogeneous with mild enhancement following gadolinium contrast material enhancement (**D** and **H**).

Differential diagnosis

- ▶ Retroperitoneal sarcoma
- ▶ Primary adrenal carcinoma

Teaching points

- ▶ Non-Hodgkin's lymphoma classically infiltrates the fascial planes rather than displacing structures by mass effect. Thus the tumor envelops vascular structures and seldom extends into the lumen of blood vessels. Confluent lymphadenopathy may be extensive.
- ▶ Retroperitoneal sarcomas are usually large, displace or invade adjacent parenchymal organs, and are commonly quite heterogeneous.
- ▶ Primary adrenal carcinomas are usually large and are centered in the adrenal fossa. The tumor invades adjacent organs and characteristically extends into the inferior vena cava and other vascular structures.

Management

- ▶ Percutaneous image-guided biopsy is indicated for definitive diagnosis. Once the diagnosis of lymphoma is established, chemotherapy can be initiated.
- ▶ Lymphoma is treated with chemotherapy, while sarcoma and adrenal carcinoma are primarily treated surgically.

Further reading

1. Bassignani MJ. Adrenal and retroperitoneal MR imaging. In: Brant WE, de Lange EE (eds), Essentials of Body MR Imaging. New York: Oxford University Press, 2012.
2. Lee FT, Jr, Thornbury JR, Grist TM, Kelcz F. MR imaging of adrenal lymphoma. Abdom Imaging 1993;18:95–96.
3. Zhang LJ, Yang GF, Shen W, Qi J. Imaging of primary adrenal lymphoma: case report and literature review. Acta Radiol 2006;47:993–997.

History

▶ 32-year-old woman with metastatic melanoma in remission presents for routine surveillance imaging.

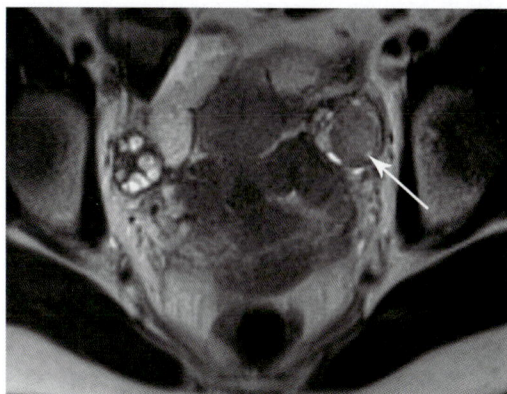

A

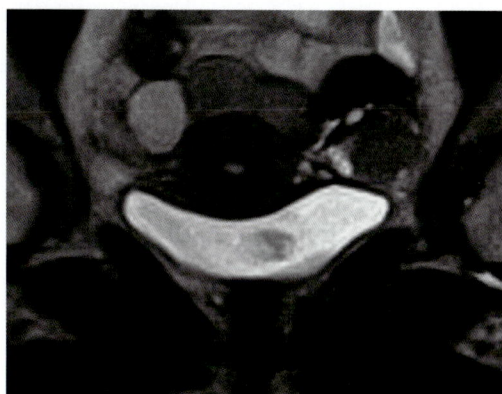

B

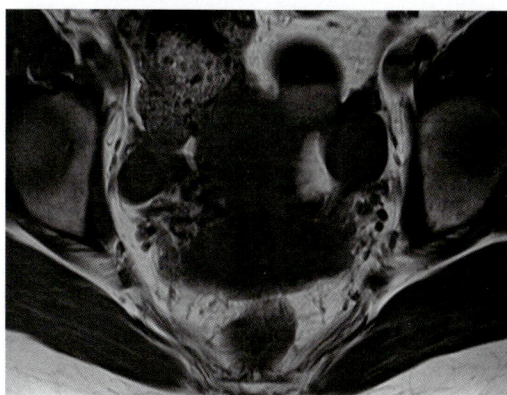

C

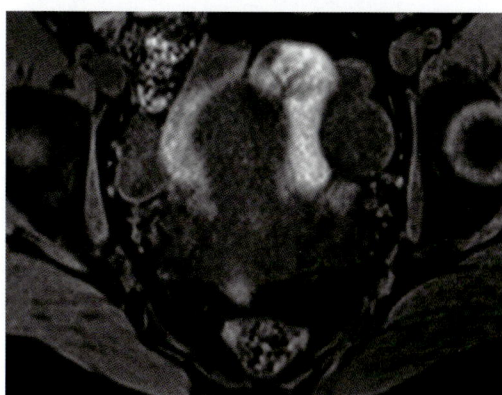

D

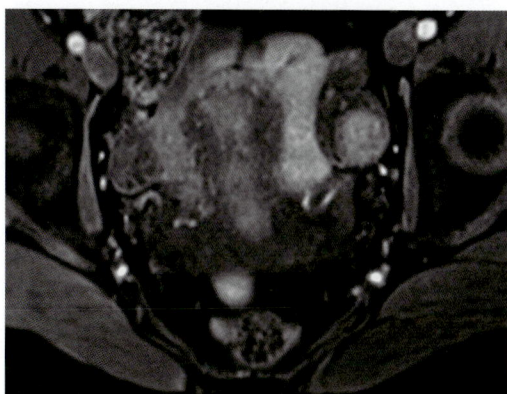

E

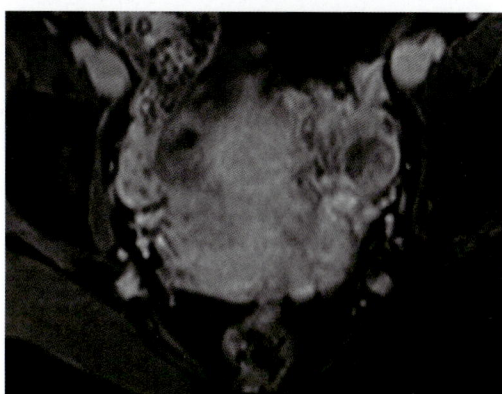

F

A. Axial and (**B**) coronal T2-weighted FSE/TSE. **C**. Axial T1-weighted spin echo. **D**. Axial pre-contrast-enhanced T1-weighted gradient echo with fat saturation. (**E**) Axial early-phase and (**F**) delayed-phase post-gadolinium contrast-enhanced T1-weighted gradient echo with fat saturation.

Case 41 Metastatic Melanoma to the Left Ovary

Findings

▶ Well-circumscribed solid mass (*arrow*) in the left ovary
▶ Mass displays intermediate-high signal intensity on fat-suppressed T1-weighted images and T2-weighted images.
▶ Avid early arterial phase enhancement and washout on delayed enhanced images

Differential diagnosis

▶ Sex-cord stromal tumor
▶ Immature teratoma
▶ Endometrioma
▶ Ovarian carcinoma

Teaching points

▶ Metastases to the ovary must be considered in the differential diagnosis of solid ovarian tumors, especially when the tumors are bilateral. Other solid adnexal lesions include fibroma, fibrothecoma, thecoma, Brenner tumor, pedunculated leiomyoma, and lymphoma.
▶ Intermediate-high signal intensity on T1- and T2-weighted images is consistent with solid mass but can also be seen with cyst containing hemorrhagic or proteinaceous material.
▶ Melanin has paramagnetic properties that can lead to increased signal intensity on T1-weighted images and variable signal intensity on T2-weighted images.
▶ Early arterial enhancement is indicative of hypervascular solid mass, including metastases from melanoma, renal cell carcinoma, and thyroid carcinoma.

Management

▶ Surgical resection
▶ Chemotherapy

Further reading

1. Kelekis NL, Semelka RC, Woosley JT. Malignant lesions of the liver with high signal intensity on T1-weighted MR images. J Magn Reson Imaging 1996;6:291–294.
2. Rajkotia K, Veeramani M, Macura KJ. Magnetic resonance imaging of adnexal masses. Top Magn Reson Imaging 2006;17:379–397.
3. Saini A, Dina R, McIndoe GA, Soutter, et al. Characterization of adnexal masses with MRI. AJR Am J Roentgenol 2005;184:1004–1009.

History

▶ 65-year-old man post bilateral nephrectomy and renal transplant for end-stage kidney disease

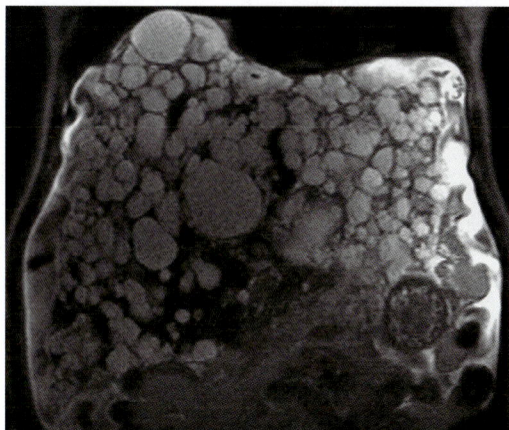

A

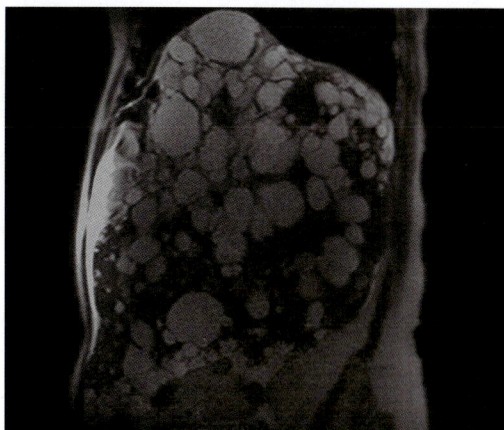

B

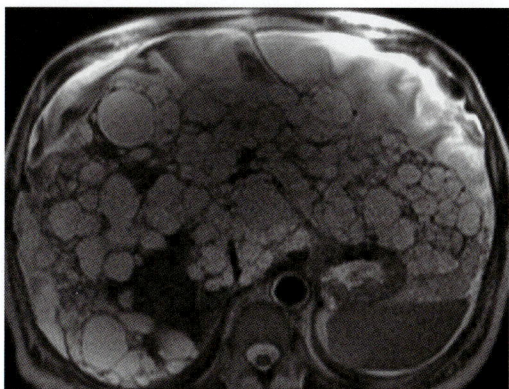

C

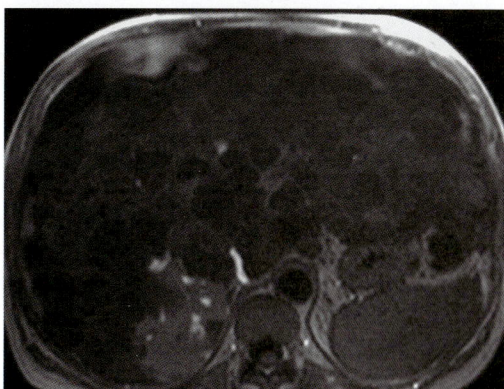

D

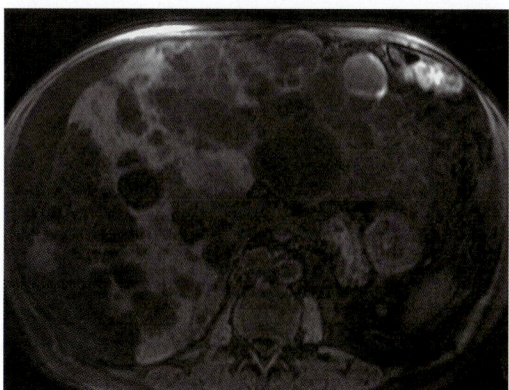

E

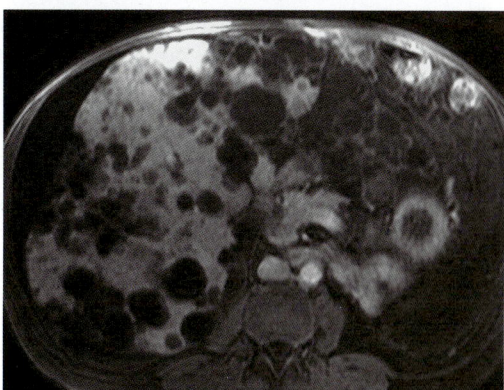

F

A. Coronal, (**B**) sagittal, and (**C**) axial T2-weighted single-shot FSE/TSE. **D**. Axial T1-weighted gradient echo. **E**. Axial pre-contrast-enhanced and (**F**) post-gadolinium contrast-enhanced gradient echo with fat saturation.

Case 42 Autosomal Dominant Polycystic Liver Disease

Findings

▶ Innumerable cysts of varying size replace most of the liver parenchyma, diffusely enlarging the liver.
▶ The cysts are thin-walled, without solid components, and show no enhancement.
▶ Both kidneys are absent as they were removed because of end-stage renal disease and their large size causing mass effect on other organs.

Differential diagnosis

▶ Caroli's disease—cysts communicate with the biliary tree
▶ Bile duct hamartomas (hamartomas)—all lesions are smaller than 1.5 cm

Teaching points

▶ Polycystic liver disease occurs in up to 40% of patients with autosomal dominant polycystic kidney disease. It is important to note that polycystic liver disease can occur in the absence of renal cysts. Progressive development and enlargement of the cysts is the usual course of disease. Patients may be asymptomatic or may have recurrent right upper quadrant pain, or symptoms related to massive hepatomegaly.
▶ In autosomal dominant polycystic liver disease the cysts have the same characteristics as benign developmental hepatic cysts, found commonly as the second most frequent hepatic mass. The cysts are thin-walled, have no solid components, and vary in size. Their shape may be affected by adjacent cysts. Hemorrhage within the cysts is the major complication. Despite the extensive liver involvement, the overall liver function is not affected in most cases. Extreme involvement may eventually result in liver failure or Budd-Chiari syndrome.
▶ MR shows well-defined cysts containing simple fluid unless hemorrhage has occurred. The cysts have uniform thin walls and contain fluid that displays uniform low signal intensity on T1-weighted images and uniform high signal intensity on T2-weighted images. No enhancement is present on dynamic post-contrast-enhanced images. MR is more sensitive than CT or ultrasound for detection of intracystic hemorrhage.

Management

▶ No treatment is required in asymptomatic patients.
▶ Patients with pain from hemorrhage may undergo surgical resection.
▶ Large cysts may be percutaneously ablated with alcohol injection.

Further reading

1. Morgan DE, Lockhart ME, Canon CL, et al. Polycystic liver disease: multimodality imaging for complications and transplant evaluation. RadioGraphics 2006;26:1655–1668.
2. Mortele KJ, Ros PR. Cystic focal liver lesions in the adult: differential CT and MR imaging features. RadioGraphics 2001;21: 895–910.
3. Vaccha B, Sun MRM, Siewart B, Eisenberg RL. Cystic lesions of the liver. AJR Am J Roentgenol 2011;196:W355–W366.

History

▶ 65-year-old woman with history of hysterectomy for leiomyomas presents with pelvic pain and pelvic mass on physical examination.

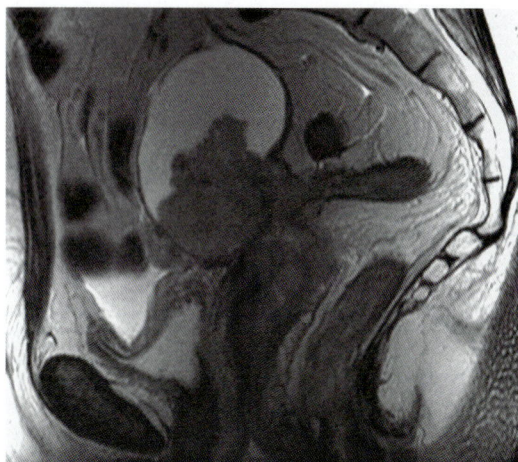

A

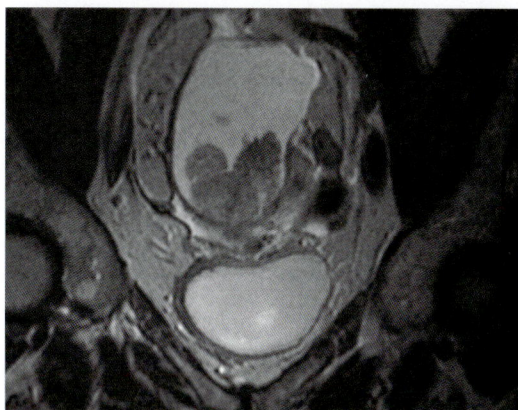

B

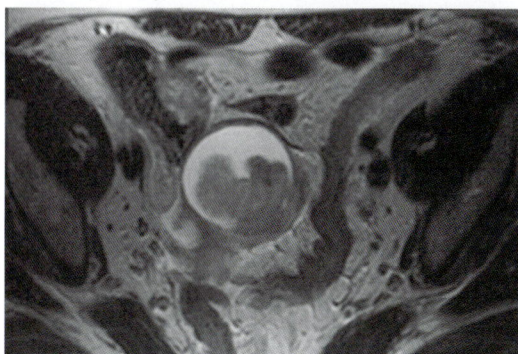

C

A. Sagittal, (**B**) coronal, and (**C**) axial T2-weighted FSE/TSE.

Case 43 Serous Cystadenocarcinoma of the Ovary

Findings

- Cystic mass in the midline of the pelvis with prominent solid components extending posteriorly and inferiorly from the mass into adjacent pelvic fat with soft-tissue involvement of the upper vagina.
- Small-volume ascites is present superior to the bladder.
- Uterus is absent.

Differential diagnosis

- This is ovarian cancer until proven otherwise.

Teaching points

- Subtypes of ovarian cancer have differing natural behavior, prognosis, and response to therapy. The four most common subtypes of ovarian cancer are serous, endometrioid, clear cell, and mucinous. Tumors are further classified into low grade, high grade, and borderline (also called tumors of low malignant potential). High-grade serous carcinoma is the most common subtype with current evidence strongly indicating that it actually arises from the epithelium of the distal fallopian tube. It is a biologically aggressive tumor with peritoneal metastases present at diagnosis in 85% of cases. Primary mucinous carcinomas are nearly always low grade and unilateral. Clear cell and endometrioid carcinomas arise in many cases from endometriosis.
- Imaging features indicative of ovarian malignancy include complex cystic mass with solid components; size larger than 5 cm; papillary projections extending from the wall of the cystic mass; nodular wall thickness greater than 3 mm; and thick nodular septations thicker than 3 mm. Ancillary findings may include ascites; peritoneal, omental, or mesenteric tumor implants; lymphadenopathy; and local extension to other pelvic organs or to the pelvic sidewall.
- With its superior tissue contrast, current high spatial resolution, and multiplanar capability MR is ideally suited for diagnosis and characterization of ovarian masses. For staging of known tumors CT and MR are comparable, with reported accuracy of each in the 70% to 90% range.

Management

- Ovarian cancer treatment is based upon surgical tumor debulking and chemotherapy.

Further reading

1. Lalwani N, Prasad SR, Vikram R, et al. Histologic, molecular, and cytogenetic features of ovarian cancers: implications for diagnosis and treatment. RadioGraphics 2011;31:625–646.
2. McCluggage WG. Morphological subtypes of ovarian carcinoma: a review with emphasis on new developments and pathogenesis. Pathology 2011;43:420–432.
3. Woodward PJ, Hosseinzadeh K, Saenger JS. Radiologic staging of ovarian carcinoma with pathologic correlation. RadioGraphics 2004;24:225–246.

History

▶ 49-year-old woman with frequent and excessive vaginal bleeding (menometrorrhagia)

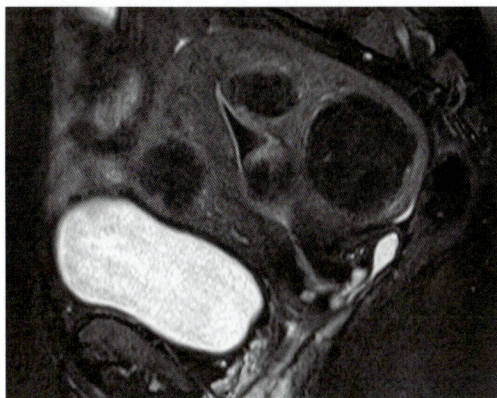
A

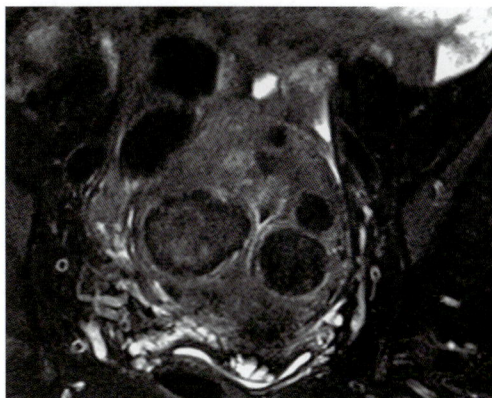
B

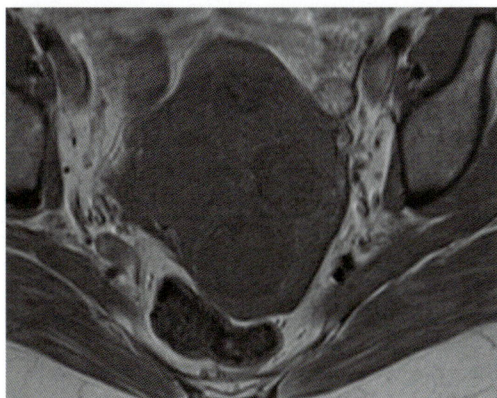
C

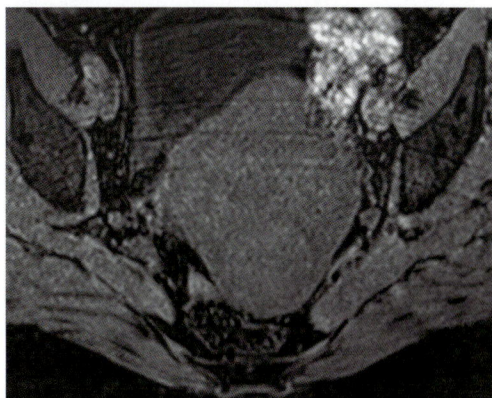
D

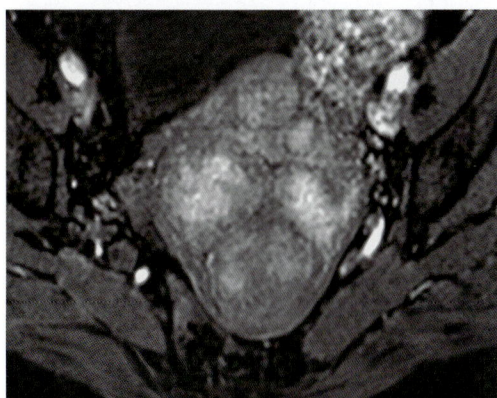
E

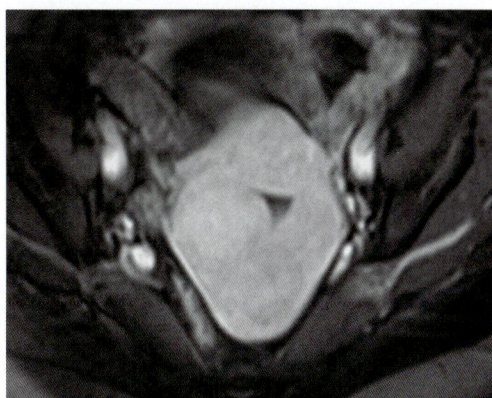
F

A. Sagittal and (**B**) oblique axial T2-weighted FSE/TSE with fat saturation. **C**. Axial T1-weighted spin echo. **D**. Axial T1-weighted gradient echo with fat saturation. **E**. Early-phase and (**F**) late-phase gadolinium contrast-enhanced axial T1-weighted gradient echo with fat saturation.

Case 44 Multiple Benign Uterine Leiomyomas

Findings

- Multiple well-defined masses arising in the myometrium
- One of the tumors shown in **A** is submucosal in origin and protrudes into and distorts the endometrial canal.
- Several of the masses are defined on T2-weighted images (**B**, **C**) by high-signal-intensity rims caused by peritumoral edema, and engorgement of the lymphatics and veins.
- T1-weighted images (**C**, **D**) show limited differentiation between the tumors and the myometrium.
- The tumors show early enhancement, becoming isointense with the myometrium on delayed post-contrast-enhanced images.

Differential diagnosis

- Adenomyosis
- Leiomyosarcoma

Teaching points

- Benign leiomyomas are tightly packed aggregates of smooth muscle cells with a variable amount of interspersed fibrous tissue. Grossly, the tumors are well defined, firm, and rubbery. Swirling of the muscle cells give the tumors a characteristic whorled appearance on MR images. A pseudocapsule of connective tissue separates the leiomyoma from the adjacent myometrium.
- Symptoms of menorrhagia, mass effect, pain, and infertility occur in 20% of patients with leiomyomas. Symptoms are related to the size, number, and location of the tumors.
- *Submucosal leiomyomas* adjacent to the endometrium may protrude into the uterine canal, eroding the endometrium and causing menometrorrhagia. Tumors may be broad-based or polypoid resembling endometrial polyps.
- *Intramural leiomyomas* are located more centrally within the myometrium.
- *Subserosal leiomyomas* protrude beyond the uterine wall. These may be pedunculated, simulating an adnexal mass, or may torse, causing acute pain.
- On MRI benign leiomyomas classically appear as well-circumscribed masses displaying low signal intensity on all sequences. A high-signal-intensity rim may or may not be present. The tumors may appear heterogeneous as a result of hyaline degeneration, cystic degeneration, hemorrhage, fat content, or coarse calcification. Post-gadolinium contrast-enhancement patterns are variable. Most enhance similar to or slightly less than the myometrium, while others show brisk hyperenhancement.

Management

- Treatment options include open surgical excision, hysterectomy, hysteroscopic excision, uterine artery embolization, and focused ultrasound ablation.

Further reading

1. Cohen DT, Oliva E, Hahn PF, et al. Uterine smooth-muscle tumors with unusual growth patterns: imaging with pathologic correlation. AJR Am J Roentgenol 2007;188:246–255.
2. DeAngelis GA. Gynecologic MR imaging. In: Brant WE, de Lange EE (eds), Essentials of Body MRI. New York: Oxford University Press, 2012.
3. Ruuskanen AJ, Hippeläinen MI, Sipola P, Manninen HI. Association between magnetic resonance imaging findings of uterine leiomyomas and symptoms demanding treatment. Eur J Radiol 2011 [Epub ahead of print].

History

▶ 54-year-old man with biliary obstruction and ductal dilatation. Both images were obtained during breath hold using the same pulse sequence and identical image parameters. Explain the difference in image quality.

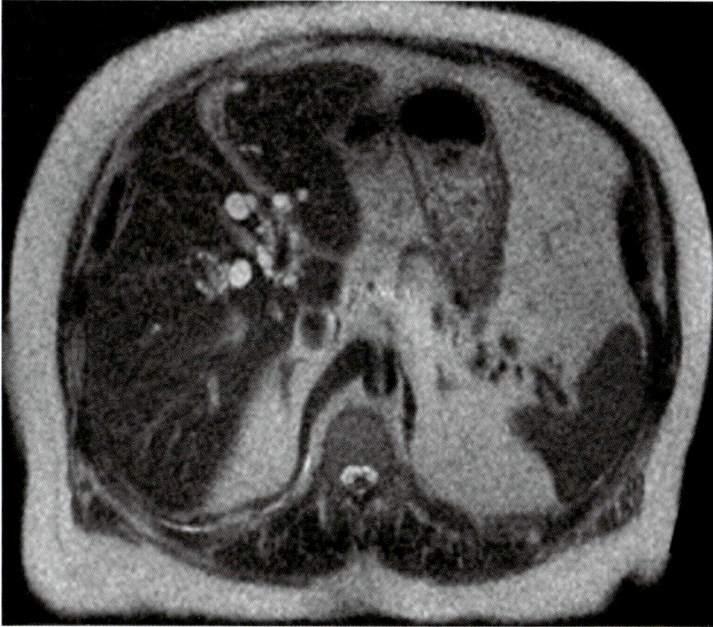

A

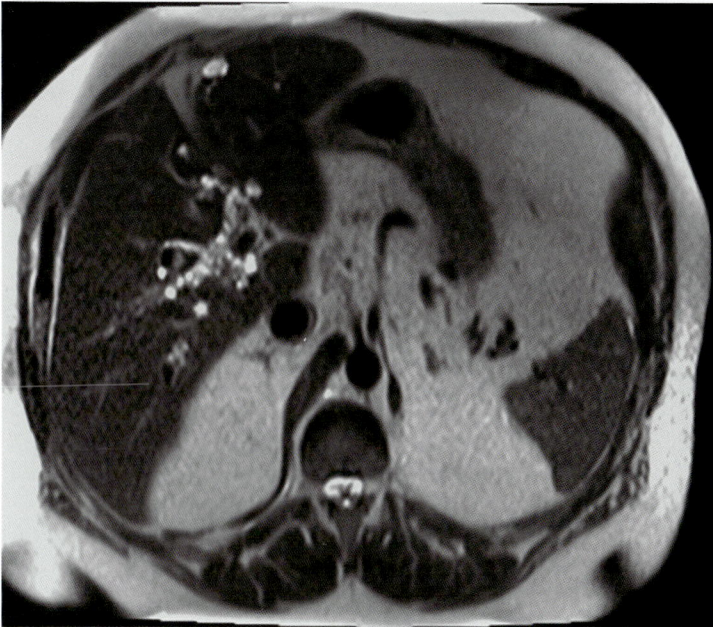

B

A and **B**. Axial single-shot FSE/TSE.

Case 45 Signal-to-Noise (SNR) versus RF Coil Type

Findings

▶ Image **A** is more grainy than **B.**

▶ SNR of image **A** is lower than that of **B.**

Teaching points

▶ Image **A** was acquired using the body radiofrequency (RF) coil, whereas a "phased-array" RF coil was used for **B.** This type of RF coil is also called a multi-channel coil or a multi-coil array, and the particular coil used for this application is also sometimes called a "body array."

▶ A phased/body-array RF coil consists of a number (at least 4 but up to 32 in more recent designs) of small-diameter coils that, combined in an array, provide a higher SNR than the body RF coil. The latter coil is part of the MR scanner itself and is located behind the surface of the magnet bore. The body coil functions to both transmit the RF pulses and receive the MR signals.

▶ The phased/body-array coil has an anterior section that is positioned over the abdomen of the patient when supine on the scanner table, and a posterior section that covers the back of the patient.

▶ With use of a phased-array coil the increase in SNR can be several times that provided by the body coil, and depends on the number and configuration of small coils within the phased/body-array system. Whereas the large body coil is sensitive to all of the noise from the large volume of tissue within the body coil, each of the smaller coils in the array is sensitive only to the noise within the small volume of tissue close to the coil. Hence, this reduced noise level provides an increased SNR. When a phased/body-array coil is used, which is generally a receive-only system, the body coil transmits the RF pulses.

▶ Use of a phased/body-array coil is preferred for obtaining high-quality MR images, especially when fast acquisition techniques are used, as in breath-hold abdominal imaging.

▶ Other causes for relatively grainy images:
  • Image obtained with high spatial resolution
  • Image obtained with small field of view
  • Image obtained using thin slices

Management

▶ Use of phased/body-array RF coil increases SNR and is preferred for obtaining good-quality images of the abdomen.

▶ In very large patients it may not be possible to use a phased/body-array coil system when there is not enough room between the patient and the wall of the scanner bore. In such cases the images are obtained using the body coil.

Further reading

1. Becerra RJ, Harsh MJ, Boskamp EB, et al. Instrumentation: Magnet, Gradients, and Coils. In: Edelman RR, Hesselink JR, Zlatkin MB, Crues JV(Eds). Clinical Magnetic Resonance Imaging. Philadelphia: Saunders, Elsevier, 3rd edition, 2006.

History

▶ 70-year-old man with history of ascending aortic aneurysm

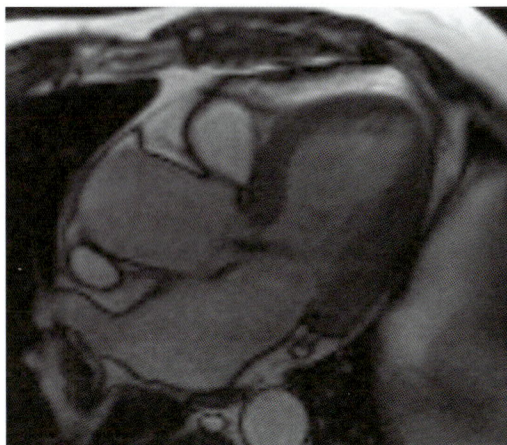

A

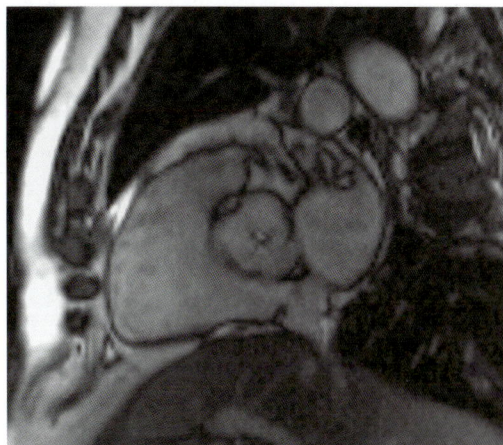

B

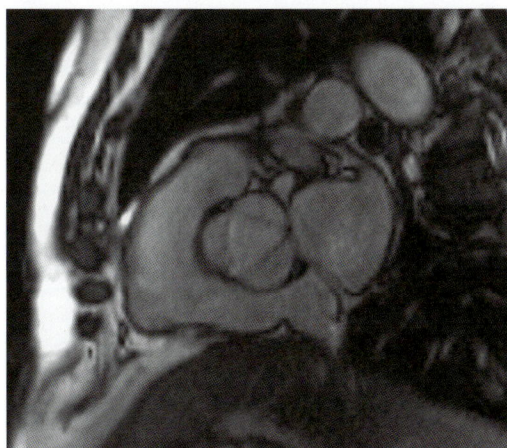

C

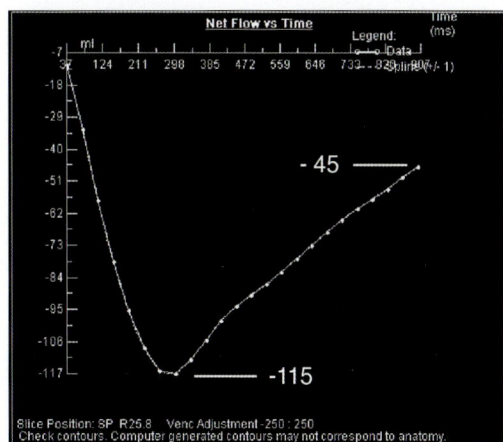

D

A. Three-chamber long-axis view balanced steady-state free precession (SSFP) during diastole. **B**. Short-axis aortic valve view during diastole and during (**C**) systole. **D**. Net flow (in mL) through the aortic valve as a function of time during the cardiac cycle (negative magnitude represents forward flow in the aorta).

Case 46   Aortic Regurgitation (AR)

Findings

▶ Central regurgitant jet within the left ventricular outflow tract on three-chamber long-axis SSFP image with mild enlargement of the aortic root

▶ Tricuspid aortic valve with poor central coaptation of the aortic leaflets on the short-axis images during diastole. The three valve leaflets are thin and normal in appearance.

▶ Sharp (downward-sloping) antegrade systolic flow with continuous retrograde flow during diastole

▶ Regurgitant fraction = Retrograde flow/Forward flow = [115 − 45]/115 = 61%, representing severe AR

Differential diagnosis

▶ Aortic stenosis

Teaching points

▶ AR results from a cusp abnormality, distortion of the aortic root, or aneurysmal dilatation of the ascending aorta.

▶ Common causes of AR include bicuspid aortic valve, bacterial endocarditis, aortic root dilatation secondary to hypertension or dissection, ankylosing spondylitis, and Marfan's disease.

▶ AR may lead to cardiogenic shock in acute cases or left ventricular dilatation and subsequent heart failure in chronic cases.

▶ AR is identified by the presence of a high-velocity retrograde jet into the left ventricle during diastole on functional cine imaging; however, the degree of regurgitation cannot be assessed by the size of the jet.

▶ Aortic stenosis demonstrates a jet directed into the aorta during systole and typically results in left ventricular hypertrophy in the early stages of the disease.

▶ Cardiac MR, as opposed to echocardiography, allows direct measurement of the regurgitant flow using velocity-encoded cine MR imaging (VENC) to grade the severity.

▶ Regurgitant fraction is the percentage of retrograde aortic flow to forward aortic flow and is graded as mild (15% to 20%), moderate (20% to 40%), and severe (>40%).

▶ Cardiac MR is useful for defining valvular anatomy, function, atrial/ventricular volumes, and aortic/pulmonary artery size, all of which are important in the timing and planning of valve surgery.

Management

▶ Dependent on the etiology of regurgitation

▶ May include valve replacement and/or medical treatment

Further reading

1. Bogaert J, Dymarkowski S, Herregods M, Taylor AM. Valvular heart disease. In: Higgins CB, de Roos A (eds), MRI and CT of the Cardiovascular System, 2nd ed. Philadelphia: Lippincott Williams & Wilkins, 2005:183.
2. Cawley PJ, Maki JH, Otto CM. Cardiovascular magnetic resonance imaging for valvular heart disease: technique and validation. Circulation 2009;119:468–478.
3. Koskenvuo JW, Jarvinen V, Parkka JP, et al. Cardiac magnetic resonance imaging in valvular heart disease. Clin Physiol Funct Imaging 2009;29:229–240.
4. Norton PT. Cardiac MR imaging. In: Brant WE, de Lange EE (eds), Essentials of Body MRI. New York: Oxford University Press, 2012.

History

▶ 37-year-old man with history of biliary colic referred to the gastroenterology service for treatment of an impacted gallstone

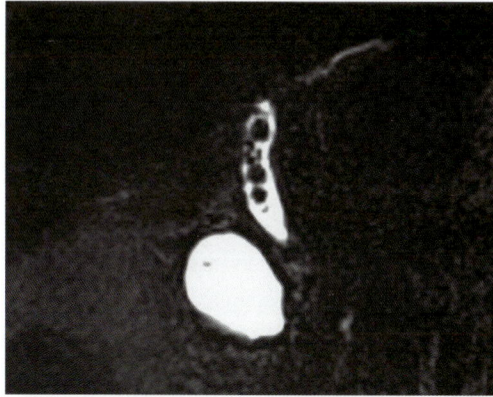

A

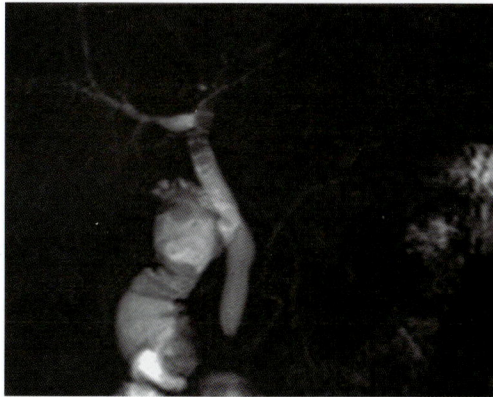

B

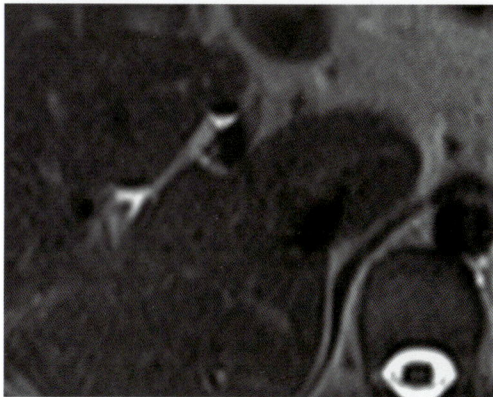

C

A. Coronal thin-slice source image of respiratory gated 3D FSE/TSE sequence for MRCP. **B**. Coronal thick-slice MRCP using single-shot FSE/TSE. **C**. Axial T2-weighted single-shot FSE/TSE.

Case 47 Air bubbles in the common bile duct in a patient who had a prior sphincterotomy

Findings

- ▶ Multiple rounded signal voids in the common bile duct
- ▶ Axial image shows the signal void with meniscus in nondependent aspect of the common bile duct, confirming that it is an air bubble.

Differential diagnosis

- ▶ Gallstones
- ▶ Blood clots
- ▶ Neoplasms

Teaching points

- ▶ Biliary stones are seen as signal voids within high-signal-intensity bile on T2-weighted images. Because most gallstones are heavier than bile they are usually seen in a dependent position of the duct with a crescent of bile outlining the anterior portion of the stone.
- ▶ Stones are often angulated and geometric in shape, and may have a lamellated appearance caused by layers of different composition.
- ▶ Stones, especially when impacted, are often associated with inflammatory changes of the bile duct including wall thickening, periductal edema, and wall enhancement with intravenous contrast material administration.
- ▶ Air bubbles within the bile duct rise to a nondependent position of the duct. The posterior portion of the air bubble may be outlined by an air–fluid level shown on T2-weighted images as a meniscus of the high-signal-intensity bile against the low-signal-intensity air (**C**).
- ▶ Susceptibility artifact showing "blooming" and increased apparent size of the air bubble may be evident on T1-weighted gradient-echo images.

Management

- ▶ None needed. The pitfall must be recognized.

Further reading

1. Irie H, Honda H, Kuroiwa T, et al. Pitfalls in MR cholangiopancreatographic interpretation. RadioGraphics 2001;21: 23–37.
2. Olazagasti J. Biliary MR imaging. In: Brant WE, de Lange EE (eds), Essentials of Body MR Imaging. New York: Oxford University Press, 2012.
3. Watanabe Y, Dohke M, Ishimori T, et al. Diagnostic pitfalls of MR cholangiopancreatography in the evaluation of the biliary tract and gallbladder RadioGraphics 1999;19:415–429.
4. Yeh BM, Liu PS, Soto JA, et al. MR imaging and CT of the biliary tract. RadioGraphics 2009;29:1669–1688.

History

▶ 66-year-old woman with history of chronic hepatitis C and recent elevation of alpha-fetoprotein

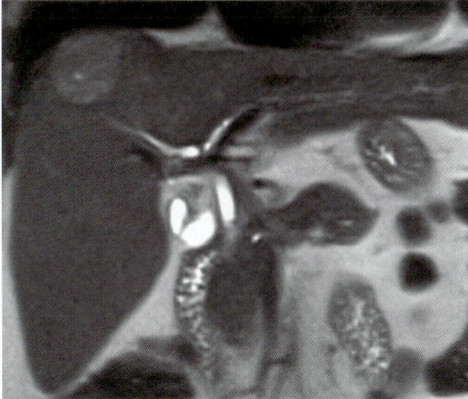

A

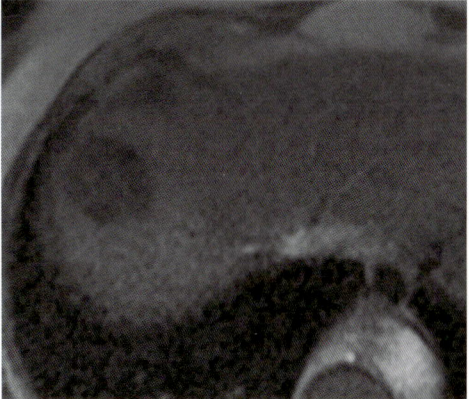

B

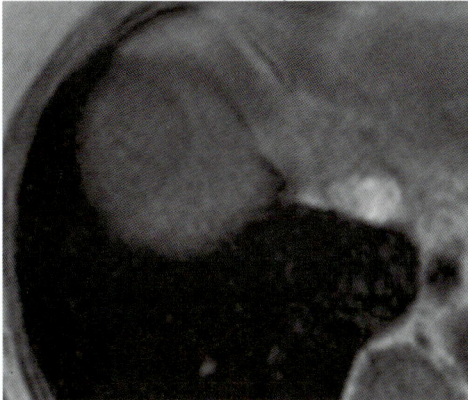

C

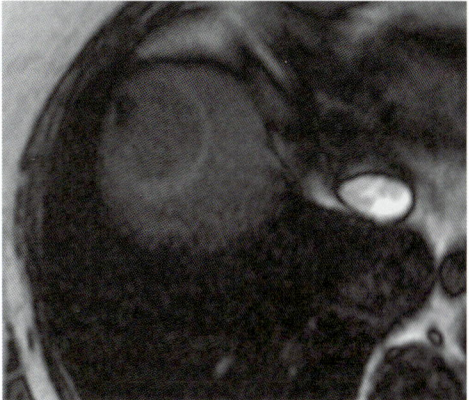

D

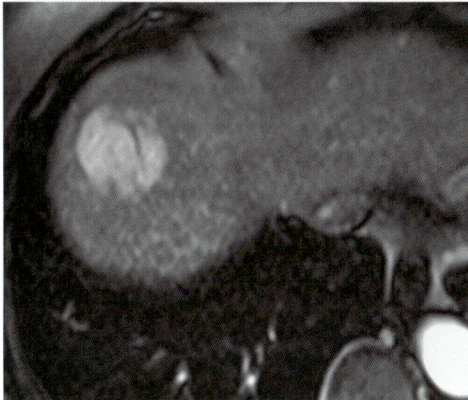

E

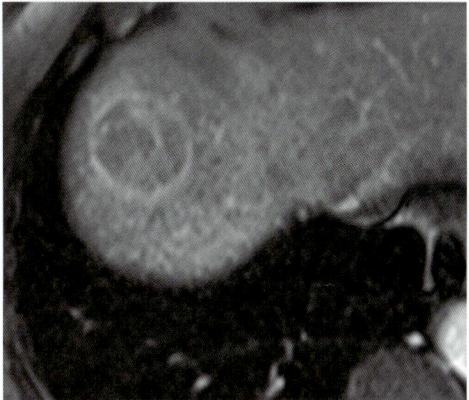

F

A. Coronal T2-weighted single-shot FSE/TSE. **B**. Axial T1-weighted gradient echo. **C**. Axial in-phase and (**D**) opposed-phase T1-weighted gradient echo. **E**. Early-phase and (**F**) delayed-phase axial T1-weighted gradient echo with fat saturation.

Case 48 Hepatocellular Carcinoma (Hepatoma)

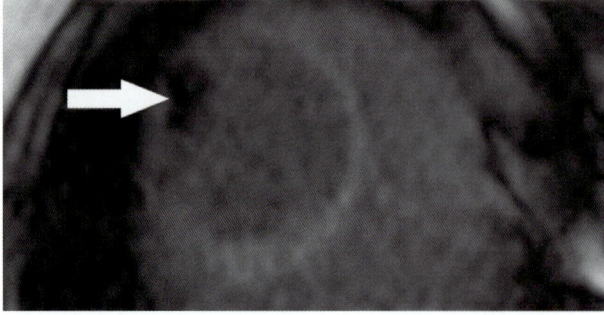

G. Opposed phase T1-weighted gradient echo image, same as **D**.

Findings

▶ A round heterogenous mass at the dome of the liver demonstrating intermediate high signal intensity on T2-weighted images and relatively low signal intensity on T1-weighted images compared to liver parenchyma.

▶ Focal signal loss (*arrow*) on out-of-phase image **D** (detailed in **G**) indicates interspersed fat along the right lateral margin.

▶ Post-contrast-enhanced imaging shows hypervascularity of the tumor with early arterial enhancement followed by early washout of contrast material on delayed post-contrast imaging.

Differential diagnosis

▶ Hepatic adenoma
▶ Focal nodular hyperplasia
▶ Hemangioma
▶ Metastases
▶ Nodular regenerative hyperplasia

Teaching points

▶ Approximately 80% of hepatocellular carcinomas develop in the setting of cirrhosis.

▶ Small lesions can have a nodule-within-a-nodule appearance. Large lesions can have interspersed fat, a heterogeneous appearance due to hemorrhage and necrosis, a fibrous capsule, and extension into adjacent parenchyma and vessels.

▶ A hyperintense lesion during the arterial phase contrast-enhanced imaging that becomes hypointense compared with adjacent liver on delayed enhanced imaging (venous washout) increases specificity for hepatocellular carcinoma, since regenerative and dysplastic nodules typically do not demonstrate these features.

Management

▶ Percutaneous tumor ablation, surgical resection, or liver transplant

Further reading

1. Bruix J, Sherman M. Management of hepatocellular carcinoma: an update. Hepatology 2011;53:1020–1022.
2. Digumarthy S, Sahani DV, Saini S. MRI in detection of hepatocellular carcinoma (HCC). Cancer Imaging 2005;5:20–24.
3. Silva AC, Evans JM, McCullough AE, et al. MR imaging of hypervascular liver masses: A review of current techniques. RadioGraphics 2009;29:385–402.

History

▶ 64-year-old man with abdominal pain and a history of melanoma was referred for MRI after ultrasound examination had revealed a mass in the gallbladder.

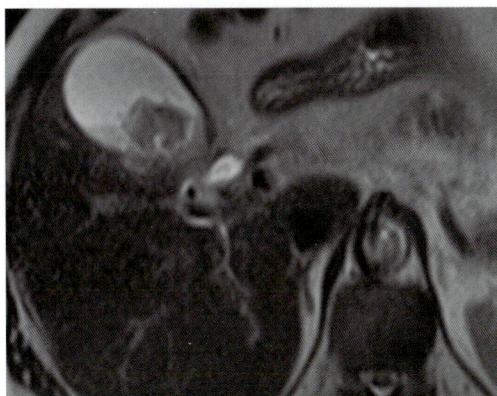

A

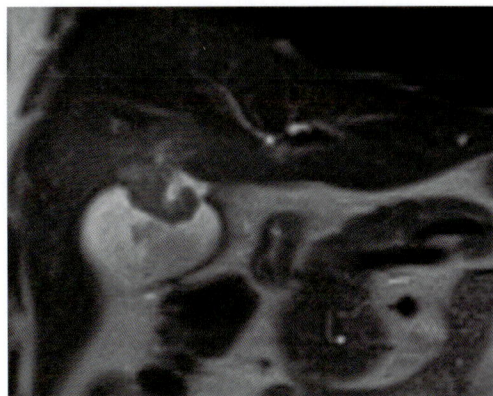

B

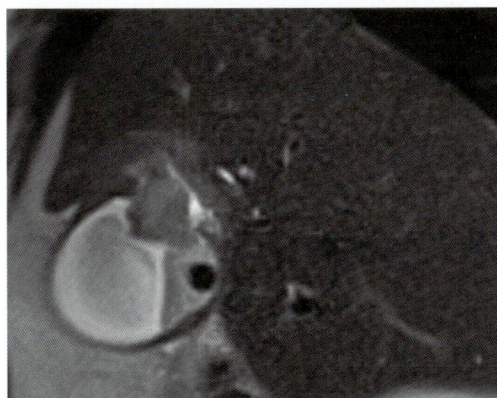

C

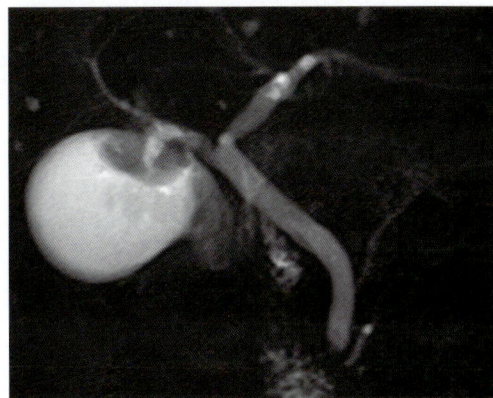

D

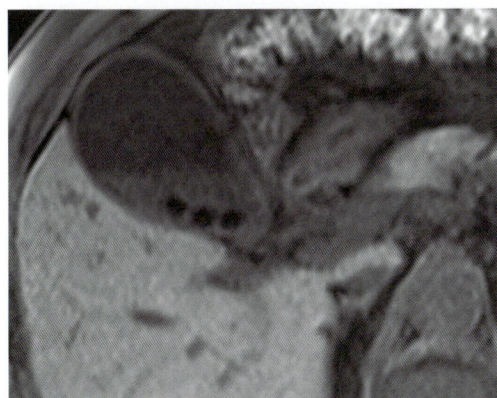

E

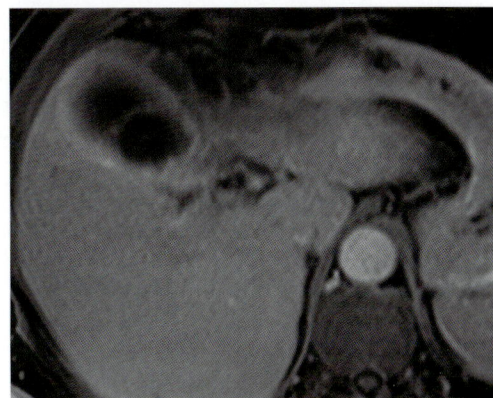

F

A. Axial, (**B**) coronal, and (**C**) sagittal T2-weighted single-shot FSE/TSE. **D**. Thick-slice MRCP obtained with single-shot FSE/TSE with fat saturation. **E**. Axial pre-contrast-enhanced and (**F**) delayed-phase post-contrast-enhanced T1-weighted gradient echo with fat saturation.

Case 49 Chronic Inflammation Mimicking Gallbladder Cancer

Findings

▶ Irregular lobulated polypoid mass projects into the lumen of the gallbladder.
▶ Coronal T2-weighted image shows the moderately high signal intensity mass to extend into the adjacent liver.
▶ Gallstones and layering sludge are present within the gallbladder lumen.
▶ Delayed-phase gadolinium-contrast-enhanced image shows persistent enhancement of the mass and the gallbladder wall.
▶ MR study was interpreted as highly indicative of gallbladder carcinoma.
▶ Surgery confirmed the findings, but histology of the specimen showed only acute and chronic cholecystitis with an organizing abscess extending into the adjacent liver. There was no evidence of cancer.

Differential diagnosis

▶ Gallbladder carcinoma
▶ Gallbladder adenomyomatosis

Teaching points

▶ Gallbladder carcinoma occurs most commonly in the elderly and is usually associated with the presence of gallstones (90%).
▶ MR findings of gallbladder carcinoma include focal or diffuse wall thickening (usually >1 cm), intraluminal polypoid mass, invasion of the adjacent liver, and soft-tissue mass replacing the gallbladder.
▶ Gallbladder cancers often show retained enhancement on delayed-phase gadolinium-contrast-enhanced images.
▶ Irregular gallbladder wall thickening, wall enhancement, intraluminal membranes and debris, pericholecystic abscess extending into the liver, and gallstones are common features of both acute and chronic cholecystitis and overlap the MR findings of gallbladder carcinoma.

Management

▶ Complete surgical excision is needed to confirm the diagnosis and to provide definitive treatment.

Further reading

1. Altun E, Semelka RC, Elias J Jr, et al. Acute cholecystitis: MR findings and differentiation from chronic cholecystitis. Radiology 2007;244:174–183.
2. Catalano OA, Sahani DV, Kalva SP, et al. MR imaging of the gallbladder: a pictorial essay. RadioGraphics 2008;28:135–155.
3. Levy AD, Murkata LA, Rohrmann CA Jr. Gallbladder carcinoma: radiologic-pathologic correlation. RadioGraphics 2001;21:295–314.

History

▶ 26-year-old man complains of severe pelvic pain.

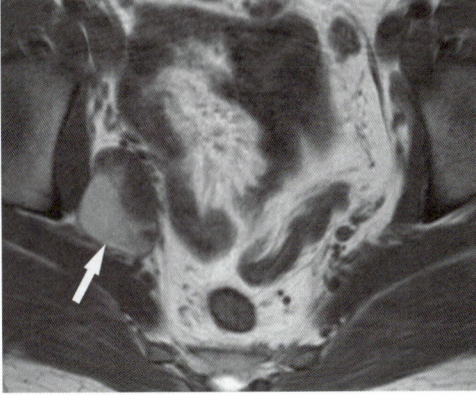

A

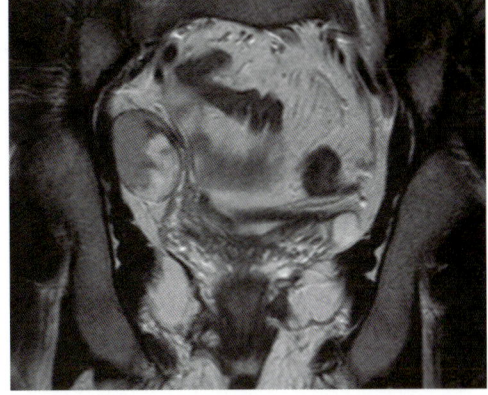

B

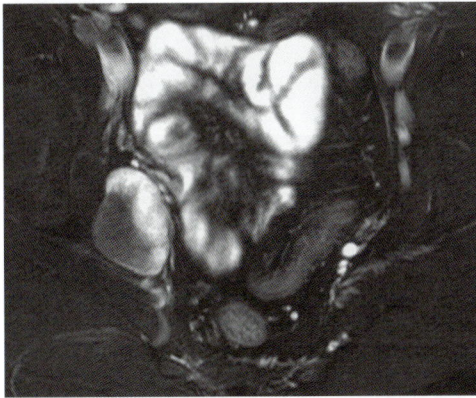

C

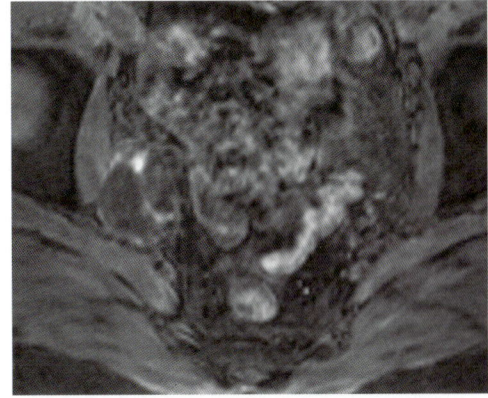

D

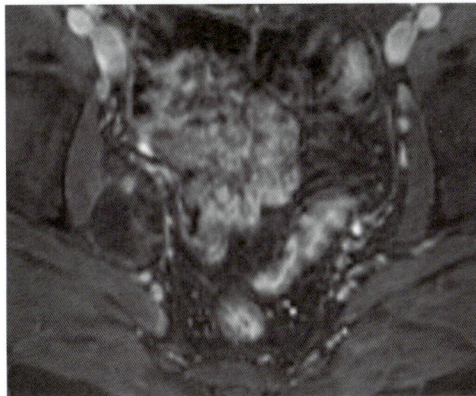

E

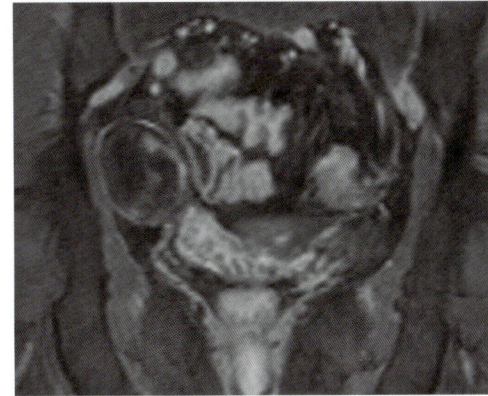

F

A. Axial T1-weighted spin echo. **B**. Coronal T2-weighted FSE/TSE. **C**. Axial T2-weighted FSE/TSE with fat saturation. **D**. Axial pre-contrast-enhanced, and (**E**) axial and (**F**) coronal post-gadolinium contrast-enhanced T1-weighted gradient echo with saturation.

Case 50 Mature Cystic Teratoma

Findings

▶ Heterogeneous well-defined mass (*arrow*) in the right pelvis

▶ Mass has a component that shows decreased signal intensity on fat-suppressed images, indicating fat.

▶ A portion of the mass shows contrast enhancement.

Differential diagnosis

▶ Well-differentiated liposarcoma

▶ Extra-adrenal myelolipoma

▶ Hibernoma

Teaching points

▶ Mature cystic teratomas occur most frequently in the ovary, but can occur in the testicle, brain, mediastinum, and peritoneum in male or female patients.

▶ Mature cystic teratoma is a benign tumor that contains at least two of the three primitive germ cell layers (endoderm, mesoderm, ectoderm).

▶ Malignant transformation is rare. When it occurs, it is usually squamous cell carcinoma. Malignant transformation is most common in the sixth or seventh decades.

▶ Immature teratomas tend to be solid.

▶ Use of fat-saturation techniques is helpful to distinguish sebaceous, fatty material from hemorrhage.

Management

▶ Surgical excision is indicated in atypical cases.

Further reading

1. Jeung M-Y, Gasser B, Gangi A, et al. Imaging of cystic masses of the mediastinum. RadioGraphics 2002;22:S79–S93.
2. Outwater EK, Siegelman ES, Hunt JL. Ovarian teratomas: tumor types and imaging characteristics. RadioGraphics 2001;21:475–490.
3. Saba L, Geurriero SL, Sulcis R, et al. Mature and immature ovarian teratomas: CT, US, MR imaging characteristics. Eur J Radiol 2009;72:454–463.

Case 51

History

▶ 74-year-old man with history of autoimmune pancreatitis and suspected autoimmune cholangiopathy, elevated liver function tests, and elevated IgG

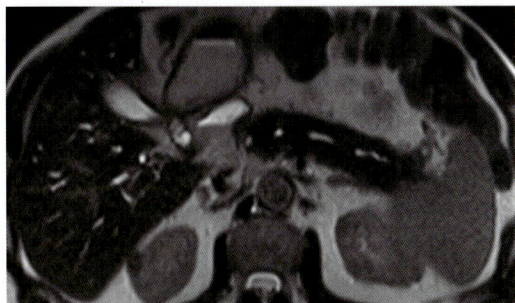
A

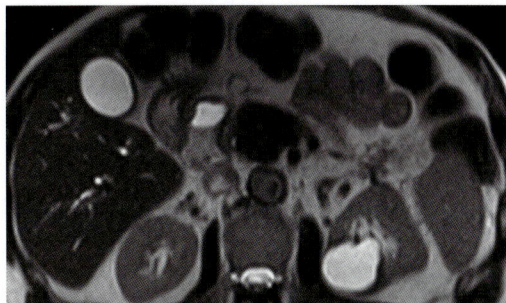
B

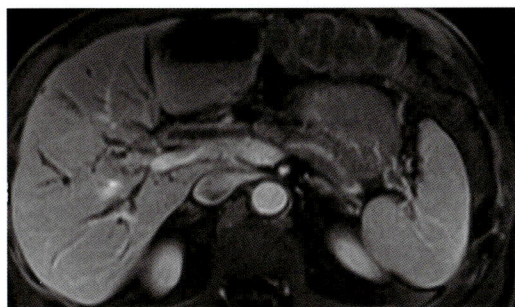
C

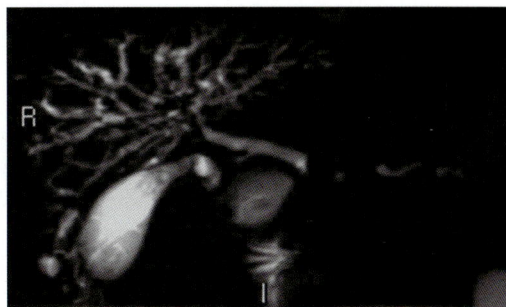
D

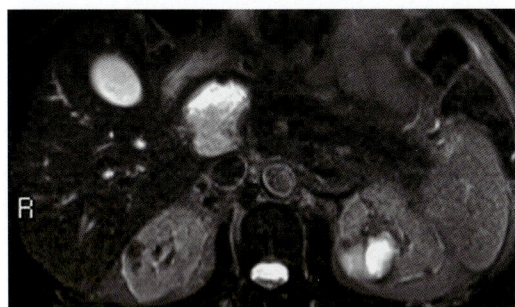
E

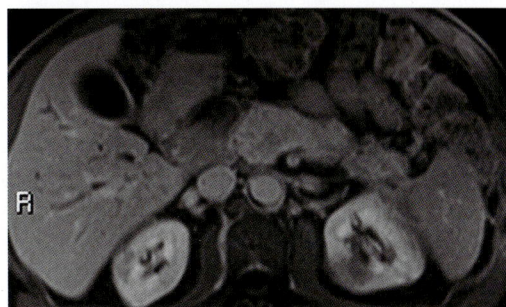
F

A, B. Axial T2-weighted single-shot FSE/TSE obtained at two different levels. **C**. Axial contrast-enhanced T1-weighted gradient echo with fat saturation. **D**. Thick-slice MRCP using single-shot FSE/TSE with fat saturation. **E**. Axial T2-weighted FSE/TSE with fat saturation. **F**. Axial contrast-enhanced T1-weighted gradient echo with fat saturation.

Case 51 IgG4-Related Sclerosing Disease—Autoimmune Pancreatitis with Associated Cholangiopathy and Renal Lesions

Findings

▶ The pancreas displays relatively low signal intensity on T2-weighted sequences and has a featureless, smooth margin with some irregularity in the caliber of the main pancreatic duct. There is no atrophy. A peripheral low-signal-intensity lesion is also noted in the right kidney.

▶ There is smooth diffuse thickening and enhancement of the walls of the common hepatic duct and common bile duct with moderate intrahepatic biliary ductal dilatation and strictures involving the right main, left main, and subsegmental branches.

▶ Larger right and smaller left low-signal-intensity lesions are noted in the kidneys bilaterally on T2-weighted images, with areas of hypoenhancement noted on the post-contrast-enhanced T1-weighted gradient-echo images.

Differential diagnosis

▶ Pancreatic adenocarcinoma for the focal form
▶ Cholangiocarcinoma and primary sclerosing cholangitis when there is biliary involvement

Teaching points

▶ Chronic pancreatitis is a major source of morbidity in the United States, although an etiology is not discovered in 30% of patients and these are classified as having idiopathic chronic pancreatitis.

▶ There is an autoimmune form, for which the accepted term is now "lymphoplasmacytic sclerosing pancreatitis" or simply "autoimmune pancreatitis." It is sometimes associated with other autoimmune disorders, and there is a strong male preponderance. Extrapancreatic involvement is not uncommon and can be a clue to the diagnosis.

▶ It is important to make the diagnosis of autoimmune pancreatitis because it is usually responsive to steroids with some recovery of pancreatic function.

▶ The diffuse form of autoimmune pancreatitis is most common showing generalized enlargement of the pancreas with minimal or no surrounding inflammatory change. The focal form, involving the pancreatic head, is less common and can be eaily confused with pancreatic carcinoma.

Management

▶ Autoimmune pancreatitis and its extrapancreatic involvement frequently respond well to steroids.

Further reading

1. Kamisawa T, Okamoto A. Autoimmune pancreatitis: proposal of IgG4-related sclerosing disease. J Gastroenterol 2006;41:613–625.
2. Sahani DV, Kalva SP, Farrell J, et al. Autoimmune pancreatitis: imaging features. Radiology 2004;233:345–352.
3. Takahashi N, Kawashima A, Fletcher JG, Chari ST. Renal involvement in patients with autoimmune pancreatitis: CT and MR imaging findings. Radiology 2007;242:791–801.

History

▶ 46-year-old woman with irregular vaginal bleeding

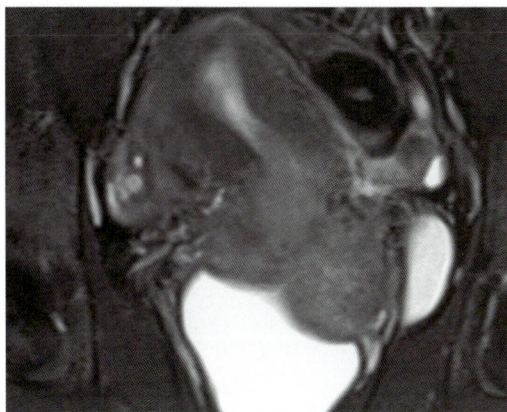

A

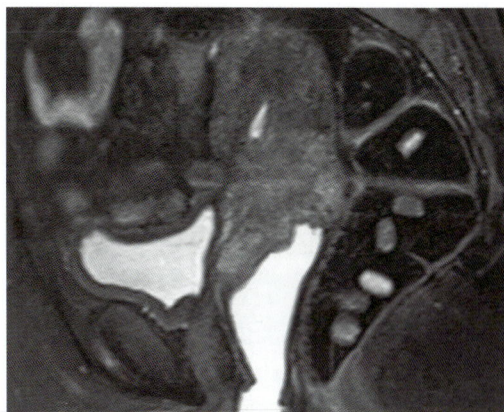

B

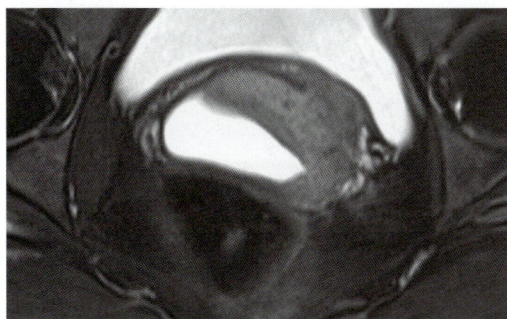

C

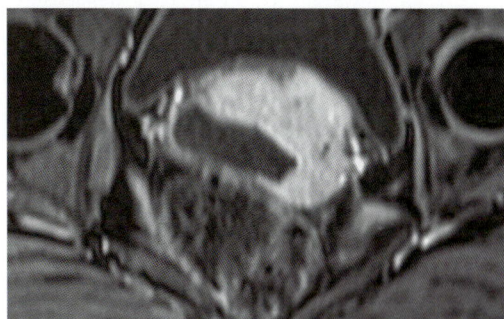

D

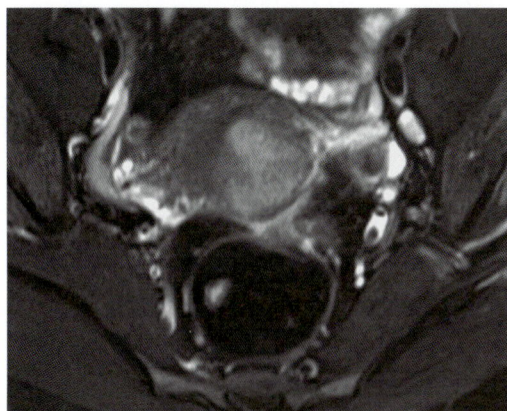

E

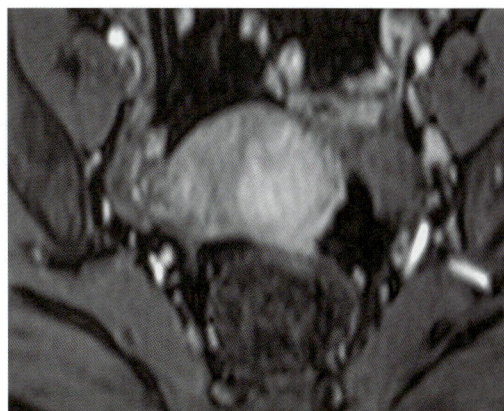

F

A. Coronal-oblique, (**B**) sagittal, and (**C**) axial T2-weighted FSE/TSE with fat saturation. **D**. Axial post-gadolinium contrast-enhanced T1-weighted gradient echo with fat saturation. **E**. Para-axial T2-weighted FSE/TSE and (**F**) post-contrast-enhanced T1-weighted gradient echo with fat saturation.

Case 52 Cervical Cancer with Uterine and Vaginal Extension (AJCC TMN Stage T2a2, FIGO Stage IIA2)

Findings

- ▶ Irregular enhancing mass centered at the cervix with extension into the uterine body and vagina
- ▶ Mass demonstrates intermediate-high signal intensity on T2-weighted images.
- ▶ Endovaginal gel was utilized to facilitate assessment of vaginal extent of the tumor.

Differential diagnosis

- ▶ Adenoma malignum
- ▶ Nabothian cyst
- ▶ Cervical polyp

Teaching points

- ▶ Cervical cancer typically arises at the squamocolumnar junction of the cervix, and the most common cell type of the tumor is squamous cell carcinoma.
- ▶ Use of intravenous gadolinium-based contrast agent is useful in determining local invasion and the presence of metastatic disease.
- ▶ The increased signal intensity of the mass on T2-weighted images is helpful in determining tumor extent as it replaces the normal low-signal-intensity cervical stroma.
- ▶ Staging of cervical cancer is done using the FIGO classification: 0, carcinoma in situ; I, involving only the cervix; II, extension beyond the cervix but not reaching the lateral pelvic wall; III, extension to the lower third of the vagina or to the lateral pelvic wall; IV, extension to the bladder or rectum, or disease outside of the pelvis (metastasis).

Management

- ▶ Noninvasive tumors are treated with electrocautery, cryo- or laser ablation, or local excision.
- ▶ Invasive lesions are treated with surgery and chemoradiation, or chemoradiation alone.

Further reading

1. Balleyguier C, Sala E, Da Cunha T, et al. Staging of uterine cervical cancer with MRI: guidelines of the European Society of Urogenital Radiology. Eur Radiol 2011;21:1102–1110.
2. Okamoto Y, Tanaka YO, Nishida M, et al. MR imaging of the uterine cervix: imaging-pathologic correlation. RadioGraphics 2003;23:425–445.

History

▶ 15-year-old boy with history of prolonged neonatal jaundice presents with pancreatitis and jaundice.

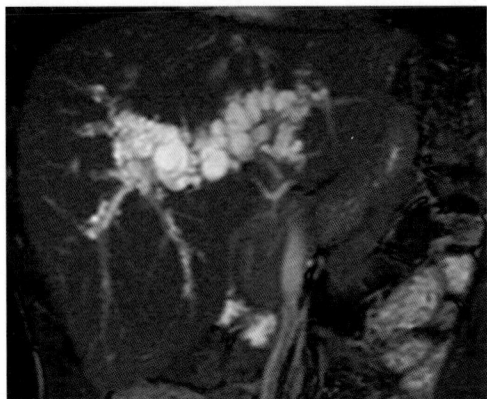

A

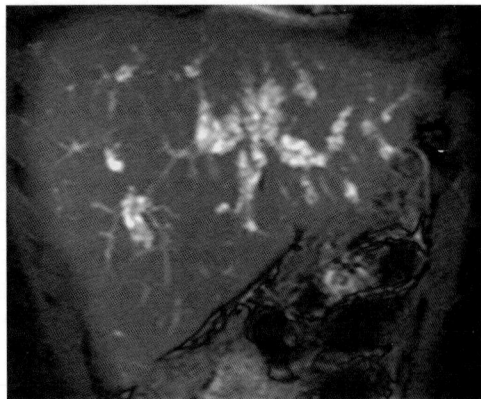

B

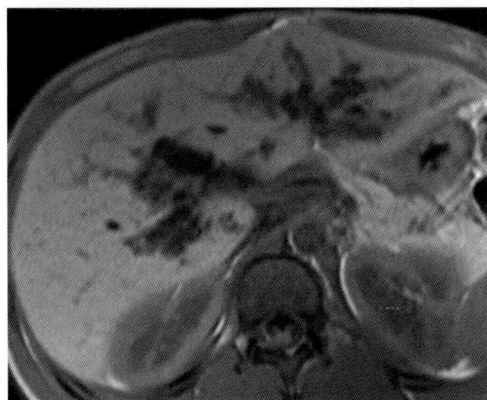

C

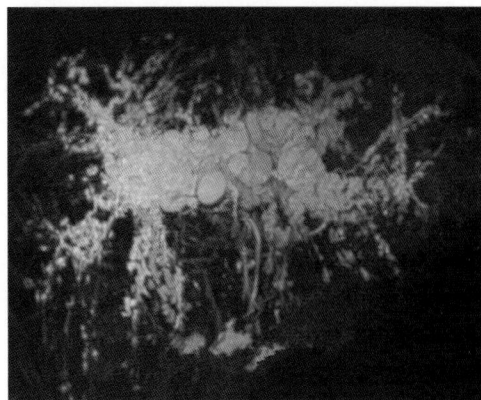

D

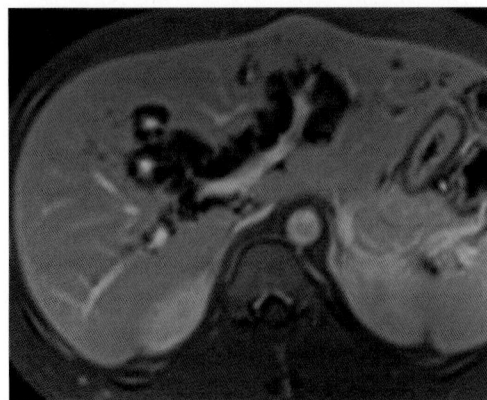

E

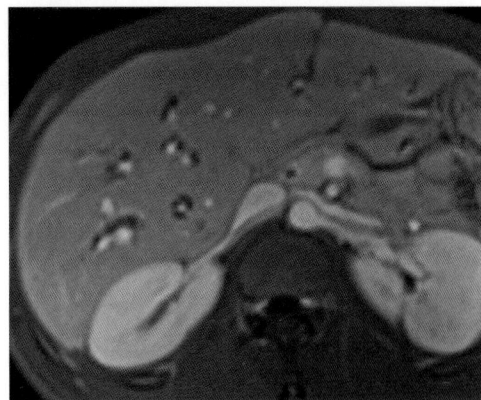

F

A, B. Coronal T2-weighted single-shot FSE/TSE. **B**. Coronal image anterior to **A** obtained with same sequence. **C**. Axial T1-weighted gradient echo with fat saturation. **D**. Maximum intensity projection MRCP image created from 3D FSE/TSE sequence **E, F**. Axial contrast-enhanced T1-weighted gradient echo with fat saturation (**F** at lower level than **E**).

Case 53 Caroli's Disease

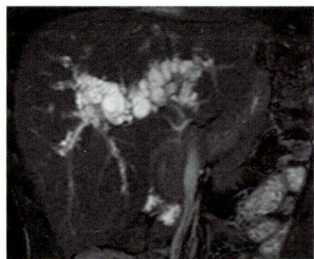

G

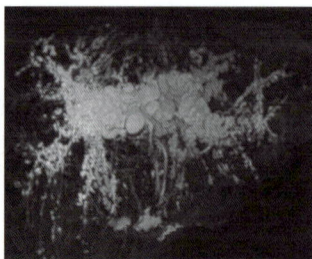

H

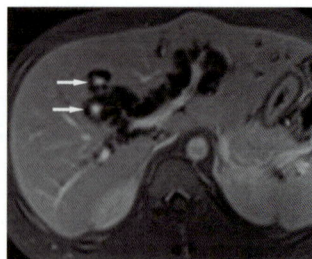

I

Findings

▶ Innumerable, beaded-appearing, abnormally dilated, and ectatic intrahepatic biliary ducts converging toward the porta hepatis in a branching fashion (**G**, **H**)

▶ The "central dot sign" (*arrows* in **I**) is evident.

Differential diagnosis

▶ Primary sclerosing cholangitis

▶ Recurrent pyogenic cholangitis

▶ Congenital hepatic fibrosis

Teaching points

▶ Caroli's disease is a rare congenital disorder characterized by saccular dilatation of the intrahepatic bile ducts resulting in biliary stasis, which predisposes to recurrent bacterial cholangitis, hepatic abscesses, and biliary calculus formation, and cancer (cholangiocarcinoma).

▶ Caroli's disease may be sporadic or inherited as an autosomal recessive trait often associated with autosomal recessive polycystic kidney disease and congenital hepatic fibrosis.

▶ On MR Caroli's disease is characterized by saccular and fusiform dilatation of the intrahepatic bile ducts up to 5 cm in diameter. The dilated ducts may contain calculi. Fusiform dilatation of the common bile duct up to 30 mm in diameter may occur.

▶ The "central dot sign," characteristic of Caroli's disease, is created by portal vein radicals partially or completely surrounded by abnormally dilated and ectatic bile ducts.

▶ Cirrhosis and portal hypertension are related to congenital hepatic fibrosis or may be secondary to biliary cirrhosis resulting from chronic biliary obstruction.

Management

▶ Progression to cirrhosis requiring liver transplant is typical.

Further reading

1. de Vries JS, de Vries S, Aronson, et al. Choledochal cysts: age of presentation, symptoms, and late complications related to Todani's classification. J Pediatr Surg 2002;37:1568–1573.
2. Kim OH, Chung HJ, Choi BG. Imaging of the choledochal cyst. RadioGraphics 1995;15:69–88.
3. Levy AD, Rohrmann CA, Murakata LA, Lonergan GJ. Caroli's disease: Radiology spectrum with pathologic correlation. AJR Am J Roentgenol 2002;179:1053–1057.

History

▶ 60-year-old man presents with abdominal pain. Outside CT was reported as showing a mesenteric mass.

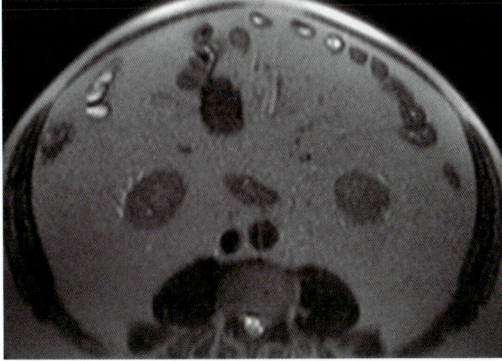

A

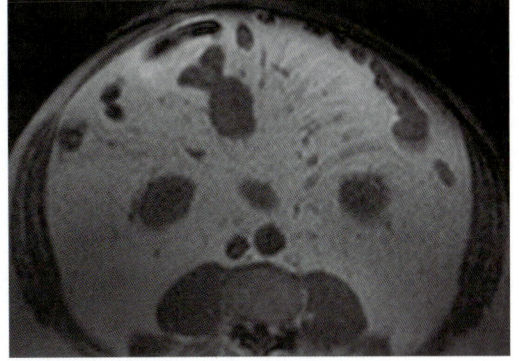

B

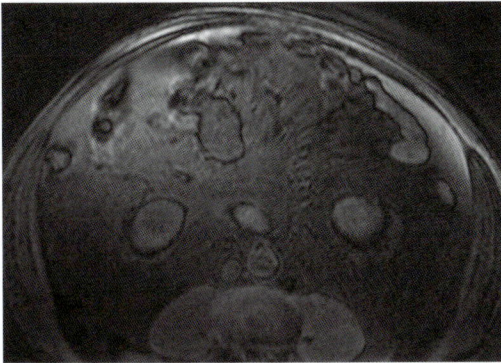

C

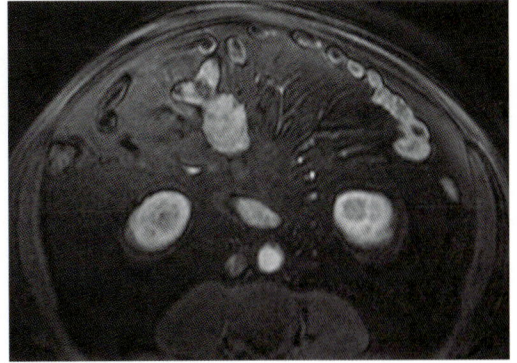

D

A. Axial T2-weighted single-shot FSE/TSE. **B**. Axial T1-weighted gradient echo. **C**. Axial pre-contrast-enhanced and (**D**) post-gadolinium contrast-enhanced T1-weighted gradient echo with fat saturation.

Case 54   Well-Differentiated Neuroendocrine Carcinoma of the Ileum (Carcinoid Tumor)

Findings
- ► Mid-abdominal mass with spiculated margins exophytic to the ileum. The mass shows avid contrast enhancement. No mesenteric lympadenopathy.

Differential diagnosis
- ► Adenocarcinoma of the ileum
- ► Gastrointestinal stromal tumor
- ► Lymphoma

Teaching points
- ► Neuroendocrine tumors account for one third of all neoplasms of the small bowel and 40% of all small bowel malignancies. Up to 90% arise in the ileum. In up to one third of cases small bowel carcinoid tumors arise at multiple primary sites. Desmoplastic reaction results in spiculated margins and mesenteric retraction. The primary tumor varies in appearance from small submucosal nodules to large intraluminal ulcerating lesions. The stellate appearance of the mesenteric reaction is most characteristic. Somatostatin-receptor scintigraphy utilizing Indium-111-octreotide, or more recently gallium-68-octreotide proton emission tomography (PET), identifies neuroendocrine tumors.
- ► Gastrointestinal stromal tumors (GISTs) may arise anywhere in the small bowel. Small bowel GISTs represent 20% to 30% of GISTs. They typically show exophytic growth with involvement of the outer muscle layer of the small bowel and with mucosal ulceration in 50%. Aggressive tumors tend to be heterogeneous with areas of necrosis and hemorrhage.
- ► Adenocarcinoma of the small bowel is most common in the duodenum (50%) and jejunum (40%), and is relatively rare in the ileum (10%). They typically cause circumferential wall thickening with luminal narrowing, or appear as an intraluminal papillary or polypoid mass with limited exophytic growth. Tumor enhancement is moderate.
- ► Small bowel lymphoma is more common in the ileum than in the duodenum or jejunum. Appearance is variable, showing as wall thickening, nodules, or large masses. Dilatation of the bowel lumen, rather than narrowing, is characteristic. The tumor tissue tends to be homogeneous with little or no contrast enhancement.

Management
- ► Surgical resection is generally required for diagnosis and treatment.

Further reading
1. Horwitz BM, Zamora GE, Gallegos MP. Gastrointestinal stromal tumor of the small bowel. RadioGraphics 2011;31:429–434.
2. Lee NK, Kim S, Kim GH, et al. Hypervascular subepithelial gastrointestinal masses: CT-pathologic correlation. RadioGraphics 2010;30:1915–1934.
3. Levy AD, Sobin LH. Gastrointestinal carcinoids: imaging features with clinicopathologic comparison. RadioGraphics 2007;27:237–257.

History

▶ 40-year-old woman presents with abdominal pain, a palpable abdominal mass, elevated liver enzymes, and 5-pound weight loss.

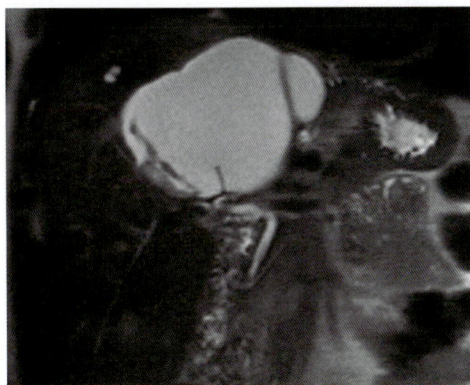

A

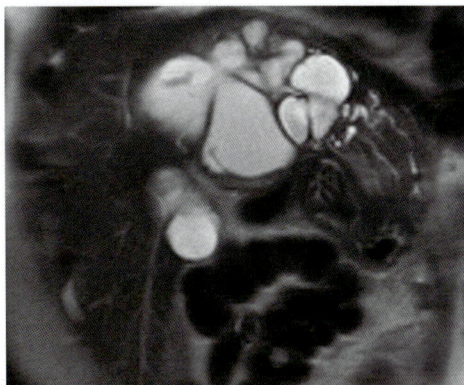

B

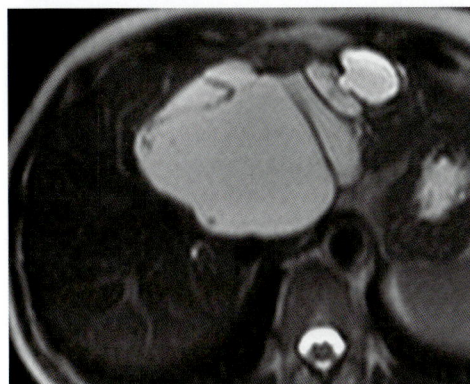

C

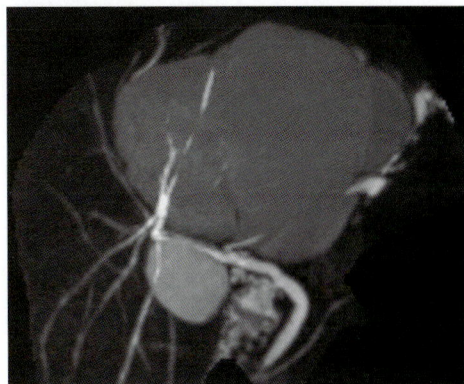

D

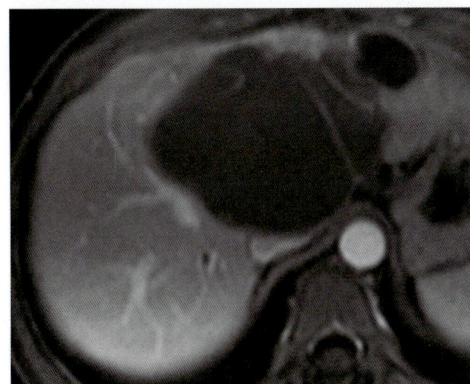

E

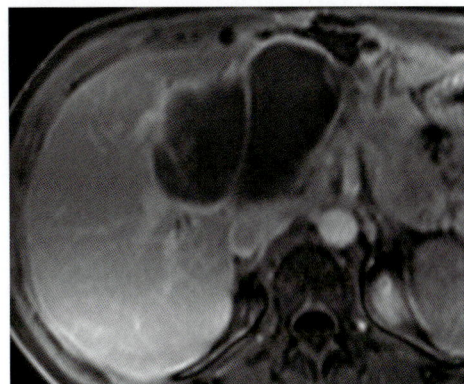

F

A and **B**. Coronal T2-weighted single-shot FSE/TSE at different levels. **C**. Axial T2-weighted single-shot FSE/TSE.
D. Maximum intensity projection MRCP image generated from 3D FSE/TSE. **E**. Relatively early and (**F**) delayed contrast-enhanced axial T1-weighted gradient echo with fat saturation.

Case 55 Biliary Cystadenoma

Findings

- A large complex multiloculated cyst measuring 12 cm in greatest dimension is present within the left lobe of the liver.
- Bile ducts are splayed and those peripheral to the lesion are dilated.
- The wall of the lesion and thin septations show enhancement after intravenous gadolinium contrast material administration.
- No distinct solid components are evident on any images obtained.

Differential diagnosis

- Abscess/hematoma/biloma/infected cyst
- Biliary cystadenocarcinoma
- Cystic or necrotic metastasis

Teaching points

- Biliary cystadenoma is a rare benign cystic biliary ductal neoplasm lined by mucin-secreting epithelium that is frequently large, up to 12 cm in diameter.
- Biliary cystadenoma is a premalignant form of biliary cystadenocarcinoma. The two neoplasms cannot be differentiated by imaging. Both occur most commonly in middle-aged women and are usually symptomatic.
- Symptoms are caused by mass effect and biliary obstruction.
- MR typically shows a well-defined thick fibrous capsule, internal septations resulting in a multilocular appearance, and mural nodularity, all of which demonstrate contrast enhancement, differentiating the neoplasm from infected cysts and hematomas.
- Fluid content, as reflected by MR signal characteristics, may be serous, mucinous, proteinaceous, gelatinous, purulent, or hemorrhagic.

Management

- Resection or cyst enucleation is generally indicated to provide definitive diagnosis, to exclude carcinoma, and to treat symptoms.

Further reading

1. Mortele KJ, Ros PR. Cystic focal liver lesions in the adult: differential CT and MR imaging features. RadioGraphics 2001;21:985–910.
2. Vachha B, Sun MRM, Siewert B, Eisenberg RL. Cystic lesions of the liver. AJR Am J Roentgenol 2011;196:W355–W366.

History

► 84-year-old woman with mass in the pancreatic tail on ultrasound examination

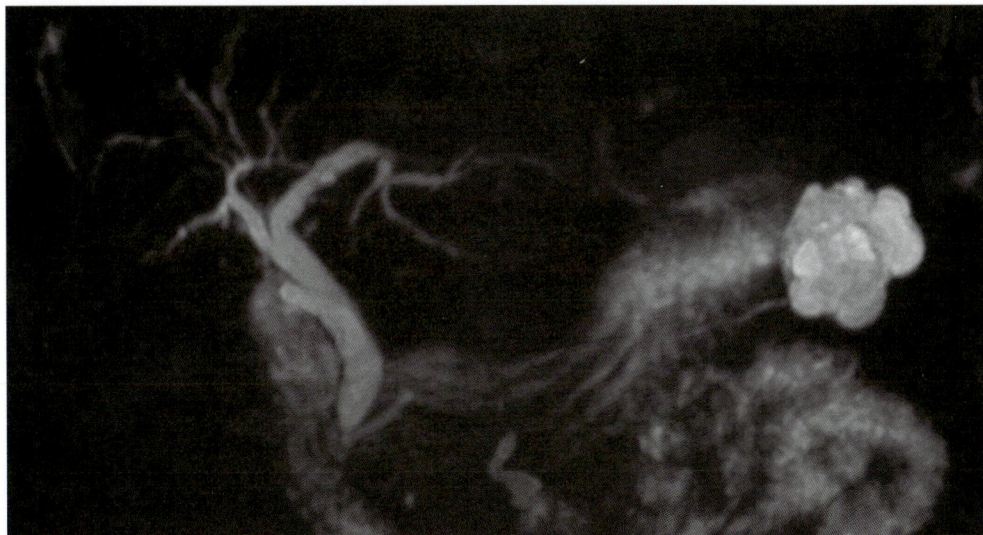

A

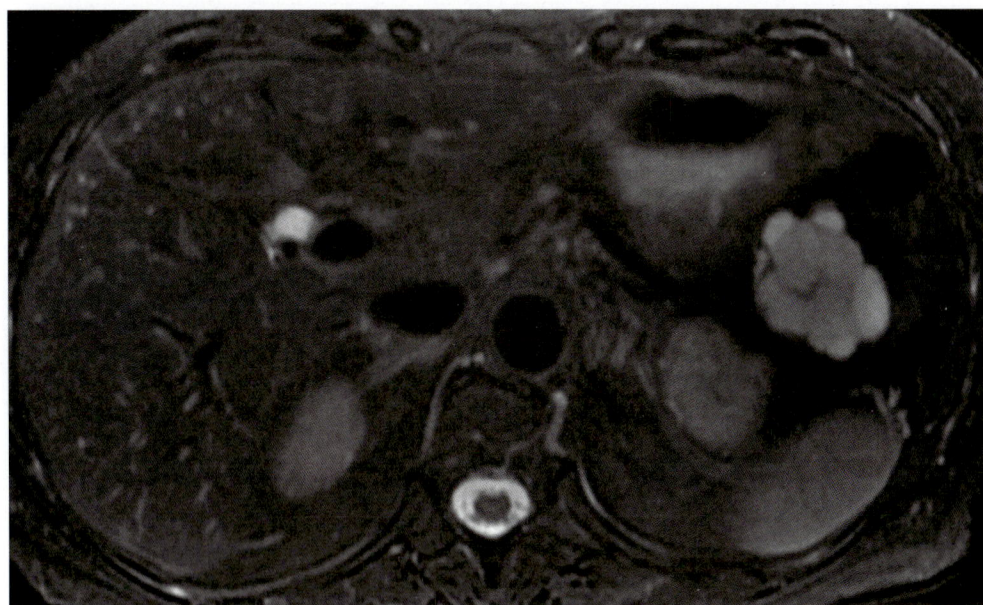

B

A. Coronal maximum intensity projection MRCP image from 3D FSE/TSE with fat saturation. **B**. Axial T2-weighted FSE/TSE with fat saturation.

Case 56   Mucinous Cystic Neoplasm (MCN) of the Pancreas (Old Term: Mucinous Cystadenoma)

Findings

- ▶ Cystic mass in pancreatic tail with few cystic spaces and intervening septa
- ▶ Pancreatic duct is not dilated.

Differential diagnosis

- ▶ Serous cystadenoma of pancreas
- ▶ Pseudocyst
- ▶ Side-branch intraductal papillary mucinous neoplasm (IPMN)
- ▶ Cystic islet cell tumor

Teaching points

- ▶ MCNs are common cystic tumors of the pancreas. Mean age at presentation is 50 years; most prevalent in females (M:F = 1:9). Patients are most often asymptomatic; MCN occasionally present with epigastric pain or rarely a palpable mass.
- ▶ The tumor is a thick-walled unilocular or multilocular low-grade malignant tumor composed of mucin-containing cystic spaces and septa. The mass demonstrates variable signal intensity based on cyst content; fluid-containing cysts are most often hypointense on T1-weighted images and hyperintense on T2-weighted images, whereas proteinaceous or hemorrhagic cysts are often hyperintense on T1-weighted images. Enhancement of the septations and cyst wall is common. The mass may cause displacement and narrowing of the pancreatic duct, leading to prestenotic ductal dilatation.
- ▶ There is a spectrum of MCNs from benign to malignant. The confident exclusion of malignancy is rarely possible on the basis of imaging findings alone.
- ▶ Differentiation from side-branch IPMN can sometimes be difficult. However, IPMN communicates with the main pancreatic duct whereas MCN does not. Further, IPMNs have no thick walls or septa.

Management

- ▶ MCNs should always be resected as they are all potentially premalignant.
- ▶ When the cyst is small in an asymptomatic patient, cyst aspiration and analysis of the cyst fluid can be helpful in differential diagnosis. Aspiration of mucin suggests MCN; however, fluid of IPMN also contains mucin, and imaging features therefore play a crucial role in diagnosis and management.

Further reading

1. Kim YH, Saini S, Sahani D, et al. Imaging diagnosis of cystic pancreatic lesions: pseudocyst versus nonpseudocyst. RadioGraphics 2005;25:671–685.
2. Sarti M. Pancreas MR imaging. In: Brant WE, de Lange EE (Eds), Essentials of Body MR Imaging. New York: Oxford University Press, 2012.

History

▶ 46-year-old man referred for MRI because of the incidental discovery of multiple liver lesions on a CT scan

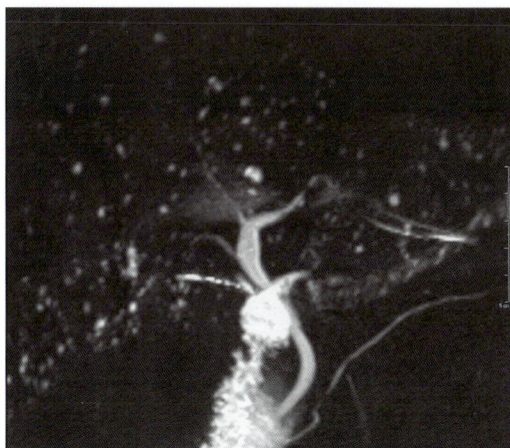

A

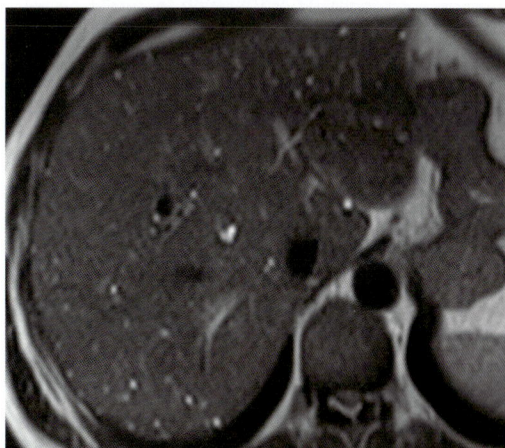

B

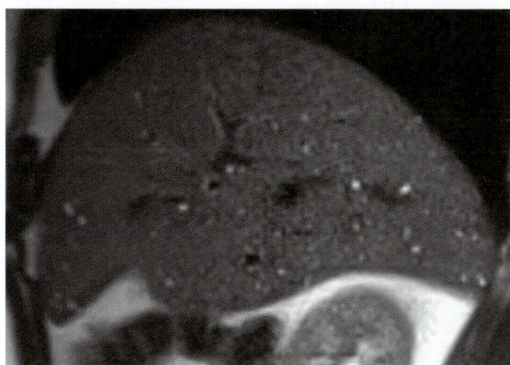

C

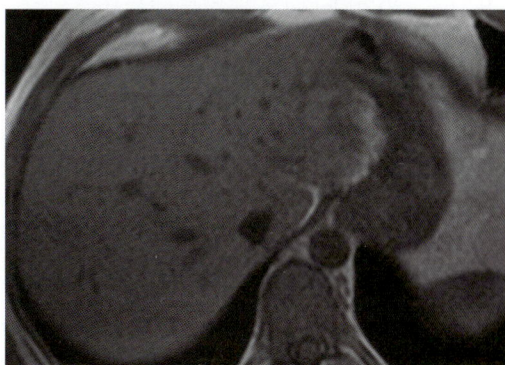

D

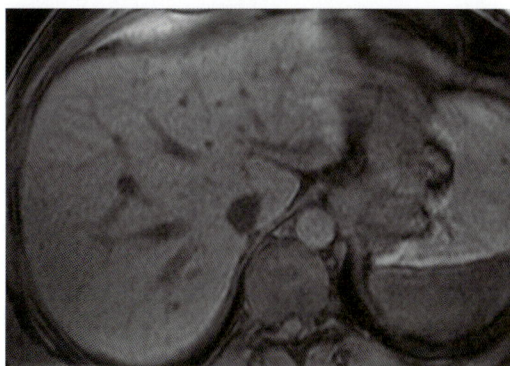

E

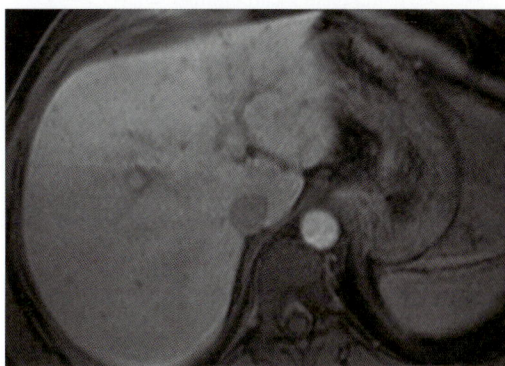

F

A. Maximum intensity projection MRCP generated from 3D FSE/TSE. **B**. Axial and (**C**) sagittal T2-weighted single-shot FSE/TSE.
D. Axial T1-weighted gradient echo. **E**. Axial pre- and (**F**) post-gadolinium contrast-enhanced T1-weighted gradient echo with fat saturation.

Case 57   Bile Duct Hamartomas

Findings

▶ Innumerable tiny lesions demonstrating high signal intensity on T2-weighted images scattered throughout the liver
▶ The lesions show no communication with the biliary system.
▶ No significant enhancement of the lesions
▶ Diagnosis of bile duct hamartomas was based on characteristic appearance and clinical findings; no pathologic proof was obtained in this case.

Differential diagnosis

▶ Caroli's disease
▶ Multiple cystic metastases
▶ Multiple liver cysts

Teaching points

▶ Bile duct hamartomas, also known as von Meyenburg complexes from the original description in 1918, arise as malformations of the ductal plate that involve small interlobular bile ducts. They are embryonic remnants of bile duct formation that fail to involute. They range in size from 2 to 15 mm and are scattered throughout the liver. They are found in 3% of autopsy studies but are much less commonly demonstrated on imaging studies.
▶ MR shows biliary hamartomas as multiple, tiny lesions uniformly distributed throughout the liver. Relative to liver parenchyma the lesions display low signal intensity on T1-weighted images and high signal intensity on T2-weighted images. The lesions do not communicate with the biliary tree and generally show no enhancement after intravenous gadolinium contrast material administration. A thin rim of contrast enhancement may be seen, likely representing compressed hepatic parenchyma.

Management

▶ Bile duct hamartomas are generally considered benign, without long-term consequences and requiring no treatment. However, several isolated case reports indicate possible degeneration of biliary hamartomas into hepatocellular carcinoma or cholangiocarcinoma.

Further reading

1. Desmet VJ. Ductal plates in hepatic ductular reactions. Hypothesis and implications. III. Implications for liver pathology. Virchows Arch 2011;458:271–279.
2. Lev-Toaff AS, Bach AM, Wechsler RJ, et al. The radiologic and pathologic spectrum of biliary hamartomas. AJR Am J Roentgenol 1995;165:309–313.
3. Tohme-Noun C, Cazals D, Noun R, et al. Multiple biliary hamartomas: magnetic resonance features with histopathologic correlation. Eur Radiol 2008;18:493–498.

Case 58

History

▶ 52-year-old woman with history of a treated pituitary tumor, ovarian cystadenoma, and four meningiomas underwent MR examination of the abdomen.

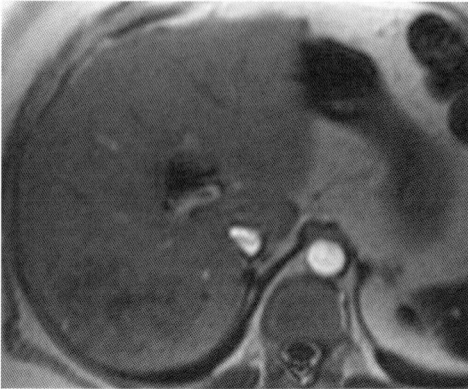

A

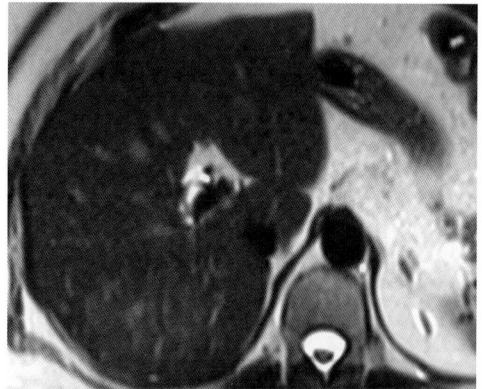

B

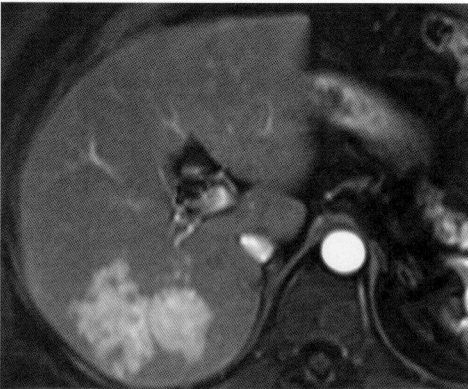

C

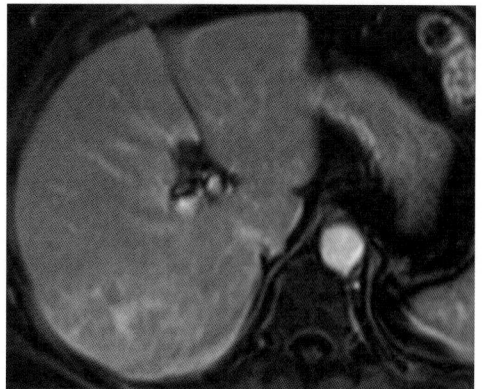

D

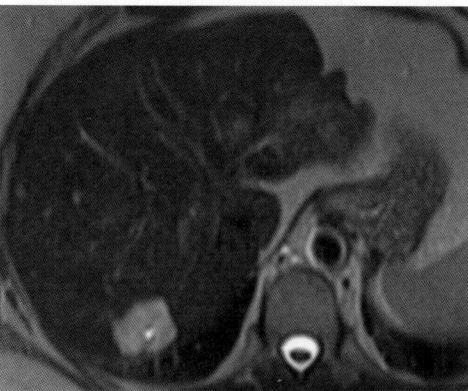

E

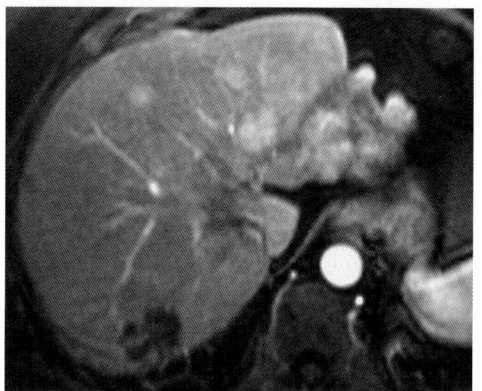

F

A. T1-weighted gradient echo, (**B**) T2-weighted single-shot FSE/TSE, (**C**) arterial- and (**D**) delayed-phase contrast-enhanced T1-weighted gradient echo with fat saturation at level 1. **E**. T2-weighted single-shot FSE/TSE and (**F**) arterial-phase contrast-enhanced T1-weighted gradient echo at level 2.

115

Case 58 Multiple Focal Nodular Hyperplasia (FNH) Syndrome

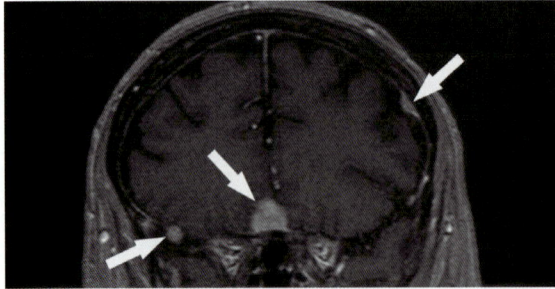

G

Findings

▶ A right lobe mass (level 1) with signal intensity relatively isointense to surrounding liver, with a central scar displaying low signal intensity on T1-weighted images and high intensity on T2-weighted images, and showing marked enhancement on arterial-phase images are the classic imaging features of focal nodular hyperplasia (FNH). Additional similar lesions of smaller size (not shown) were also present.

▶ A 2-cm right lobe lesion (level 2) in the same patient displays relatively high signal intensity on T2-weighted images and a very-high-signal-intensity central focus. There is focal, nodular arterial-phase enhancement and delayed meshlike enhancement (not shown). These features are atypical for FNH but are indicative of hemangioma.

▶ Coronal gadolinium contrast-enhanced T1-weighted gradient-echo image of the brain (G) in the same patient shows multiple meningiomas (*arrows*).

Differential diagnosis

▶ Multiple hypervascular metastases
▶ Multiple or multifocal hepatocellular carcinoma
▶ Multiple hepatic adenomas

Teaching points

▶ Multiple FNH syndrome is defined as consisting of two or more foci of FNH in combination with hepatic hemangiomas, vascular malformations, or intracranial tumors.

▶ Other neoplasias, including meningiomas, astrocytomas, pheochromocytomas, and gastrointestinal stromal tumors, are also associated. The link creating the syndrome may be angiogenic growth factors, including estrogen.

▶ Multiple FNH lesions are found in 20% to 25% of patients without FNH syndrome.

▶ When FNH lesions are multiple, the lesions often show atypical imaging features.

Management

▶ A patient with multiple FNH syndrome may need close monitoring for the development of additional neoplasia.

Further reading

1. Finley AC, Hosey JR, Noone TC, et al. Multiple focal nodular hyperplasia syndrome: diagnosis with dynamic, gadolinium-enhanced MRI. Magn Reson Imag 2005;23:511–513.
2. Hussain SM, Terkivatan T, Zondervan PE, et al. Focal nodular hyperplasia: findings at state-of-the-art MR imaging, US, CT, and pathologic analysis. RadioGraphics 2004;24:3–17.
3. Wariless IR, Albrecht S, Bilbao J, et al. Multiple focal nodular hyperplasia of the liver associated with vascular malformations of various organs and neoplasia of the brain: a new syndrome. Mod Pathol 1989;2:456–462.

History

▶ 55-year-old asymptomatic woman presents for MR evaluation of an incidental finding seen on CT.

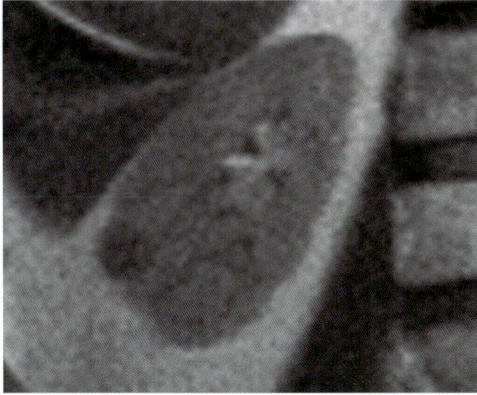

A

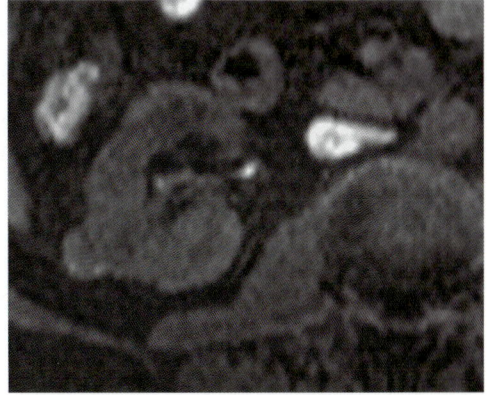

B

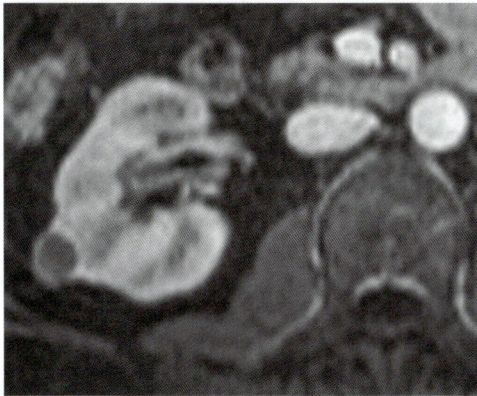

C

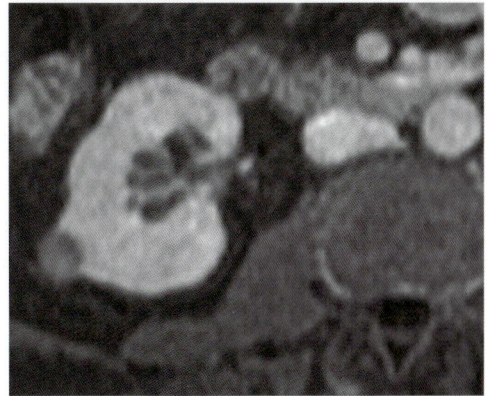

D

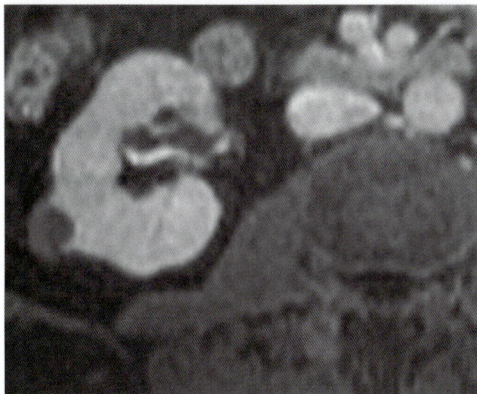

E

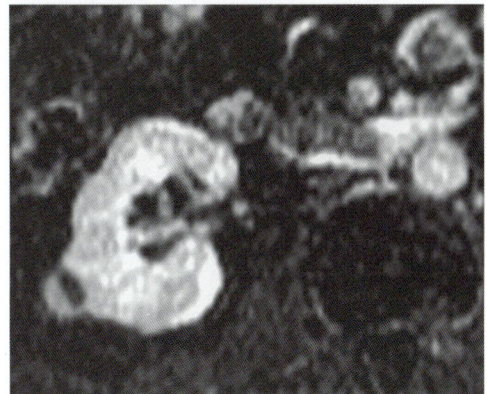

F

A. Coronal T2-weighted single-shot FSE/TSE. **B**. Axial T1-weighted gradient echo with fat saturation pre-contrast. **C**. Axial contrast-enhanced T1-weighted gradient echo with fat saturation, early enhancement (cortical) phase, (**D**) late enhancement (nephrogram) phase, and (**E**) delayed enhancement (pyelogram) phase. **F**. Subtraction image of nephrogram enhancement phase.

Case 59 Renal Cell Carcinoma, Papillary Type

Findings

▶ A small exophytic mass in the inferior pole of the right kidney demonstrates uniform intermediate/low signal intensity on T2-weighted images and heterogeneous intermediate/low signal intensity on T1-weighted images compared to the adjacent renal parenchyma.

▶ Peripheral enhancing nodule is most evident on the post-contrast-enhanced subtraction image (**F**).

▶ Rapid contrast material washout is evident on the pyelogram-phase image (**E**).

▶ The tumor invaded the perirenal fat but did not involve Gerota's fascia (stage pT3a).

Differential diagnosis

▶ Hemorrhagic cyst

▶ Metastatic disease

Teaching points

▶ With heterogeneous signal intensity on T1-weighted images and low signal intensity on T2-weighted images this lesion could be mistaken for a benign hemorrhagic cyst.

▶ The necessity for administration of intravenous contrast agent to show tumor enhancement is emphasized.

▶ Post-contrast-enhanced subtraction images increase the conspicuity of contrast enhancement.

▶ The papillary subtype of renal cell carcinoma is typically hypovascular and can be mistaken for a cyst because it demonstrates little enhancement.

▶ MR cannot accurately differentiate stage I tumor (confined by the renal capsule) from stage II disease (tumor spread through the renal capsule into the perirenal fat).

Management

▶ The clinical choices are imaging follow-up to assess growth, percutaneous renal tumor ablation, or surgical excision.

Further reading

1. Beer AJ, Dobritz M, Zantl N, et al. Comparison of 16-MDCT and MRI for characterization of kidney lesions. AJR Am J Roentgenol 2006;186:1639–1650.
2. Poghosyan T. Urinary tract MR imaging. In: Brant WE, de Lange EE (Eds), Essentials of Body MRI. New York: Oxford University Press, 2012.
3. Remzi M, Özsoy M, Klingler H-C, et al. Are small renal tumors harmless? Analysis of histopathological features according to tumors 4 cm or less in diameter. J Urol 2006;176:896–899.

History

▶ 72-year-old man with claudication, congestive heart failure, and chronic renal insufficiency

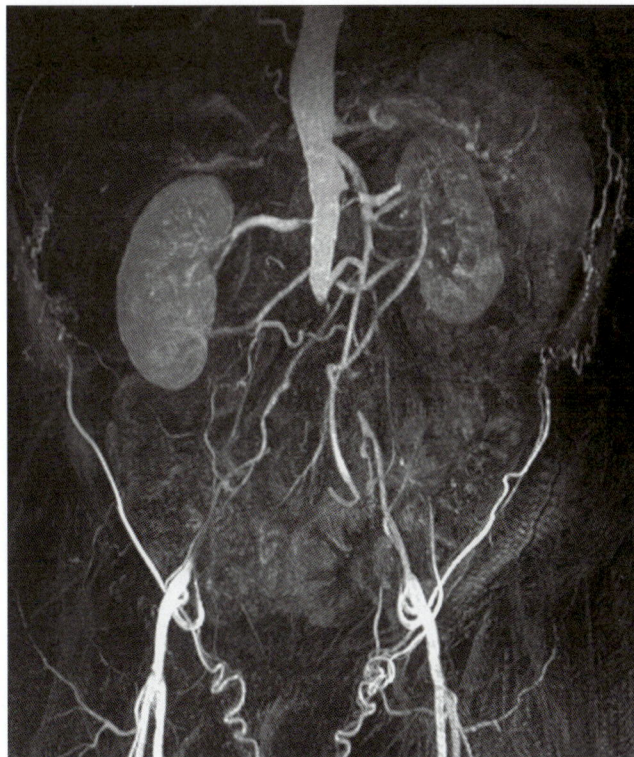

A

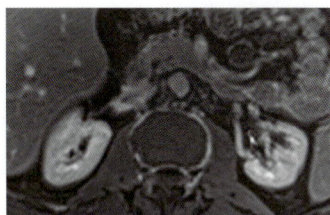

B

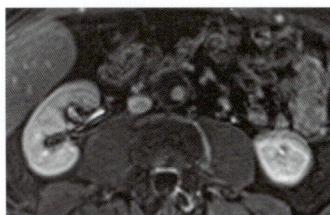

C

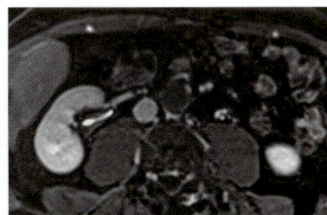

D

A. Coronal maximum intensity projection MRA image generated from gadolinium-contrast-enhanced 3D gradient echo with fat saturation. **B**. Axial contrast-enhanced T1-weighted gradient echo with fat saturation obtained at the level of the superior infrarenal abdominal aorta, (**C**) mid infrarenal abdominal aorta, and (**D**) distal infrarenal abdominal aorta.

Case 60 Chronic Aortic Occlusive Disease

Findings

► Occlusion of the infrarenal abdominal aorta
► Iliac arteries reconstitute from enlarged inferior epigastric and circumflex iliac arterial collaterals.
► High-grade stenosis of the superior left renal artery

Differential diagnosis

► Vasculitis
► Aortic dissection
► Aortic trauma
► Endovascular sarcoma (rare)

Teaching points

► Chronic occlusion is caused by progressive narrowing of the aorta resulting from atherosclerotic disease. The presence of hypertrophied collateral vessels indicates chronic disease.
► Acute occlusion of the aorta is rare and can result from atherosclerotic plaque rupture and aortic thrombosis or from large emboli, most often from the heart.
► If acute, look for high-signal-intensity thrombus on T1- and T2-weighted images occluding the aorta and signal voids within the aorta.
► Acute occlusion presents with pain, pallor, cool extremities, and absent distal pulses, with or without signs of mesenteric ischemia.
► Chronic occlusion classically presents with Leriche syndrome (absent femoral pulses, claudication, impotence) or simply with lower-extremity claudication.
► Depending on the extent of occlusion, flow in chronic occlusion is supplied by collateral pathways that include the inferior mesenteric artery to the internal iliac artery via the rectal arteries, the internal mammary arteries to the inferior epigastric arteries, and the intercostal and lumbar arteries to the superficial circumflex iliac arteries.

Management

► Acute occlusion is a surgical emergency. Treatment options include endovascular thrombolysis and surgical bypass.
► Chronic disease is treated first by optimizing medical management, which includes smoking cessation, exercise, and platelet inhibitors.
► In cases of rest pain or tissue loss, surgical management with bypass remains the treatment of choice, though options for endovascular treatment are increasing.

Further reading

1. Morita S, Masukawa A, Suzuki K, et al. Unenhanced MR angiography: techniques and clinical applications in patients with chronic kidney disease. RadioGraphics 2011;31:E13–E33.
2. Ruehm SG, Weishaupt D, Debatin JF. Contrast-enhanced MR angiography in patients with aortic occlusion (Leriche syndrome). J Magn Reson Imaging 2000;11:401–410.

History

▶ 58-year-old woman with a history of alcohol-related cirrhosis underwent screening MR for hepatocellular carcinoma as part of her workup for liver transplant. An outside MR was reported to show a questionable lesion.

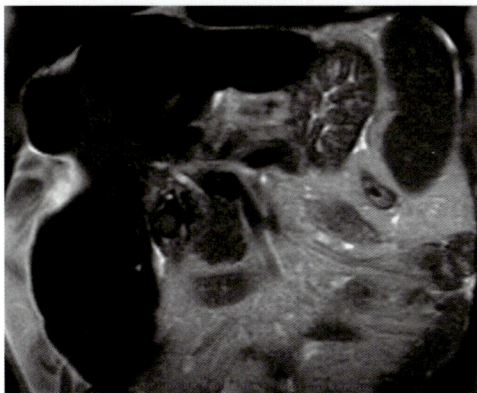

A

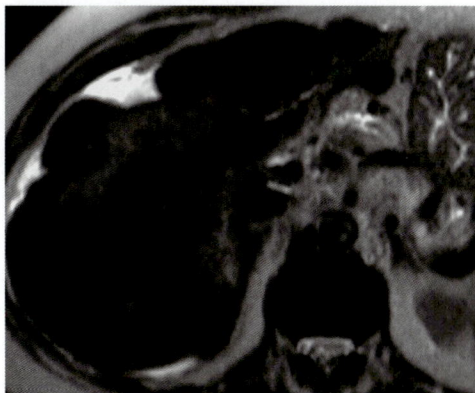

B

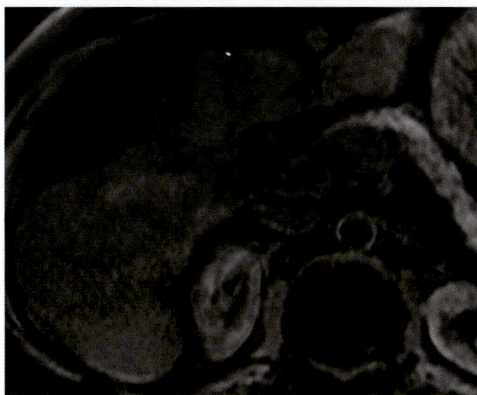

C

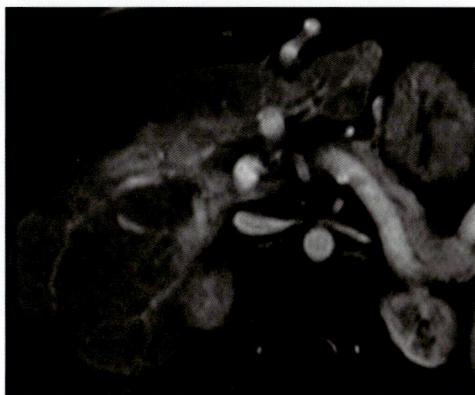

D

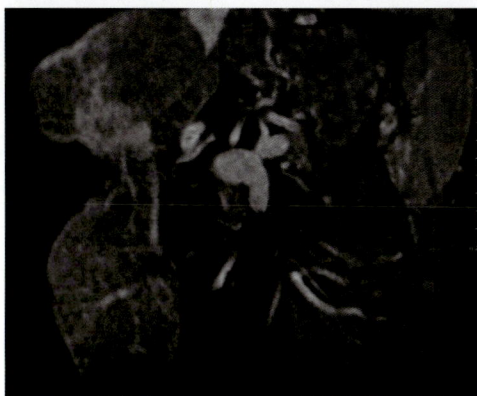

E

A. Coronal and (**B**) axial T2-weighted single-shot FSE/TSE. **C**. Axial pre-contrast-enhanced, and (**D**) axial and (**E**) coronal post-gadolinium contrast-enhanced T1-weighted gradient echo with fat saturation.

Case 61   Confluent Hepatic Fibrosis

Findings

▸ The liver has diffuse nodular changes and heterogeneous parenchyma indicative of cirrhosis.

▸ T2-weighted images show a region of increased signal intensity involving the anterior segment of the right lobe and the medial segment of the left lobe. This lesion extends from the porta hepatis to the retracted liver capsule.

▸ On non-contrast-enhanced T1-weighted images the region shows decreased signal intensity compared with that of the background liver.

▸ With intravenous gadolinium-based contrast enhancement the tissue shows relative hypo-enhancement on early-phase contrast-enhanced images, progressive increased enhancement on portal-venous-phase images, and marked persistent enhancement on delayed-phase images.

Differential diagnosis

▸ Neoplasm: hepatocellular carcinoma, cholangiocarcinoma

▸ Injury: infarction or scar, post-treatment effects of chemotherapy, post-embolization

Teaching points

▸ Confluent hepatic fibrosis is present in up to 15% of patients with cirrhosis. For unclear reasons, the entity occurs more commonly in alcoholic cirrhosis than in other forms of cirrhosis. The lesion represents thick bands of fibrous tissue with atrophic parenchyma within it. Confluent fibrosis may present as a mass-like lesion, but the characteristic appearance that helps differentiate it from a true mass is that it is wedge-shaped radiating from the porta hepatis to the capsular surface where the extent is widest. There is associated parenchymal atrophy with capsular retraction over the lesion.

▸ The anterior segment of the right lobe and the medial segment of the left lobe, or both, are most commonly involved.

▸ Confluent fibrosis, like most fibrotic tissue, displays intermediate high signal intensity on T2-weighted images and relatively low signal intensity on T1-weighted images. Rare arterial-phase contrast enhancement is reported, but more typically, there is progressive increased enhancement at the portal venous phase with strong persistent enhancement on delayed-phase images, features that mimic cholangiocarcinoma. Confluent fibrosis may not demonstrate delayed enhancement when gadolinium chelates predominantly designed for biliary excretion are employed.

Management

▸ Confluent fibrosis, per se, does not change management of typical hepatocellular carcinoma screening of cirrhotic patients. When the diagnosis of tumor remains in the differential, follow-up imaging may be useful because confluent fibrosis will continue to retract, whereas neoplasm will continue to grow.

Further reading

1. Faria SC, Ganesan K, Mwangi I, et al. MR Imaging of liver fibrosis: current state of the art. RadioGraphics 2009;29:1615–1635.

History

▶ 52-year-old man underwent repeated CT evaluation for jaundice at an outside hospital. An MR was requested to further evaluate biliary obstruction. Only images of the kidneys from that examination are shown.

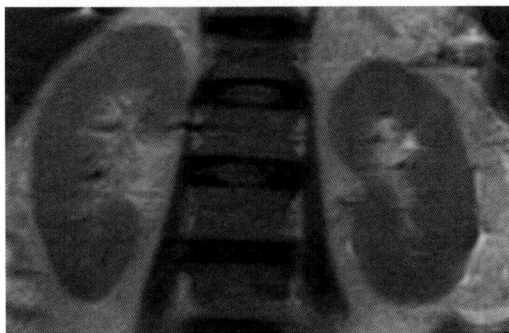

A

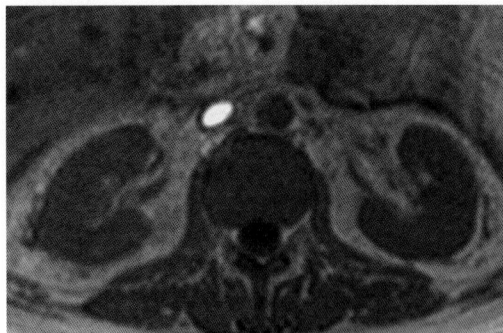

B

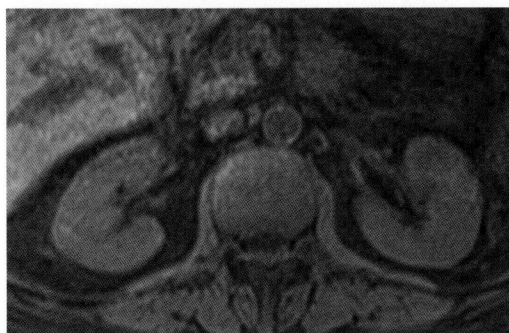

C

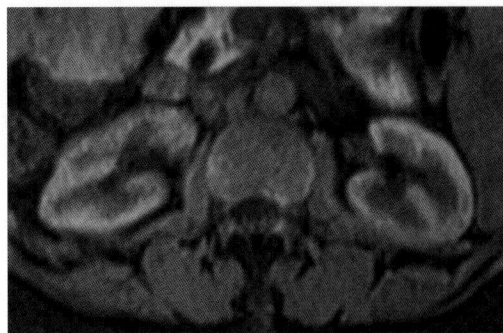

D

A. Coronal T2-weighted single-shot FSE/TSE. **B**. Axial T1-weighted gradient echo without and (**C**) with fat saturation. **D**. Image obtained in a different patient using same technique as **C**. No gadolinium contrast material was given.

Case 62 Acute Renal Failure

Findings

▶ Absence of corticomedullary differentiation on T1- and T2-weighted images. At the time of the MR examination the patient had a serum creatinine of 9 mg/dL with a calculated glomerular filtration rate (GFR) of 6 mL/min/1.73 m^2. Gadolinium-containing contrast material was not administered because of the risk of inducing nephrogenic systemic sclerosis.

▶ For comparison, the normal kidneys from a healthy subject are shown in image **D** showing normal corticomedullary differentiation.

▶ Acute renal failure was probably induced by repeated intravenous administration of large-doses of iodinated contrast material.

Differential diagnosis

▶ Loss of corticomedullary differentiation is a nonspecific finding of diffuse renal disease that may be seen with acute or chronic renal dysfunction due to any cause, including pyelonephritis, glomerulonephritis, dehydration, hydronephrosis, and acute renal allograft rejection.

Teaching points

▶ Normal kidneys in well-hydrated patients show corticomedullary differentiation on T1-weighted images, with the cortex showing higher signal intensity than the medulla. Corticomedullary differentiation is best shown on unenhanced T1-weighted fat-suppressed gradient-echo images.

▶ Patients with chronic renal failure who have a serum creatinine level above 3.0 mg/dL will show loss of corticomedullary differentiation on MR.

▶ In acute renal failure corticomedullary differentiation may be preserved for at least two weeks following the onset of renal failure, even if renal function impairment is severe.

Management

▶ Observation of absent corticomedullary differentiation on MR images may be early clinical evidence of diffuse renal disease that will require further evaluation.

Further reading

1. Chung JJ, Semelka RC, Martin DR. Acute renal failure: common occurrence of preservation of corticomedullary differentiation on MR images. Magn Reson Imaging 2001;19:789–793.
2. Jeong JY, Kim SH, Lee HJ, Sim JS. Atypical low-signal intensity renal parenchyma: causes and patterns. RadioGraphics 2002;22:833–846.
3. Semelka RC, Corrigan K, Ascher SM, et al. Renal corticomedullary differentiation: observation in patients with differing serum creatinine levels. Radiology 1994;190:149–152.

History

▶ Incidental finding on MR performed for other indication.

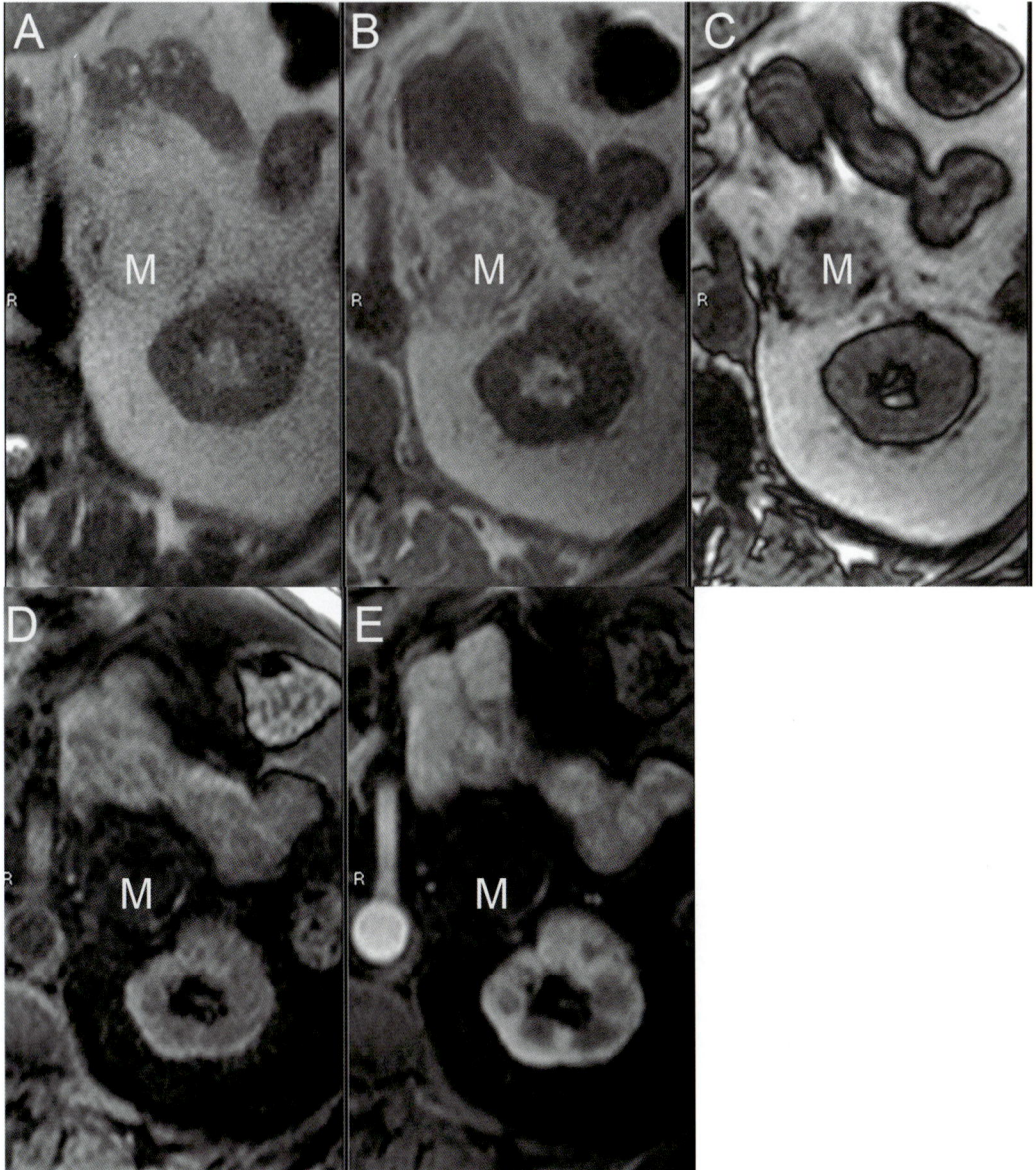

A. Axial T2-weighted single-shot FSE/TSE. **B**. Axial in-phase and (**C**) opposed-phase T1-weighted gradient echo. **D**. Axial pre- and (**E**) post-contrast-enhanced T1-weighted gradient echo with fat saturation.

Case 63 Adrenal Myelolipoma

Findings

- A fatty mass (*M*) arises from the left adrenal gland.
- The mass does not decrease in signal intensity on the opposed-phase gradient-echo image (**C**) when compared with the in-phase image (**B**).
- The mass follows the signal of retroperitoneal fat on all sequences (**C** and **D**).
- The mass demonstrates markedly decreased signal on fat-suppressed images, similar as that of the fat surrounding the kidney, consistent with an adrenal mass composed of macroscopic (adipose) fat.
- Only a rim of tissue enhances following gadolinium contrast enhancement (**E**).

Differential diagnosis

- Findings are pathognomonic for adrenal myelolipoma.

Teaching points

- Myelolipoma is an uncommon benign adrenal tumor that consists of hematopoietic bone marrow tissue including mature adipose tissue. The presence of mature fat within the lesion is diagnostic of myelolipoma. Fat-suppressed MR imaging best demonstrates the adipose fat of myelolipomas, while in-phase/opposed-phase (chemical shift) MR imaging best demonstrates the intracellular fat characteristic of benign adrenal adenomas.
- To definitively diagnose an adrenal myelolipoma, the mass must be shown to arise from the adrenal gland.
- If the fatty mass arises in the retroperitoneum separate from the adrenal gland or if it invades the adrenal gland, liposarcoma should be considered

Management

- Myelolipomas are benign neoplasms of the adrenal gland and should be left alone.
- Spontaneous hemorrhage is a rare complication that may require angiographic embolization.

Further readings

1. Han M, Burnett AL, Fishman EK, Marshall FF. The natural history and treatment of adrenal myelolipoma. J Urol 1997;157:1213–1216.
2. Olobatuyi FA, Maclennan GT. Myelolipoma. J Urol 2006;176:1188.
3. Rao P, Kenney PJ, Wagner BJ, Davidson AJ. Imaging and pathologic features of myelolipoma. RadioGraphics 1997;17:1373–1385.
4. Sanders R, Bissada N, Curry N, Gordon B. Clinical spectrum of adrenal myelolipoma: analysis of 8 tumors in 7 patients. J Urol 1995;153:1791–1793.

► 56-year-old man had right liver lobe transplant from living donor for cirrhosis and hepatocellular carcinoma three years ago. Follow-up clinical examination revealed increasing blood alpha-fetoprotein levels and a lung mass at MR imaging.

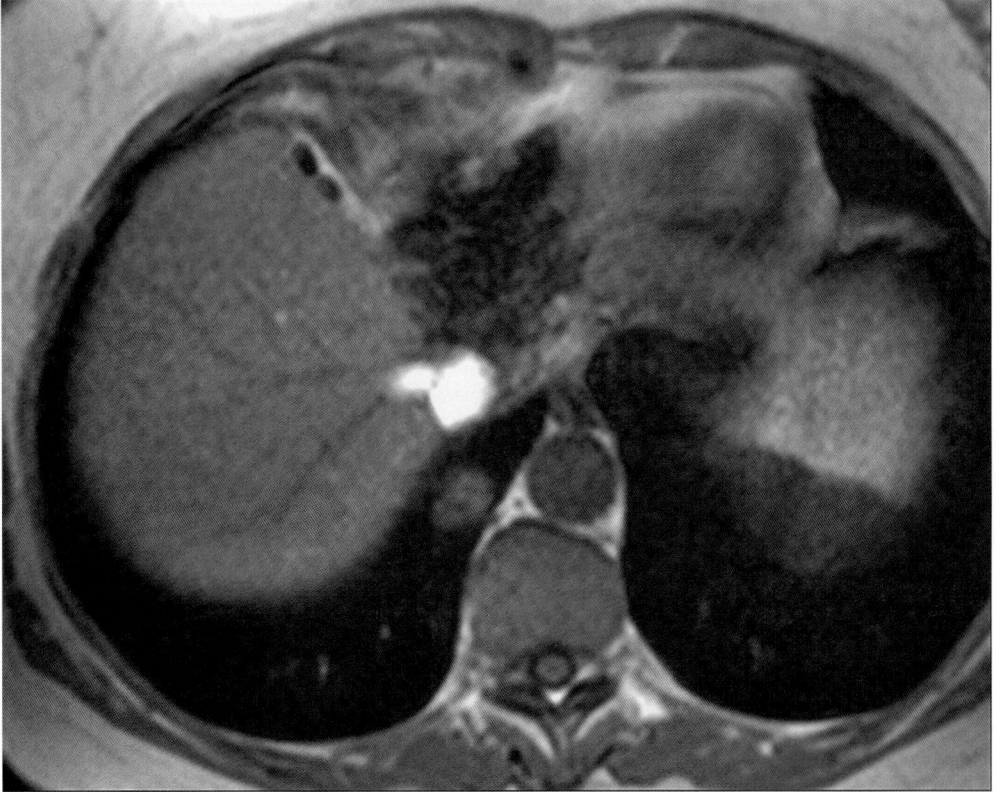

A. T1-weighted gradient-echo image

Case 64 Ghost Artifact from Flowing Blood

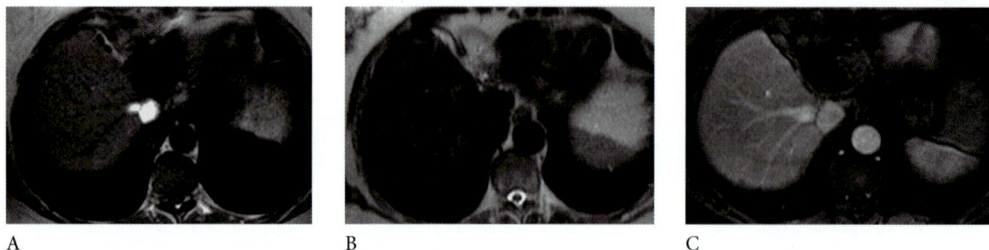

A

B

C

Findings:

▶ Mass-like lesion in right lower lung on T1-weighted gradient-echo image (**A**)

▶ No mass on corresponding T2-weighted (**B**) image and post-gadolinium contrast-enhanced T1-weighted gradient-echo (**C**) image.

Differential diagnosis

▶ Primary lung carcinoma

▶ Lung metastasis

Teaching points

▶ The inferior vena cava (IVC) shows high signal intensity from blood flowing in the caudiocranal direction into the most inferior slice of an image set that includes contiguous two-dimensional T1-weighted gradient-echo images (**A**).

▶ Inflow enhancement is strong as blood, with longitudinal magnetization at thermal equilibrium, flows from outside the imaging volume into the slice. The degree of inflow enhancement varies during the acquisition due to pulsatility of flow in the IVC, leading to concomitant modulation of the signal during the acquisition, which produces a flow (ghost) artifact.

▶ The artifact appears as signal displaced from the IVC along the phase-encoding direction, with shape as the IVC.

▶ Aortic inflow enhancement is not seen because a spatial presaturation RF pulse was placed cranial to the most superior slice of the image set to suppress the signal from aortic blood flowing in the craniocaudal direction.

▶ No flow artifacts are seen in **B** because the blood that flows into the slice during the echo train of the sequence did not experience the 90° excitation RF pulse that initiates the echo train and, hence, provides no signal contribution.

▶ In image **C**, ghost artifacts from inflowing blood are essentially absent because the T1 relaxation time for blood is shortened substantially by the gadolinium-containing contrast agent. For a very short T1, the longitudinal magnetization associated with the gadolinium-contaning blood relaxes to nearly thermal equilibrium between repetitions of the gradient-echo pulse sequence, and thus blood that has experienced one or more excitation RF pulses yields approximately the same signal as that from "fresh" blood flowing into the slice. As a result, the signal from the IVC does not vary significantly due to pulsatile flow, and flow artifacts are substantially reduced or may be fully suppressed.

Further reading

1. de Lange EE, Mugler JP. MR acquisition techniques & practical considerations for abdominal imaging. In: Brant WE, de Lange EE (Eds), Essentials of Body MR Imaging. New York: Oxford University Press, 2012.

History

▶ 40-year-old woman developed portal and splenic vein thrombosis as a complication of cholangitis 3 years earlier. She complains of diffuse abdominal pain for the past two weeks.

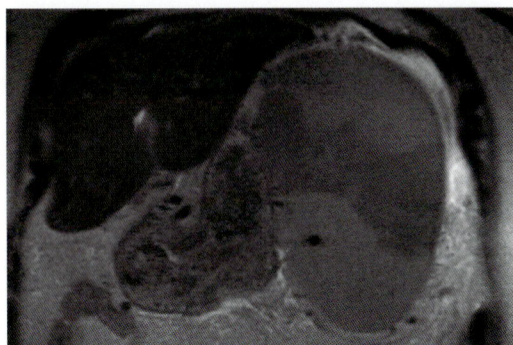

A

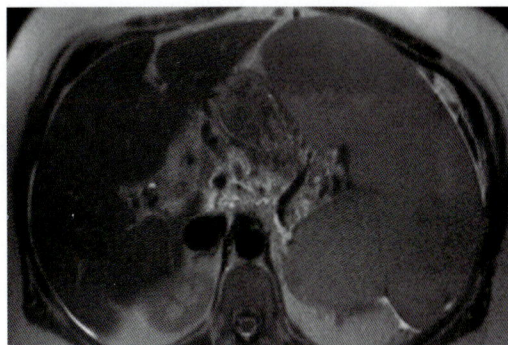

B

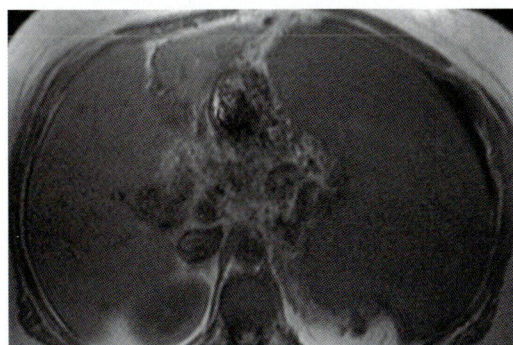

C

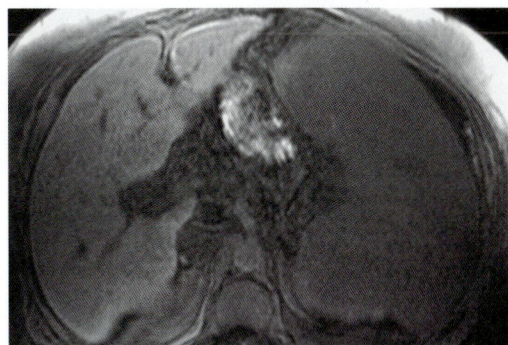

D

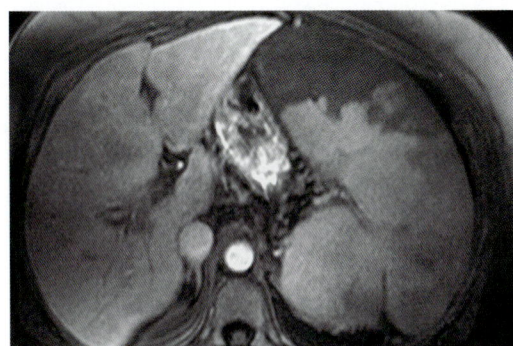

E

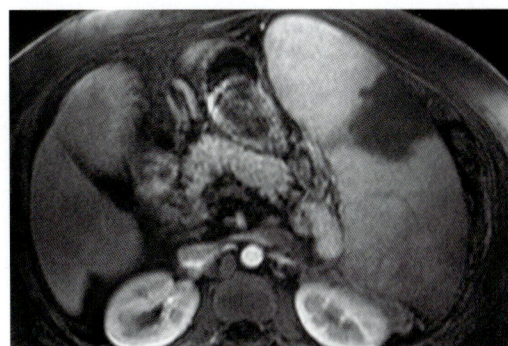

F

A. Coronal and (**B**) axial T2-weighted single-shot FSE/TSE. **C.** Axial T1-weighted gradient echo. (**D**) Pre- and (**E**) post-gadolinium contrast-enhanced axial T1-weighted gradient echo with fat saturation. **F**. Same technique as in **E** but obtained at lower level through the spleen.

Case 65 Multiple Splenic Infarctions

Findings

▶ The spleen is markedly enlarged. Trace ascites is present. Neither the splenic nor the portal vein is well demonstrated. Collateral vessels are seen in the splenic hilum and gastrohepatic ligament.

▶ Multiple geographic low-signal-intensity flow defects are seen in the spleen. The defects extend to the periphery of the spleen abutting the splenic capsule. Some defects are wedge-shaped.

▶ The splenic defects are best seen on T2-weighted and post-gadolinium contrast-enhanced images, and are poorly demonstrated on unenhanced T1-weighted images.

Differential diagnosis

▶ Multifocal splenic lymphoma is typically near-isointense to splenic parenchyma on T1- and T2-weighted images and is best seen as minimally enhancing lesions on post-contrast-enhanced MR. The lesions are mass-like and rarely demonstrate a wedge-shaped, broad base abutting the splenic capsule.

▶ Metastatic disease appears as mass lesions that are hyperintense on T2-weighted images and show variable enhancement following gadolinium contrast material administration depending on the nature of the primary tumor.

▶ Extramedullary hematopoiesis may produce a splenic mass and may be associated with multiple splenic infarctions. Active lesions display intermediate to high signal intensity on T1- and T2-weighted images and show mild enhancement. Old infarcts show low signal intensity on all sequences and do not enhance.

Teaching points

▶ Splenic infarction occurs as a result of occlusion of the splenic artery causing parenchymal ischemia and necrosis. The infarctions may be focal or segmental or involve the entire spleen.

▶ Infarction occurs most commonly in the setting of diseases of the spleen and in splenomegaly.

▶ Predisposing conditions include leukemia, lymphoma, myelofibrosis, venous thrombosis, embolic disorders, trauma, pancreatitis, and autoimmune vascular disorders.

▶ Infarctions show as low-signal-intensity foci on T1- and T2-weighted images and do not enhance following intravenous gadolinium contrast material administration. They characteristically show a broad base that abuts the splenic capsule.

Management

▶ Splenic infarction is treated with pain control. Splenectomy may be indicated for complications such as splenic rupture, bleeding, or abscess.

Further reading

1. Elasyes KM, Narra VR, Mukundan G, et al. MR imaging of the spleen: spectrum of abnormalities. RadioGraphics 2005;25:967–982.

History

▶ 35-year-old otherwise healthy woman presents with several months of vague abdominal pain and increased abdominal girth.

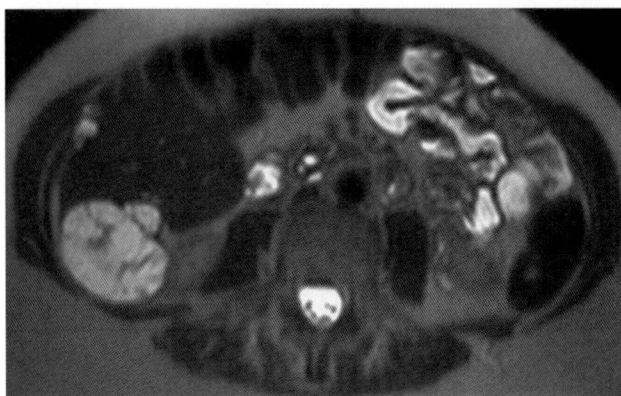

A

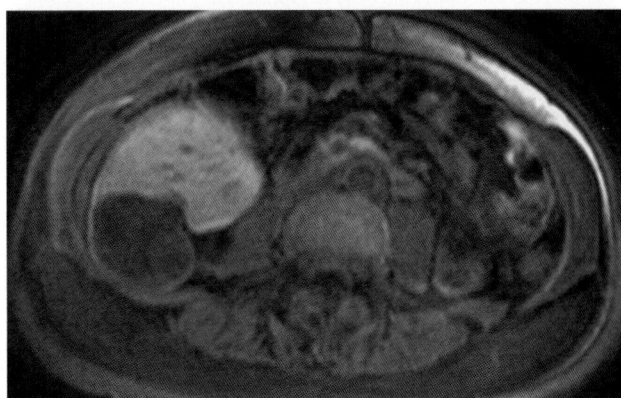

B

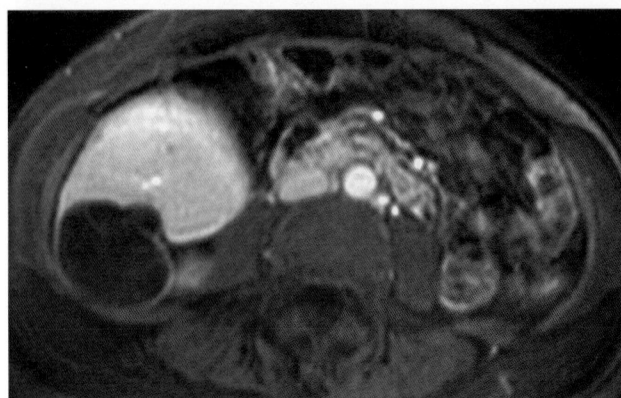

C

A. Axial T2-weighted single-shot FSE/TSE. **B**. Unenhanced and (**C**) gadolinium contrast-enhanced T1-weighted images with fat saturation.

Case 66 Pseudomyxoma Peritonei

Findings

▶ Figure **A** demonstrates a lesion with internal septations adjacent to the right lobe of the liver displaying relative high signal intensity on T2-weighted images. This lesion leads to scalloping of the liver.

▶ Figures **B** and **C** demonstrate the lesion with low signal intensity on T1-weighted images and with no evidence of contrast enhancement.

Differential diagnosis

▶ Peritoneal carcinomatosis
▶ Tuberculosis peritonitis
▶ Peritoneal sarcomatosis

Teaching points

▶ Pseudomyxoma peritonei is a rare entity consisting of mucinous peritoneal implants and gelatinous ascites.

▶ The presentation is variable. Some patients present with vague abdominal pain and bloating while others present with an acute abdomen secondary to bowel obstruction. It is often an unexpected finding at the time of laparotomy.

▶ Pseudomyxoma peritonei is often initially misdiagnosed as an ovarian neoplasm.

▶ The most diagnostic feature is scalloping of the liver or spleen caused by the peritoneal implant.

Management

▶ The mainstay of treatment is surgical excision and debulking.

▶ Adjuvant trials with hyperthermic intraperitoneal chemotherapy, systemic chemotherapy, and intraperitoneal nuclear isotope-based therapy are currently being explored.

Further reading

1. Hinson FL, Ambrose NS. Pseudomyxoma peritonei. Br J Surg 1998;85:1332–1339.
2. Jarvinin P, Lepisto A. Clinical presentation of pseudomyxoma peritonei. Scand J Surg 2010;99:213–216.

History

▶ 56-year-old man with severe hypertension was referred for MR imaging to determine the presence of renal artery stenosis

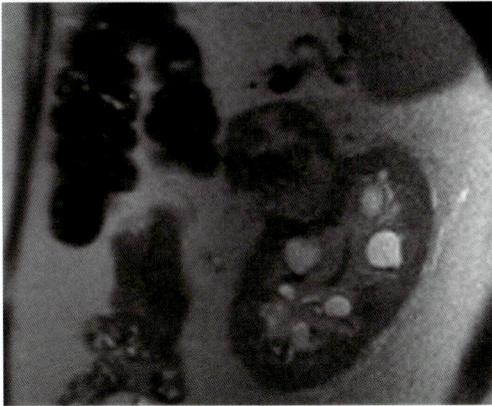

A

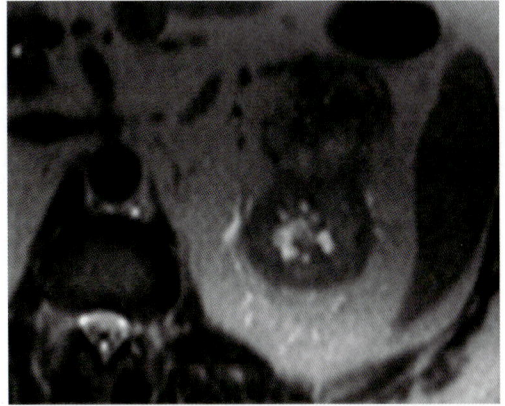

B

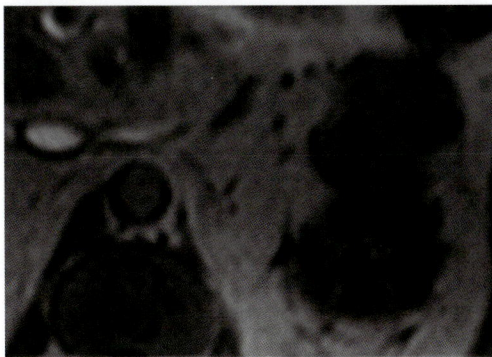

C

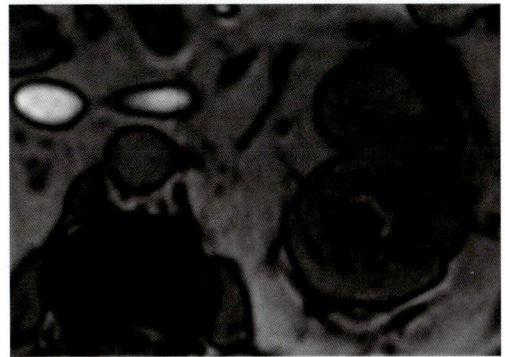

D

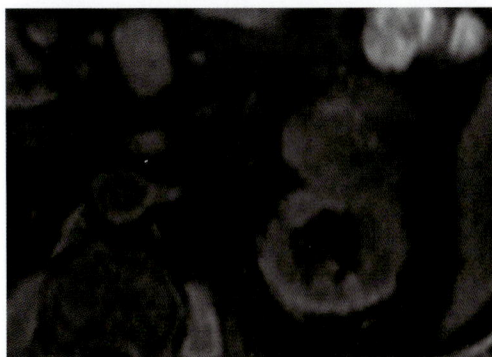

E

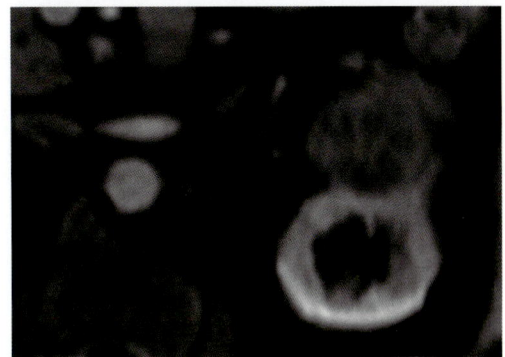

F

A. Sagittal and (**B**) axial T2-weighted single-shot FSE/TSE. **C**. Axial in-phase and (**D**) opposed-phase T1-weighted gradient echo. **E**. Unenhanced and (**F**) post-gadolinium contrast-enhanced axial T1-weighted gradient echo with fat saturation.

Case 67 Papillary Renal Cell Carcinoma (RCC) with Oncocytic Features

Findings

▶ A complex mass arises anteriorly from the upper pole of the left kidney. The mass contains foci of high signal intensity similar to fat on T2-weighted images.

▶ Chemical shift gradient-echo imaging shows no signal intensity loss on the opposed-phase compared to the in-phase images, effectively excluding the presence of intracellular fat within the renal tumor. In addition, the absence of the low intensity signal ("India ink" artifact) at the interface between the tumor and renal parenchyma on the opposed-phase images excludes the presence of bulk fat within the tumor abutting the renal parenchyma.

▶ The lesion shows distinct enhancement, somewhat less than that of the renal cortex, on post-contrast enhanced images, indicating renal cell carcinoma as the most likely diagnosis.

▶ The mass contained copious hemorrhage and cystic areas at pathologic examination.

Differential diagnosis

▶ Angiomyolipoma

▶ Oncocytoma

Teaching points

▶ The presence of bulk (adipose) fat is most reliably demonstrated on MR by comparing two sets of images acquired using the same pulse sequence technique but with one set with and the other set without fat-suppression.

▶ The presence of intracellular (microscopic) fat within the water-containing tumor tissue is most reliably demonstrated by using opposed-phase gradient-echo imaging showing loss of signal compared to in-phase images (chemical shift imaging). Intracellular fat may be present in up to 60% of RCC cases, especially of the clear cell type.

▶ Papillary RCC is second to clear cell as the most common type of RCC. The classic MR appearance of papillary RCC is that of a well-encapsulated mass that displays homogeneous low signal intensity on T2-weighted images and shows homogeneous low-level enhancement that is less than that of the renal cortex on post-contrast-enhanced images. A second classic appearance of papillary RCC is that of a cystic mass with papillary projections.

▶ The lesion shown here, though classified pathologically as a papillary RCC, is atypical because of the presence of hemorrhage and multiple cystic areas.

Management

▶ Radical or partial nephrectomy

Further reading

1. Pedrosa I, Sun MR, Spencer M, et al. MR imaging of renal masses: correlation with findings at surgery and pathologic analysis. RadioGraphics 2008;28:985–1003.
2. Poghosyan T. Urinary tract MR imaging. In: Brant WE, de Lange EE (Eds), Essentials of Body MR Imaging. New York: Oxford University Press, 2012.
3. Vikran R, Ng CS, Tamboli P, et al. Papillary renal cell carcinoma: radiologic-pathologic correlation and spectrum of disease. RadioGraphics 2009;29:741–757.

Case 68

History

▶ 78-year-old man underwent CT for evaluation of constipation. A cystic abdominal mass was discovered.

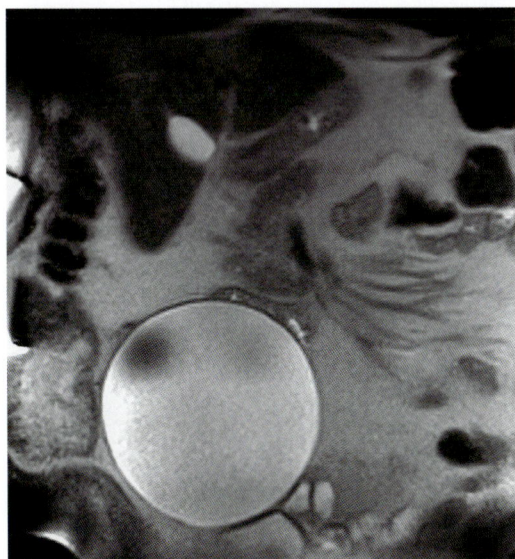

A

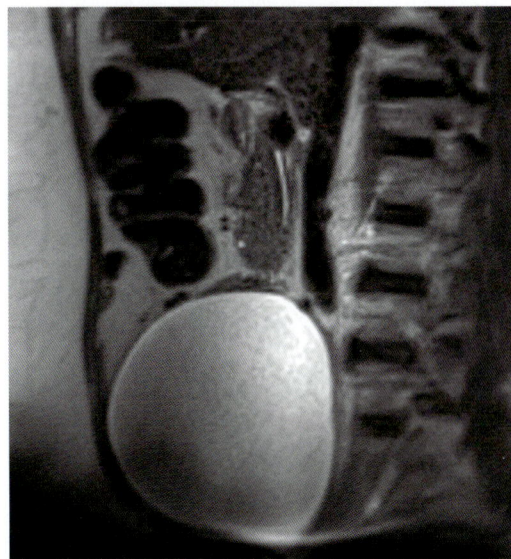

B

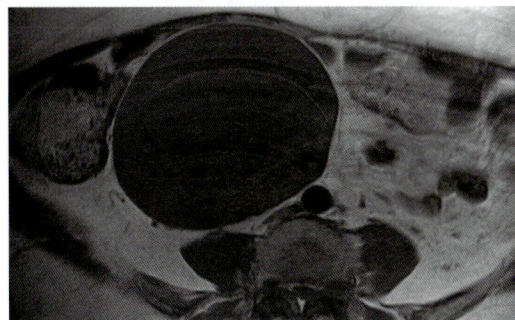

C

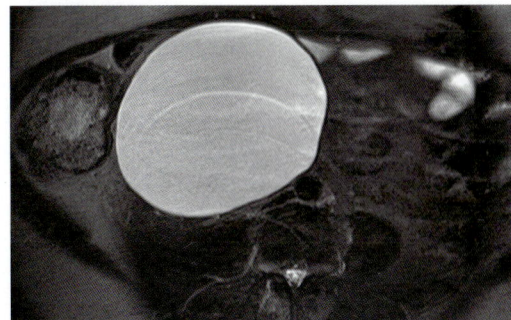

D

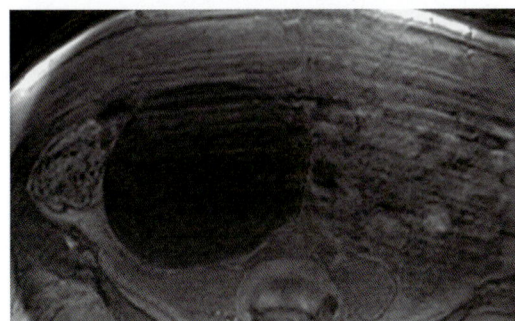

E

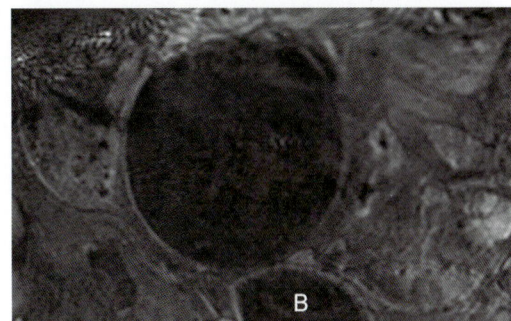

F

A. Coronal and (**B**) sagittal T2-weighted single shot. **C**. Axial T1-weighted spin echo. **D**. Axial T2-weighted FSE/TSE with fat saturation. **E**. Axial unenhanced and (**F**) coronal contrast-enhanced T1-weighted gradient echo. *B*, bladder.

Case 68 Mesenteric Cyst

Findings

▶ A large thin-walled cystic mass is seen within the mesentery on multiplanar imaging. Bowel and mesenteric vessels are displaced but do not appear involved by the mass.

▶ Cyst fluid is simple based upon low signal intensity on T1-weighted images and high signal intensity on T2-weighted images.

▶ The cyst wall shows minimal contrast enhancement. Cyst contents shows no enhancement.

▶ Endoscopic ultrasound-guided aspiration yielded white cloudy proteinaceous fluid with a few benign lymphocytes present.

Differential diagnosis

▶ Cystic lymphangioma
▶ Enteric duplication cyst
▶ Pancreatic or non-pancreatic pseudo cyst
▶ Cystic teratoma
▶ Mucinous or serous cystadenoma
▶ Abscess

Teaching points

▶ The classification of cystic masses of the mesentery is controversial. Most authorities state that cystic lymphangioma is primarily an entity found in children and young adults (mean age 10, up to 75% male), while mesenteric cyst is found in all age groups (mean age 44). Cystic lymphangiomas may be proliferative and invasive, and cause abdominal pain, whereas mesenteric cysts have a benign, usually indolent, course.

▶ Cystic lymphangioma is a congenital malformation of the lymphatic system resulting from a lack of communication of small bowel lymphatic vessels with the lymphatic system. Contents are usually chylous but may be serous or hemorrhagic. Imaging shows a multiloculated cystic mass with complex fluid. Lymphatic endothelial cells line the cyst.

▶ Mesenteric cysts are of mesothelial origin and are lined by benign mesothelium. They are thin-walled and unilocular and contain serous fluid.

▶ Enteric duplication cysts are lined by intestinal epithelium and are usually thick-walled with serous contents. The walls consist of mucosa, circular and longitudinal muscular layers, and mesenteric plexus.

Management

▶ Endoscopy with endoscopic ultrasound-guided fluid aspiration is indicated to confirm the diagnosis by obtaining fluid for analysis.

▶ Surgical enucleation should be considered as rare malignant degeneration of cystic lymphangioma has been reported in adults, though never in children.

Further reading

1. de Perrot M, Bründler M, Tötsch M, et al. Mesenteric cysts. Toward less confusion? Dig Surg 2000;17:323–328.
2. Stoupis C, Ros P, Abbitt PL, et al. Bubbles in the belly: imaging of cystic mesenteric or omental masses. RadioGraphics 1994;14:729–737.

History

▶ 81-year-old woman with a history of cholelithiasis presents with obstructive jaundice and palpable right upper quadrant mass.

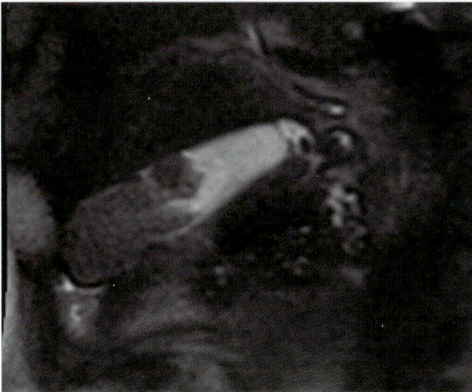

A

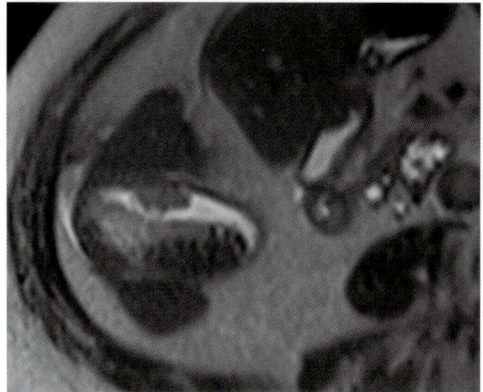

B

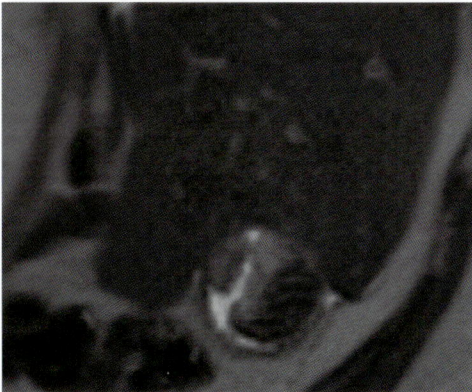

C

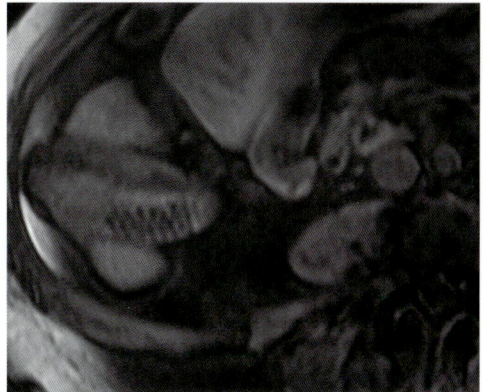

D

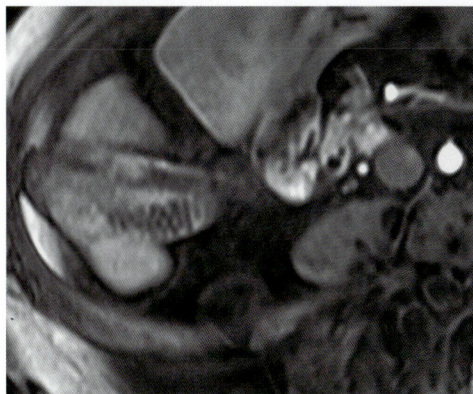

E

A. Coronal, (**B**) axial, and (**C**) sagittal T2-weighted single-shot FSE/TSE. **D**. Axial pre- and (**E**) post-contrast-enhanced T1-weighted gradient echo with fat saturation.

Case 69 Adenocarcinoma of the Gallbladder

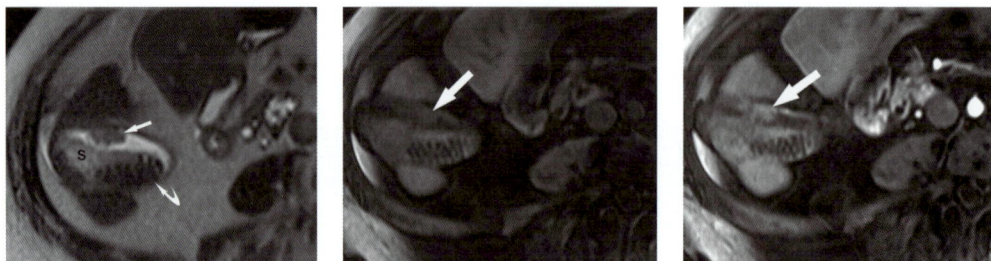

Findings

▶ The gallbladder contains layering gallstones (*curved arrow*) and sludge (S).

▶ A polypoid mass is suspended from the nondependent anterior wall of the gallbladder.

▶ The gallbladder polyp shows distinct low-grade enhancement following intravenous contrast material administration.

Differential diagnosis

▶ Complicated cholecystitis

▶ Metastatic disease

▶ Adenomyomatosis

▶ Lymphoma

Teaching points

▶ Imaging patterns of gallbladder carcinoma include:
  ▪ Mass replacing the gallbladder (40% to 65%)
  ▪ Focal or diffuse thickening of the gallbladder wall (20% to 30%)
  ▪ Intraluminal polypoid mass (15% to 25%)

▶ Patterns of disease spread include:
  ▪ Direct extension into the liver and adjacent organs
  ▪ Extension into the biliary tree causing biliary obstruction
  ▪ Lymph node metastases
  ▪ Hematogenous metastases: lung, bone, pancreas, adrenal, brain

Management

▶ Complete surgical resection if feasible

Further reading

1. Levy AD, Murakata LA, Rohrmann CA. Gallbladder carcinoma: Radiologic-pathologic correlation. RadioGraphics 2001;21:295–314.
2. Olazagasti J. Biliary tree MR imaging. In: Brant WE, de Lange EE (Eds), Essentials of Body MRI. Oxford University Press, New York. 2012

History

▶ 70-year-woman with biopsy-proven chronic hepatitis C cirrhosis underwent MR imaging to screen for hepatocellular carcinoma.

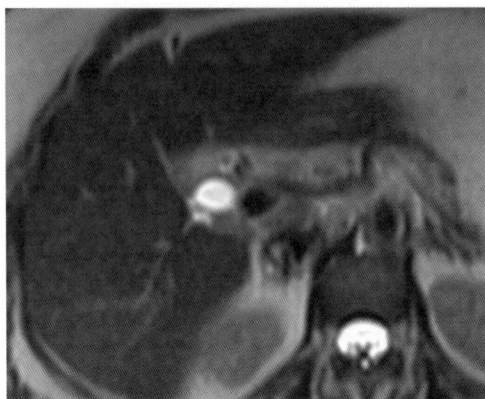

A

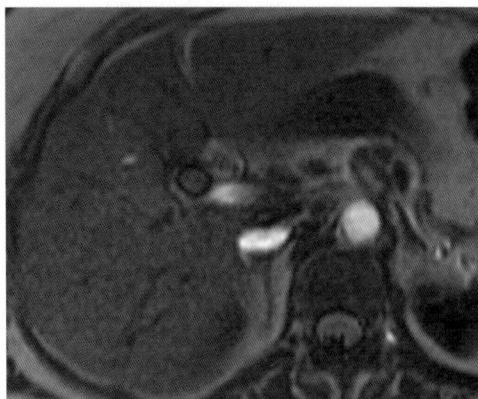

B

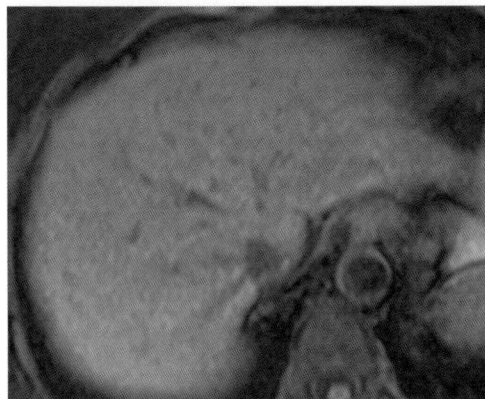

C

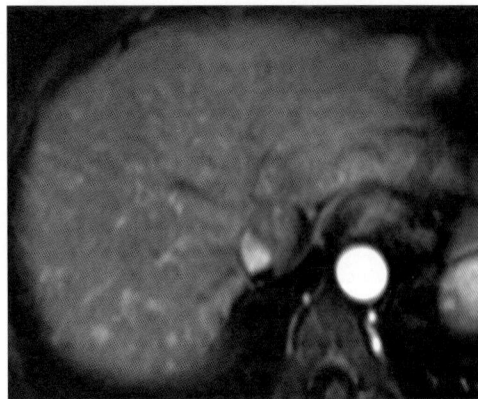

D

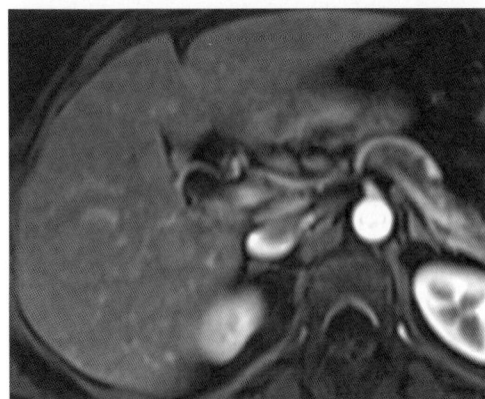

E

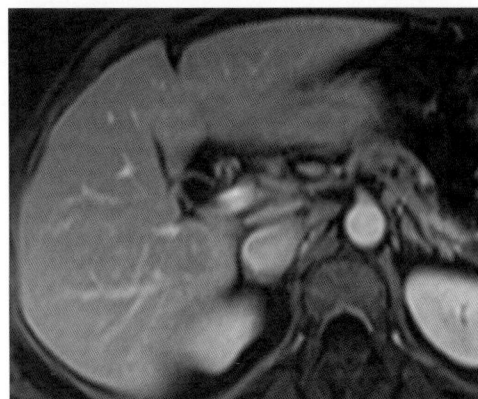

F

A. Axial T2-weighted single-shot FSE/TSE. **B**. T1-weighted magnetization-prepared gradient echo. **C**. Pre-contrast-enhanced T1-weighted gradient echo with fat saturation and (**D**) arterial-phase, (**E**) early portal venous-phase, and (**F**) delayed-phase post-gadolinium contrast-enhanced T1-weighted gradient echo with fat saturation.

Case 70 Numerous Hepatic Arterial-Phase Enhancing (HAPE) Lesions, Presumed to be Benign

Findings

► Multiple small hyperenhancing foci are seen in early arterial-phase images. The most prominent is seen in the posterior right lobe beneath the capsule. None of these foci measures more than 20 mm. No corresponding focal signal abnormalities are seen on delayed-phase contrast-enhanced images and any other sequences, including T2- and non-contrast-enhanced T1-weighted imaging.

Differential diagnosis

► Arterial-portal venous shunting
► Regenerative or dysplastic nodules
► Hepatocellular carcinoma
► Peliosis hepatis

Teaching points

► Although the diagnosis of hepatocellular carcinoma (HCC) can often be confidently made on imaging alone, smaller tumors may present only as foci of early arterial enhancement without the expected increased signal on T2-weighted images. These small (<20 mm) foci of early arterial enhancement without signal abnormalities on other sequences are known as HAPE-only lesions. Diagnostic considerations of HAPE-only lesions include benign entities (arterial-portal venous shunts, regenerative nodules, and peliosis) as well as malignant/premalignant neoplastic lesions (HCC and dysplastic nodules).
► The presence or absence of HCC, even small cancers, carries major implications for patient management, especially regarding the decision to offer transplant. A study by Holland et al. evaluated the histopathology of explanted cirrhotic livers that were known to contain HAPE-only lesions. A prevalence of 35% was reported in this series of 46 pretransplant cirrhotic livers. They found that 93% of the HAPE-only lesions were benign even in livers with simultaneous pathologically proven HCC located remotely from the HAPE-only lesion.

Management

► Given the high likelihood most HAPE-only lesions are benign, continued screening at normal intervals for detecting HCC is appropriate management. An alternative modality such as CT or catheter angiography could be useful. Biopsy is unlikely to yield useful results considering the small size of the lesions.

Further reading

1. Holland AE, Hecht EM, Hahn WY, et al. Importance of small (≤20-mm) enhancing lesions seen only during the hepatic arterial phase at MR imaging of the cirrhotic liver: evaluation and comparison with whole explanted liver. Radiology 2005;237:938–944.
2. Silva AC, Evans JM, McCullough AE, et al. MR imaging of hypervascular liver masses: a review of current techniques. RadioGraphics 2009;29:385–402.

History

▶ 42-year-old woman with increased abdominal girth, shortness of breath, and history of "pancreatic cysts"

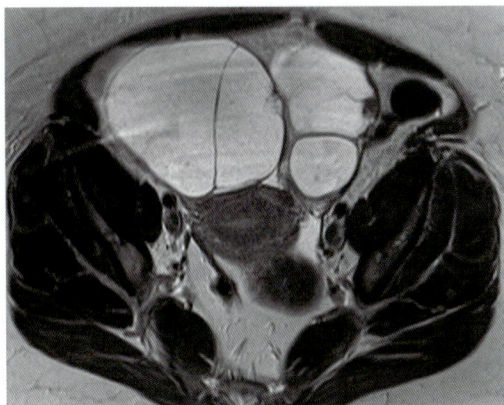

A

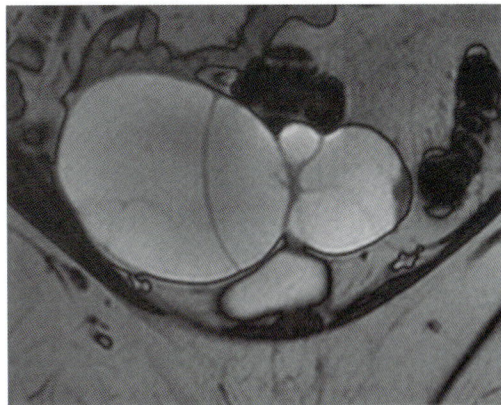

B

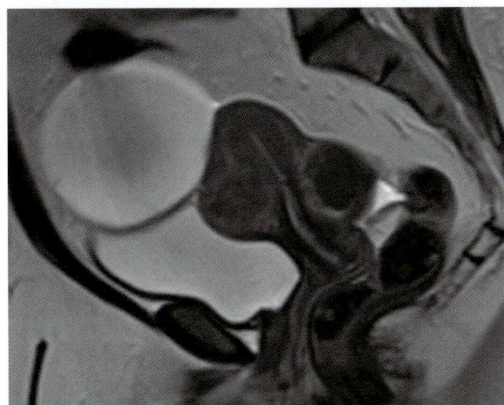

C

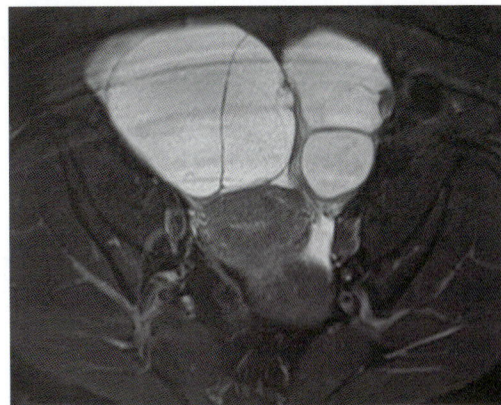

D

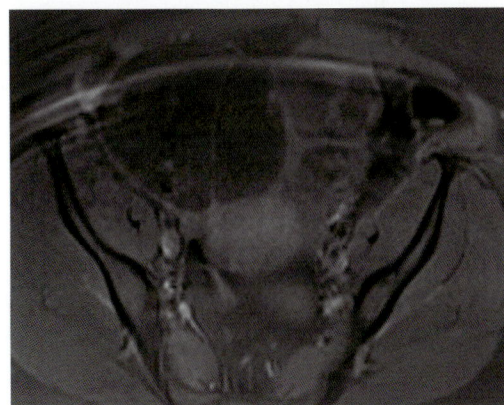

E

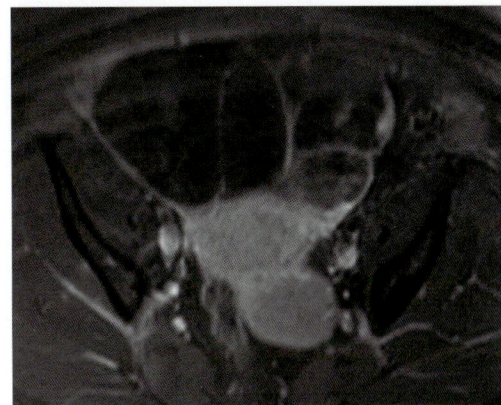

F

A. Axial, (**B**) coronal, and (**C**) sagittal T2-weighted FSE/TSE. **D**. Axial T2-weighted FSE/TSE with fat saturation. **E**. Axial pre-contrast-enhanced and (**F**) post-gadolinium contrast-enhanced T1-weighted spin echo with fat saturation.

Case 71   Metastatic Adenocarcinoma to the Ovaries from a Primary Pancreatic Mucinous Cystic Adenocarcinoma

Findings

▶ A 11 × 10 × 10-cm right cystic ovarian mass and a 10 × 8 × 7-cm left cystic ovarian mass
▶ The right ovarian mass demonstrates multiple septations and is thin-walled, with a 3-cm enhancing mural nodule.
▶ The left ovarian mass demonstrates multiple septations and a 2.7-cm enhancing mural nodule.
▶ Additional findings: a subserosal uterine leiomyoma and a left intramural leiomyoma

Differential diagnosis

▶ Primary ovarian cancer—mostly multilocular cystic appearance (in contrast to mixed solid and cystic secondary ovarian malignancies)
▶ Lymphoma of the ovaries—homogeneous, minimally enhancing solid masses (hypointense on T1-weighted images and mildly hyperintense on T2-weighted images) with extensive lymphatic involvement

Teaching points

▶ Metastasis to ovaries occurs via direct extension or peritoneal spread. Metastases account for 10% to 15% of the ovarian cancers. The most common primary tumor is colon cancer. Other common primary tumors include stomach, breast, lung, and pancreas.
▶ Krukenberg tumors are specific metastatic ovarian tumors from gastric carcinoma consisting of mucin-filled signet-ring cells in a cellular stroma.
▶ Typical ovarian metastases are often bilateral, solid, and strongly enhancing. However, ovarian metastases can have cystic and necrotic components, which complicate differentiation from primary ovarian cancers. Imaging findings of primary and secondary ovarian tumors often overlap. Correlation with the clinical findings as well as the imaging features of the primary tumor may provide helpful information.
▶ MRI shows solid components on T1-weighted images with intermediate signal intensity. Solid components have heterogeneous signal intensity on T2-weighted images, whereas cystic and necrotic components have high signal intensity. There is heterogeneous enhancement of the solid components on post-contrast-enhanced T1-weighted images.

Management

▶ Tumor-reductive surgery (in this case distal pancreatectomy with splenectomy and bilateral salpingo-oophorectomy)
▶ There is usually poor response to chemotherapeutic agents

Further reading

1. Chang WC, Meux MD, Yeh BM, et al. CT and MRI of adnexal masses in patients with primary nonovarian malignancy. AJR Am J Roentgenol 2006;186:1039–1045.
2. de Waal YR, Thomas CM, Oei AL, et al. Secondary ovarian malignancies: frequency, origin, and characteristics. Int J Gynecol Cancer 2009;19:1160–1165.
3. Meriden Z, Yemelyanova AV, Vang R, et al. Ovarian metastases of pancreaticobiliary tract adenocarcinomas: analysis of 35 cases, with emphasis on the ability of metastases to simulate primary ovarian mucinous tumors. Am J Surg Pathol 2011;35:276–288.
4. Yemelyanova AV, Vang R, Judson K, et al. Distinction of primary and metastatic mucinous tumors involving the ovary: analysis of size and laterality data by primary site with reevaluation of an algorithm for tumor classification. Am J Surg Pathol 2008;32:128–138.

History

▶ 68-year-old man with history of liver disease

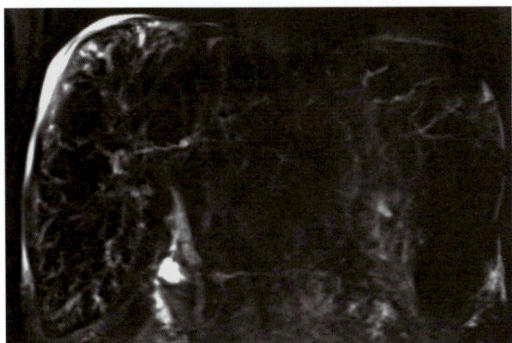

A

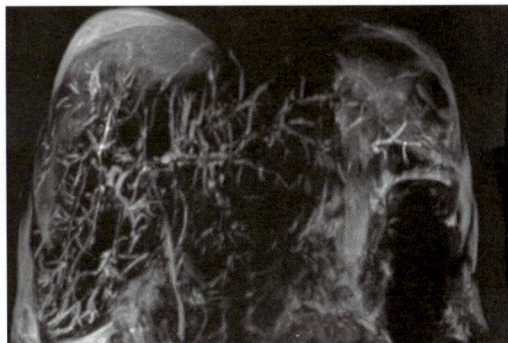

B

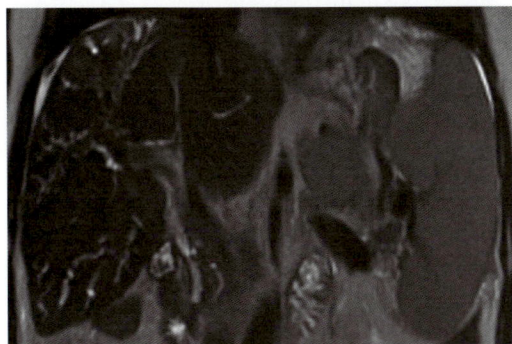

C

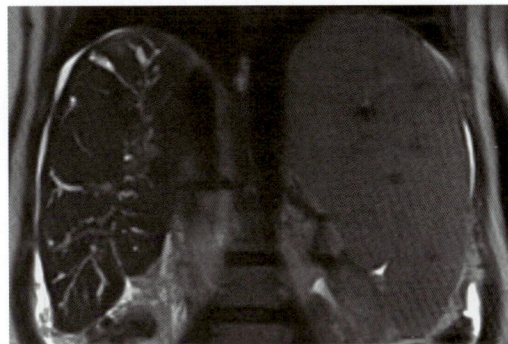

D

A. Thick-slice MRCP obtained with single-shot FSE/TSE with fat saturation. **B**. MRCP reconstructed from respiratory-gated 3D FSE/TSE with fat saturation. **C**. Coronal T2-weighted single-shot FSE/TSE through common bile duct and (**D**) at a level posterior to **C**.

Case 72 Primary Sclerosing Cholangitis with Cirrhosis and Portal Hypertension

Findings

▶ Diffuse dilatation of the intrahepatic biliary tree with multifocal segments of uneven dilatation and narrowing of the bile ducts
▶ Cirrhosis, splenomegaly, ascites

Differential diagnosis

▶ Primary biliary cirrhosis
▶ Recurrent pyogenic cholangitis
▶ AIDS cholangiopathy

Teaching points

▶ Primary sclerosing cholangitis (PSC) is a chronic progressive disease characterized by inflammation and fibrosis of the biliary tree. Progressive fibrosis obliterates the small, medium, and large bile ducts, leading to chronic cholestasis that results in cirrhosis and liver failure. The cause is unknown.
▶ PSC is strongly associated with inflammatory bowel disease, both ulcerative colitis and Crohn's disease, one of which is present in 71% of cases with PSC.
▶ Cirrhosis resulting from PSC typically is of the macronodular variety with wedge-shaped areas of parenchymal atrophy. Large regenerative nodules are most characteristic. Progression to end-stage liver disease is typical.
▶ Cholangiocarcinoma occurs in 10% to 15% of patients with PSC.
▶ Characteristic findings at MRCP include randomly distributed, circumferential, short-segment (1 to 3 mm) strictures alternating with normal or mildly dilated bile duct segments. As the disease progresses the peripheral bile ducts become obliterated and are no longer visualized. A key feature is random and uneven distribution of biliary strictures.

Management

▶ Progressive cirrhosis leads to liver transplantation.

Further reading

1. Bader TR, Beavers KL, Semelka RC. MR imaging features of primary sclerosing cholangitis: patterns of cirrhosis in relationship to clinical severity of disease. Radiology 2003;226:675–685.
2. Dave M, Elmunzer BJ, Dwamena BA, Higgins PD. Primary sclerosing cholangitis: a meta-analysis of diagnostic performance of MR cholangiopancreatography. Radiology 2010;256:387–396.
3. Vitellas KM, Keogan MT, Freed KS, et al. Radiologic manifestations of sclerosing cholangitis with emphasis on MR cholangiopancreatography. RadioGraphics 2000;20:959–975.

History

▶ 42-year-old woman with history of cirrhosis and acute and chronic renal failure underwent an MR angiogram to evaluate her renal transplant. She had an abdominal MR and an MR angiogram two years prior during which she received 40 cc gadodiamide injected intravenously. At the time of the MR shown here the patient was confined to a wheelchair with continuing complaints of muscle aches, weakness, joint pain and stiffness, dry skin, and hair loss.

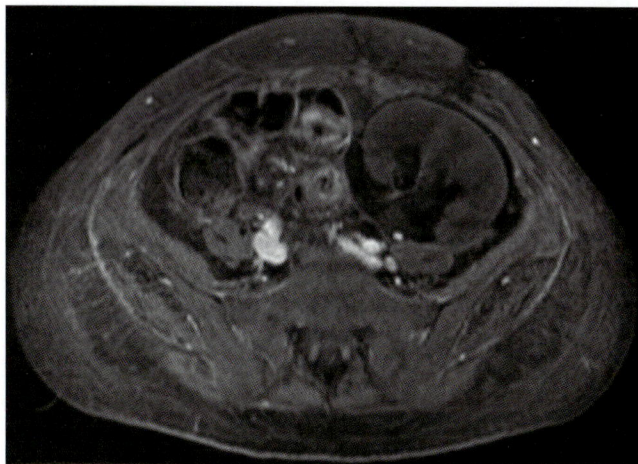

A

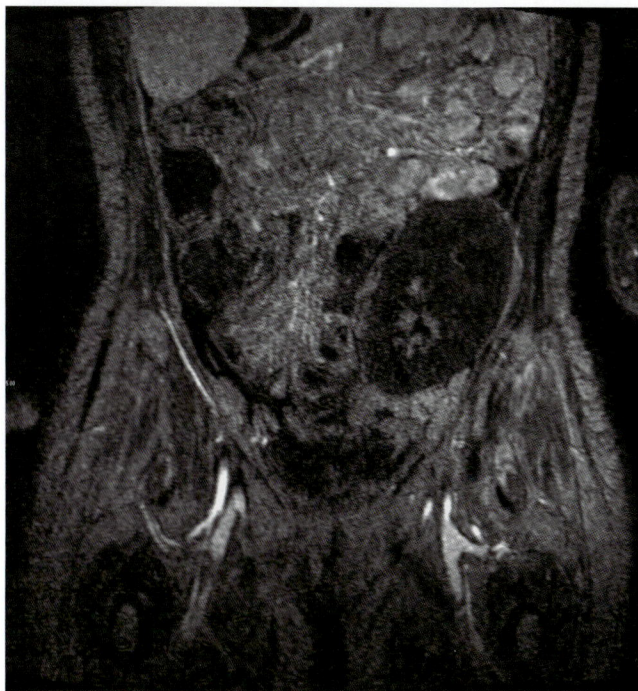

B

A. Axial gadolinium-contrast-enhanced T1-weighted gradient echo with fat suppression. **B**. Coronal source image from contrast-enhanced 3D T1-weighted gradient-echo sequence for MRA.

Case 73   Nephrogenic Systemic Fibrosis (NSF)

Findings

▶ The skin is thickened and the subcutaneous tissues, muscles, and fascia are diffusely edematous.

▶ The transplanted kidney does not enhance. Doppler US and catheter angiography confirmed complete thrombosis of the renal artery to the transplanted kidney.

Teaching points

▶ NSF was first described in the United States in 1997, was thought to be confined to the skin, and was called "nephrogenic fibrosing dermopathy."

▶ Clinical findings are most prominent in the extremities with induration, thickening, and hardening of the skin, mild pitting edema, and progressive hair loss. Skin thickening results in progressive flexion contractures, especially of the hands. The trunk may be involved with a *peau d'orange* appearance of involved skin. Pain and intense pruritus are prominent features. Visceral organ fibrosis and vascular thrombosis are part of the disease. Diagnosis is confirmed by skin biopsy. At present, there is no effective treatment for NSF, though stabilizing or reversing renal failure limits the progression of disease.

▶ MR findings include skin thickening and edema in the subcutaneous fat, intramuscular fascia, and muscles. Symmetrical involvement is typical.

▶ In 2006 and 2007 NSF was linked to the use of high-dose gadolinium-based contrast agents, especially gadodiamide (Gd-DTPA-BMA, Omniscan®), in patients with severe progressive renal failure.

Management

▶ Proposed guidelines for use of gadolinium contrast agents in patients with renal failure include:

   ▪ Measure serum creatinine and calculating glomerular filtration rate (GFR) in all patients 60 years and older as well as in all patients at risk for renal disease.

   ▪ Limit the maximum dose of gadolinium contrast agent to 20 mL for all patients with calculated GFR lower than 60 mL/min/1.73 m^2.

   ▪ Prohibit use of any gadolinium-based contrast agent in patients with calculated GFR lower than 30 mL/min/1.73 m^2, and in those on dialysis, except in emergency situations.

   ▪ Many experts also advise against the use of gadodiamide in any patients.

▶ Using these guidelines a study of 52,954 examinations, including 6,454 patients with GFR in the 30-to-59 range and 36 with GFR below 30, reported no new cases of NSF.

Further reading

1. Altun E, Semelka RC, Cakit C. Nephrogenic systemic fibrosis and management of high-risk patients. Acad Radiol 2009;16:897–905.
2. Morris MF, Zhang Y, Zhang H, et al. Features of nephrogenic systemic fibrosis on radiology examinations. AJR Am J Roentgenol 2009;193:61–69.
3. Prince MR, Zhang HL, Prowda JC, et al. Nephrogenic systemic fibrosis and its impact on abdominal imaging. RadioGraphics 2009;29:1565–1574.
4. Wang Y, Alkasab TK, Narin O, et al. Incidence of nephrogenic systemic fibrosis after adoption of restrictive gadolinium-based contrast agent guidelines. Radiology 2011;260:105–111.

History

▶ 52-year-old man with a history of multiple myeloma complains of chest tightness and palpitations with activity.

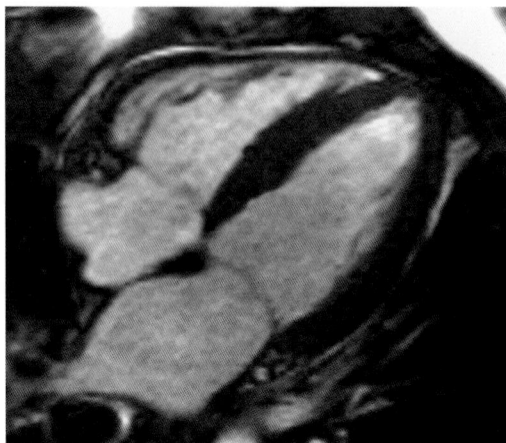

A

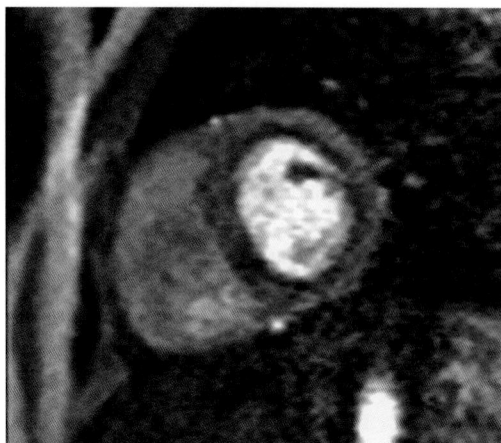

B

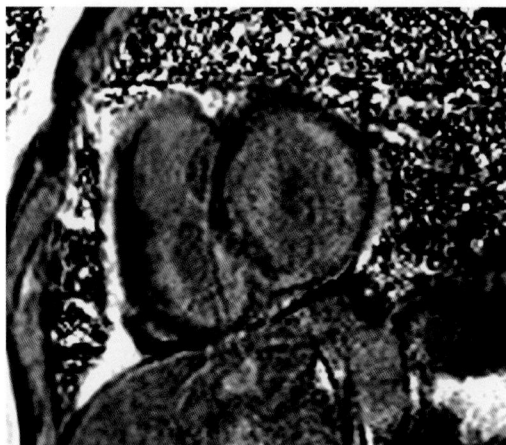

C

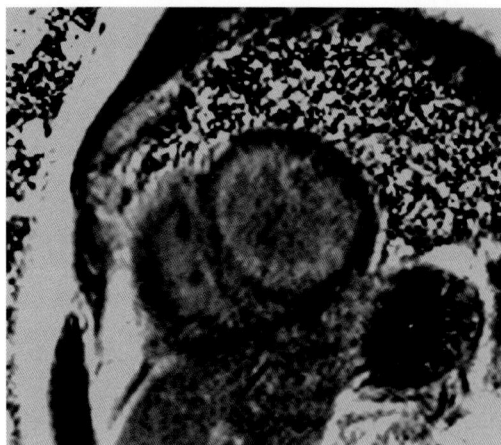

D

A. Horizontal long-axis (4-chamber) balanced steady-state free precession (SSFP) at end-diastole. **B**. Short-axis first-pass rest perfusion imaging using T1-weighted gradient echo with segmented echo planar readout. **C**. Basal short-axis and (**D**) apical short-axis late gadolinium enhancement (LGE) phase-sensitive inversion recovery (PSIR).

Case 74 Cardiac Amyloidosis

Findings
▶ Diffuse thickening of the left ventricular myocardium measuring up to 17 mm (**A**)
▶ Circumferential subendocardial perfusion defect on short-axis rest imaging (**B**)
▶ Diffuse, circumferential subendocardial late gadolinium enhancement (LGE) (**C, D**)

Differential diagnosis
▶ Myocardial infarction

Teaching points
▶ Amyloidosis is the result of extracellular deposition of malformed protein.
▶ Classification is based on the type of protein deposited. The most common form is systemic amyloid light-chain (AL) amyloidosis, in which up to 90% of patients have cardiac involvement.
▶ AL amyloidosis is associated with multiple myeloma and has a high risk for sudden death.
▶ Physiologic consequences of protein fibril deposition in the heart include diffuse myocardial thickening, impaired contractility, diastolic dysfunction, and restrictive physiology.
▶ MR imaging characteristics include >6 mm thickening of the intra-atrial septum or free wall and LGE in the distribution of protein deposition, most often affecting the subendocardium in a global distribution that does not follow vascular territories (differentiating amyloid from myocardial infarction).
▶ A characteristic feature of amyloidosis is rapid washout of gadolinium from myocardium and blood pool, which may result in difficulty selecting the appropriate inversion time for LGE imaging due to the unusually dark blood pool. The rapid washout suggests the diagnosis of amyloidosis if observed in the setting of other previously described imaging features.

Management
▶ Untreated systemic AL amyloidosis with cardiac involvement is a rapidly fatal disorder.
▶ Treatment depends on the type of disease. AL amyloidosis is treated with chemotherapeutics and novel agents, and occasionally heart transplant.

Further reading
1. Kapoor P, Thenappan T, Singh E, et al. Cardiac amyloidosis: a practical approach to diagnosis and management. Am J Med 2011;124:1006–1015.
2. Sparrow PJ, Merchant N, Provost YL, et al. CT and MR imaging findings in patients with acquired heart disease at risk for sudden cardiac death. RadioGraphics 2009;29:805–823.

History

▶ 80-year-old man presents with recurrent gallstone pancreatitis.

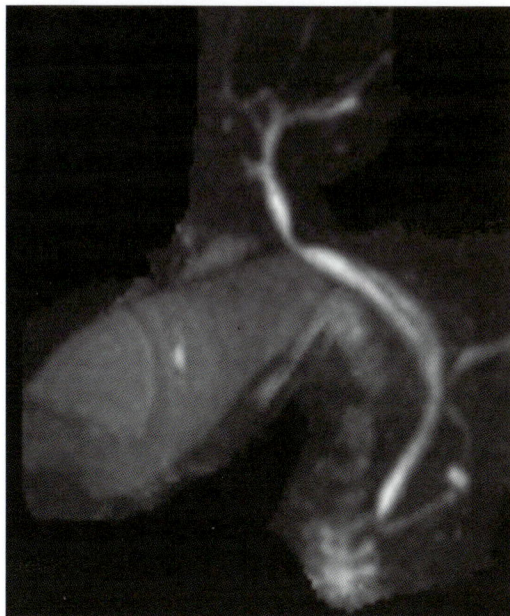

A

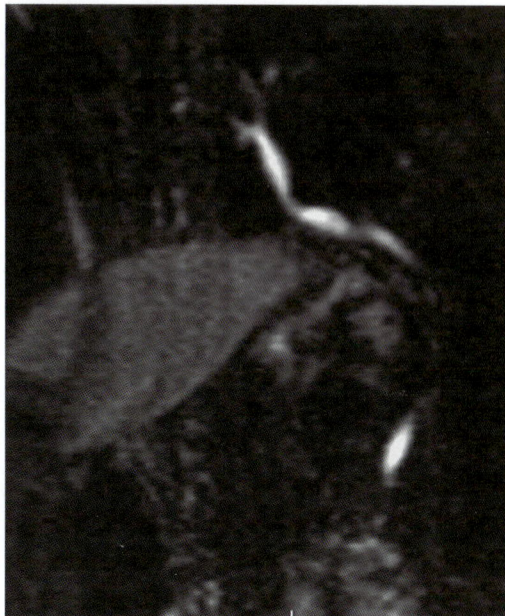

B

A. Maximum intensity projection MRCP image generated from 3D FSE/TSE. **B**. Source image from same sequence.

Case 75 Pseudostenosis of the Common Hepatic Duct Caused by the Right Hepatic Artery Crossing the Duct

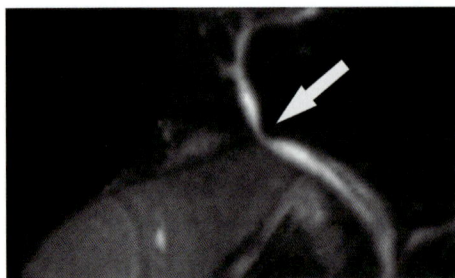

C

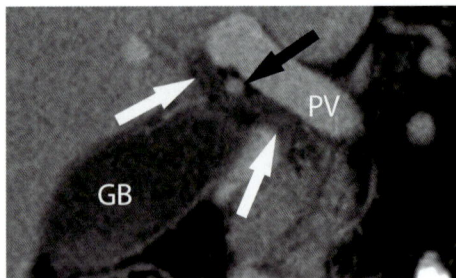

D

Findings

- ▶ MRCP image (**C**) demonstrates narrowing (*arrow*) of the common hepatic duct (CHD).
- ▶ Coronal reconstructed contrast-enhanced CT image (**D**) demonstrates the right hepatic artery (*black arrow*) causing mild narrowing of the CHD (low density structure outlined by *white arrows*). *PV* = main portal vein. *GB*, gallbladder.

Differential diagnosis

- ▶ Biliary stricture
- ▶ Tumor (cholangiocarcinoma)

Teaching points

- ▶ The branches of the common hepatic artery are closely related to the extrahepatic bile ducts anatomically. The right hepatic artery commonly passes immediately posterior to the proximal portion of the CHD.
- ▶ The extrahepatic bile duct is susceptible to extrinsic pulsatile compression where the artery crosses the bile duct. The right hepatic artery is the most common cause of this pseudo-stenosis, but other common hepatic artery branches, including the gastroduodenal artery and cystic artery, can cause similar artifact.
- ▶ Maximum intensity projection reconstructed MRCP images can overestimate the extent of biliary narrowing.
- ▶ The absence of prestenotic dilatation of the CHD is a key finding indicating that there is no true stenosis and hence that an obstructing stone or bile duct stricture is unlikely.
- ▶ Differentiation between pseudo-stenosis and true stenosis can be best made by closely examining coronal T2-weighted images, and by determining whether prestenotic biliary dilatation is present.

Management

- ▶ Recognizing narrowing of the CHD by arterial pulsatile compression artifact should prevent incorrect diagnosis of stone or stricture on MRCP images.
- ▶ When biliary stenosis is strongly suspected clinically, further examination with ERCP may be necessary.

Further reading

1. Izuishi K, et al. Compression of the common hepatic duct by the right hepatic artery. J Clin Imaging 2005;29:342–344.
2. Miashita K, et al. The right hepatic artery syndrome. World J Gastroent 2005;11:3008–3009.
3. Watanabe Y, et al. Pseudo-obstruction of the extrahepatic bile ducts due to artifact from arterial pulsatile compression: A diagnostic pitfall of MR holangiopancreatography. Radiology 2000;214:856–860.

History

▶ 55-year-old woman with a history of melanoma arising on the shoulder. MRI was requested for restaging.

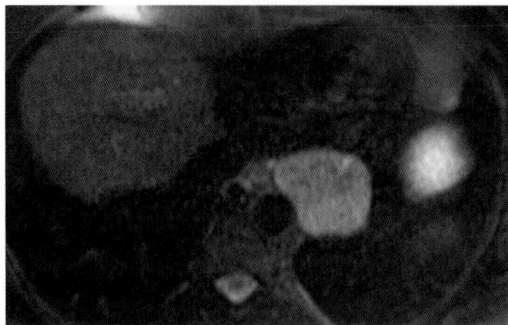

A

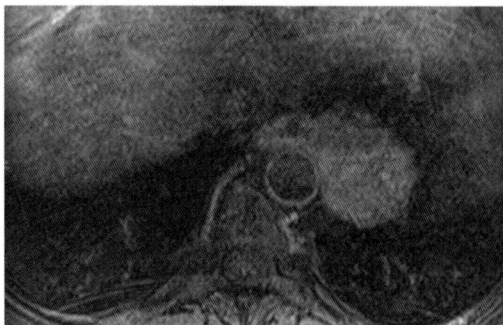

B

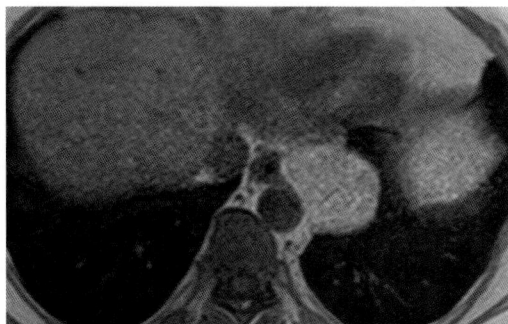

C

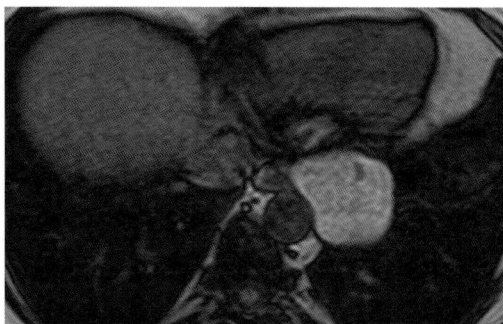

D

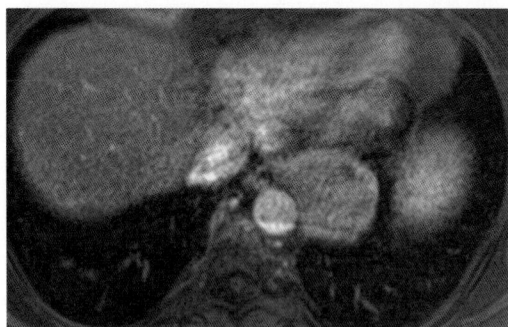

E

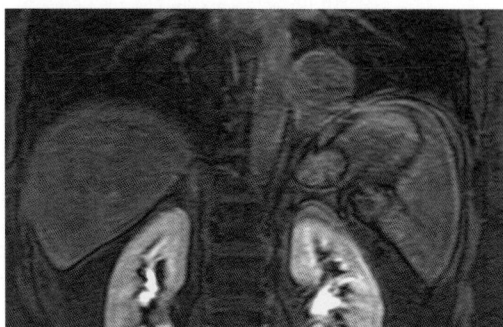

F

A. Axial T2-weighted FSE/TSE with fat saturation. **B**. Axial T1-weighted gradient echo with fat saturation. **C** Axial in-phase and (**D**) opposed-phase T1-weighted gradient echo. **E**. Axial and (**F**) coronal gadolinium-contrast enhanced gradient echo with fat saturation.

Case 76 Esophageal Duplication Cyst

Findings

► Cystic mass in the lower middle mediastinum abuts the esophagus.
► The mass displays high signal intensity on both T1- and T2-weighted images and shows no enhancement following gadolinium contrast material administration.
► The diagnosis was based on characteristic appearance on MRI, CT, and endoscopic ultrasound, and stability of the finding for 1 year.

Differential diagnosis

► Bronchogenic cyst
► Pericardial cyst

Teaching points

► Esophageal duplication cysts are developmental in origin, classified as foregut or bronchopulmonary duplications. The primitive foregut gives rise to both the upper gastrointestinal tract and the lower respiratory tract. Mediastinal cysts are classified as esophageal duplication cysts if they abut the esophagus, have two muscle layers, and are lined by ciliated epithelium. Many are asymptomatic.
► Symptoms associated with esophageal duplication cysts include dysphagia and chest or epigastric pain. Ectopic gastric mucosa within the duplication may cause hemorrhage. Additional complications include obstruction, infection, perforation, and very rarely, malignancy arising within the cyst.
► Ultrasound is the most specific imaging modality used to confirm the diagnosis and demonstrates the characteristic bowel composition of the cyst wall consisting of echogenic inner mucosa/submucosa surrounded by a hypoechoic muscle layer.
► Gastrointestinal duplication cysts are of two general types: A cystic duplication (approximately 80% of cases) which is spherical and without communication with the gastrointestinal tract, and a tubular duplication (20% of cases) which communicates directly with the bowel lumen.

Management

► Symptomatic esophageal duplication cysts are removed by thoracotomy or thorascopic excision

Further reading

1. Herbella FA, Tedesco P, Muthusamy R, Patti MG. Thorascopic resection of esophageal duplication cysts. Dis Esophagus 2006;19:132–134.
2. Jeung M-Y, Gasser B, Gangi A, et al. Imaging of cystic masses of the mediastinum. RadioGraphics 2002;22:S79–S93.
3. Lee NK, Kim S, Jeon TY, et al. Complications of congenital and developmental abnormalities of the gastrointestinal tract in adolescents and adults: evaluation with multimodality imaging. RadioGraphics 2010; 30:1489–1507.

History

▶ 73-year-old man with urinary frequency, hesitancy, and dribbling

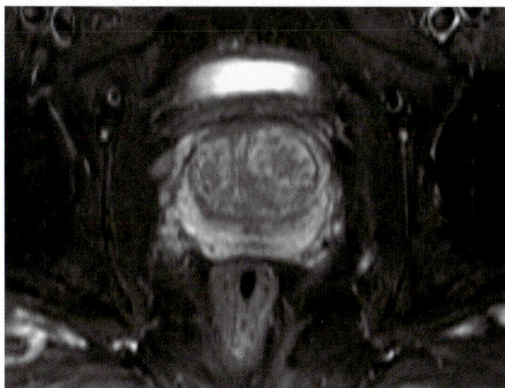

A

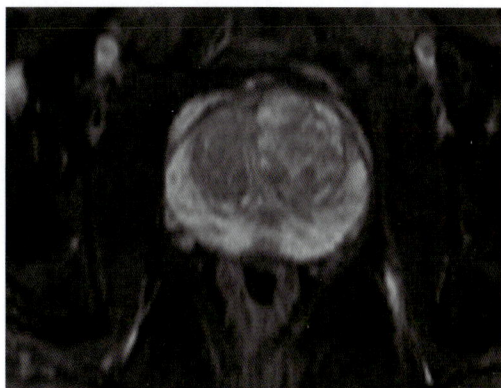

B

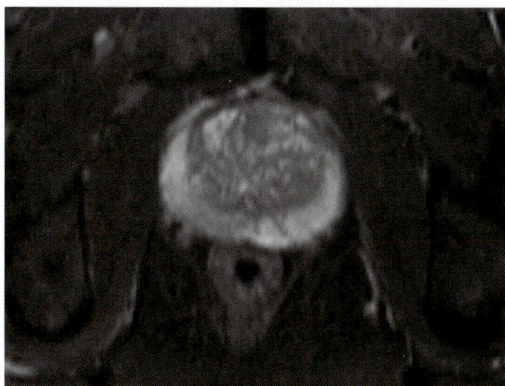

C

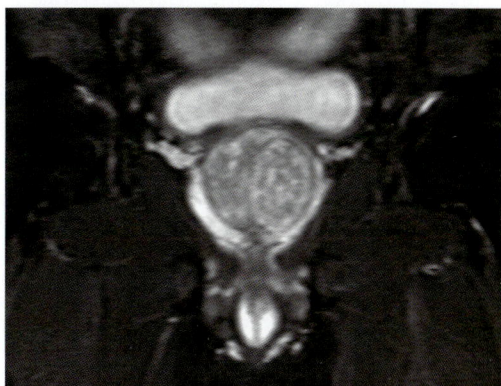

D

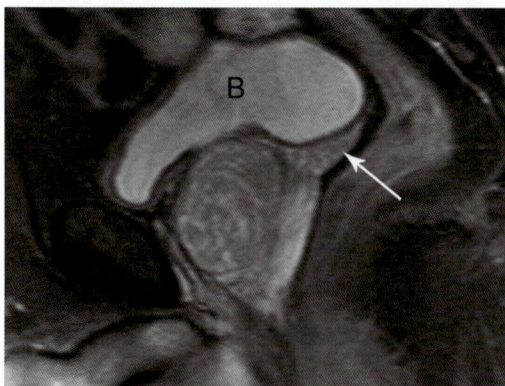

E

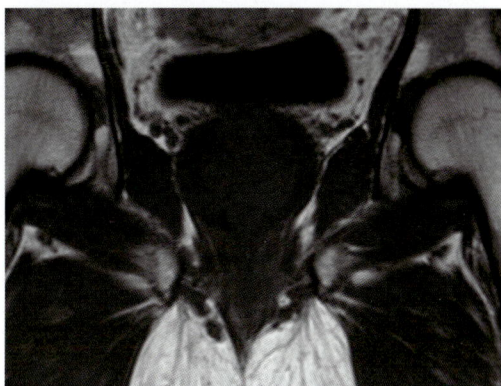

F

A, B, C. Consecutive (cranial–caudal) axial T2-weighted FSE/TSE images with fat saturation. **D**. Coronal and (**E**) sagittal T2-weighted FSE/TSE with fat saturation. **F**. Coronal T1-weighted spin echo. *B*, bladder. *Arrow*, seminal vesicle.

Case 77   Benign Prostatic Hypertrophy

Findings

- On T2-weighted images the central gland is seen to be enlarged and contains multiple nodules of heterogeneous high signal intensity. The normal high signal intensity of the peripheral zone is preserved. The normal high signal intensity of the seminal vesicles is evident.
- The enlarged prostate mildly elevates the bladder base. The wall of the bladder is mildly thickened.
- T1-weighted images fail to clearly demonstrate the zonal anatomy of the prostate gland as the entire gland displays low signal intensity. On these images the hypertrophied central gland tissue is only slightly higher in signal intensity than the peripheral zone.

Differential diagnosis

- Prostate carcinoma involving the central gland

Teaching points

- Benign prostatic hypertrophy (BPH) refers to hyperplasia of the glandular and stromal elements of the prostate gland predominantly occurring in the periurethral transitional zone. The condition is so common that many consider it to be part of the normal aging process, affecting 90% of men by age 85.
- Typical clinical symptoms involve voiding dysfunction with urinary frequency, urgency, decreased force of the urine stream, and sensation of incomplete emptying.
- T2-weighted images optimally show the zonal anatomy of the prostate gland. The characteristic appearance of BPH with glandular hyperplasia is that of multiple nodules in the central gland showing heterogeneous central high signal intensity on T2-weighted images with peripheral low signal intensity. Cystic components are common.
- Stromal hyperplasia results in foci of intermediate or low signal intensity in the central gland on T2-weighted images.
- Marked BPH may compress the peripheral zone and protrude into the bladder base.
- BPH is commonly associated with thickening of the bladder wall.

Management

- Treatment options include a wide variety of medications or transurethral resection of part of the prostate.

Further reading

1. Bonekamp D, Jacobs MA, El-Khouli R, et al. Advancements in MR imaging of the prostate: from diagnosis to interventions. RadioGraphics 2011;31:677–703.

History

▶ 49-year-old man who had recent liver transplantation.

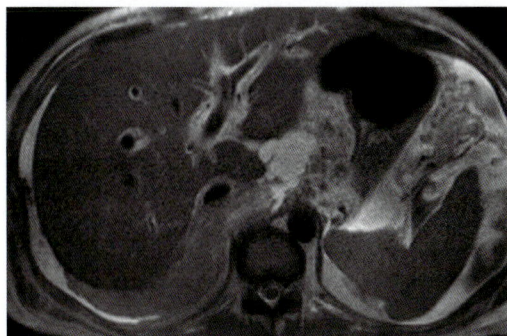
A

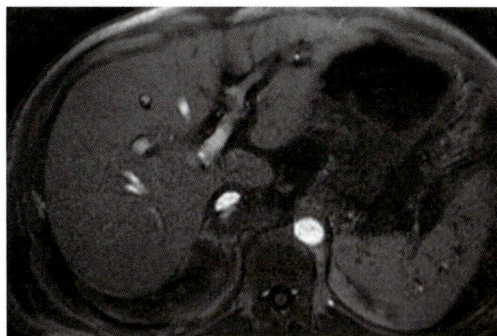
B

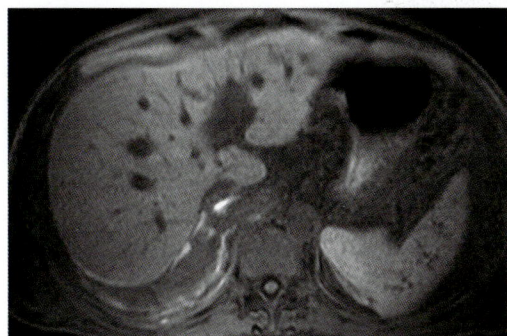
C

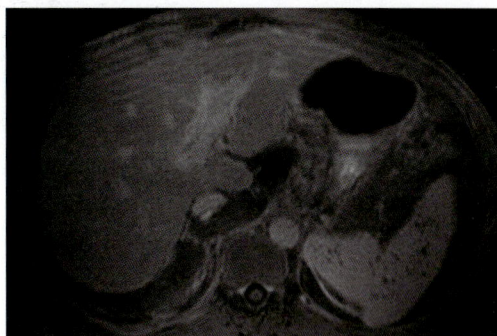
D

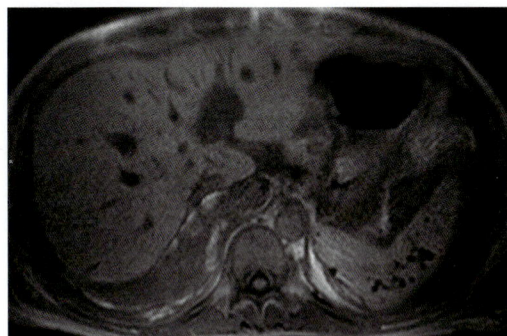
E

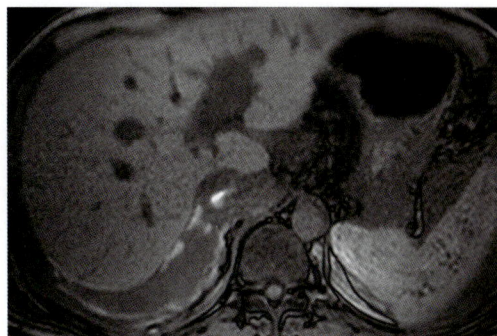
F

A. Axial T2-weighted single-shot FSE/TSE. **B**. Axial T1-weighted magnetization-prepared gradient echo. **C**. Axial pre-contrast-enhanced and (**D**) late-phase gadolinium-contrast-enhanced T1-weighted gradient echo with fat saturation. **E**. Axial in-phase and (**F**) opposed-phase T1-weighted gradient echo.

Case 78 Intraperitoneal Hemorrhage

Findings

▶ Crescentic, slightly heterogenous, collection posterior to the transplanted liver. Collection appears lower in signal intensity than liver on T1-weighted images, and higher in signal intensity than liver on T2-weighted images. The collection does not significantly enhance after intravenous gadolinium contrast administration. No signal loss is evident on out-of-phase imaging, signifying the absence of intracellular fat.

▶ Gamna-Gandy bodies are evident in the spleen.

Differential diagnosis

▶ Hepatic necrosis

Teaching points

▶ Hematomas vary in appearance based on age of blood at time of imaging.

▶ Acute hematomas (less than 48 hours) may have a nonspecific signal intensity.

▶ At 2 to 3 days, hemorrhagic fluid tends to be homogenous, and appears hypointense on T1-weighted images relative to the liver and markedly hypointense on T2-weighted images, due to intracellular deoxyhemoglobin.

▶ At 3 to 5 days, hematoma is hyperintense on T1-weighted images and hypointense on T2-weighted images, due to intracellular methemoglobin.

▶ One may see so-called "hematocrit effect," referred to as a cellular-fluid level, with the dependent portion demonstrating increased signal on T1-weighted images compared with the supernatant, with the signal intensity reversed on T2-weighting.

	Blood products	T1 signal	T2 signal
Hyperacute	Oxyhemoglobin/Serum	Intermediate	High
Acute	Deoxyhemoglobin	Intermediate	Low
Subacute, early	Intracellular methemoglobin	High	Low
Subacute, late	Extracellular methemoglobin	High	High
Chronic	Hemosiderin	Low	Low

Further reading

1. Balci N, Semelka R, Noone T. Acute and subacute liver-related hemorrhage: MRI findings. Mag Reson Imaging 1999;17:207–211.
2. Caiado AHM, Blasbalg R, Marcelino ASZ, et al. Complications of liver transplantation: multimodality imaging approach. RadioGraphics 2007;27:1401–1417.
3. de Lange EE, Mugler JP. MR acquisition techniques & practical considerations for abdominal imaging. In: Brant WE, de Lange EE (Eds), Essentials of Body MR Imaging. New York: Oxford University Press, 2012.

History

▶ 32-year-old pregnant woman in whom MRI was performed because of abnormal finding at ultrasound. She had a history of a cesarean section for the previous pregnancy, at which time a leiomyoma of the right broad ligament was reported.

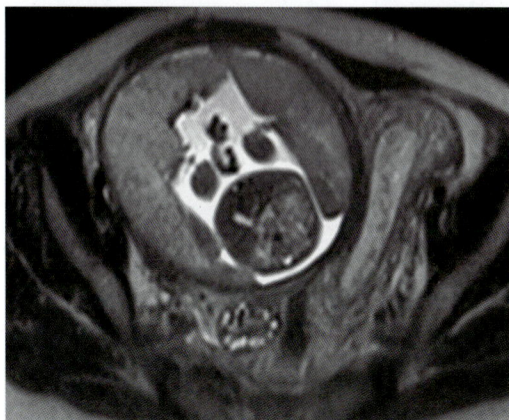

A

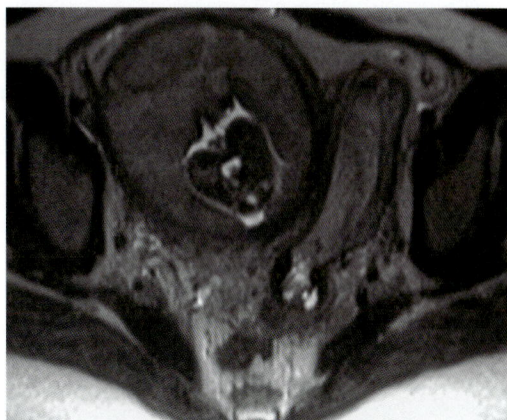

B

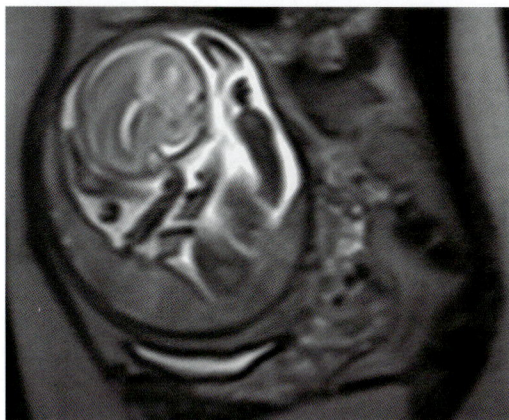

C

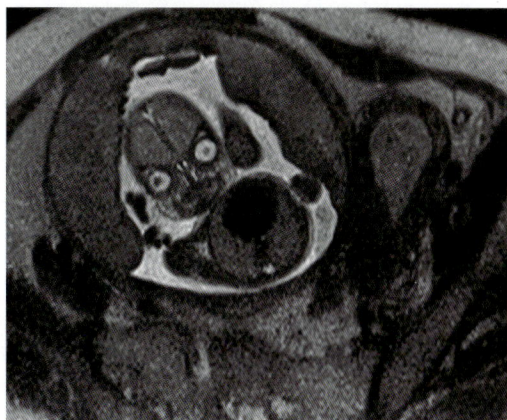

D

A, B. Axial T2-weighted single-shot FSE/TSE obtained at different levels. **C**. Sagittal and (**D**) axial T2-weighted single-shot FSE/TSE.

Case 79 Unicornuate Uterus with Cornual Ectopic Pregnancy

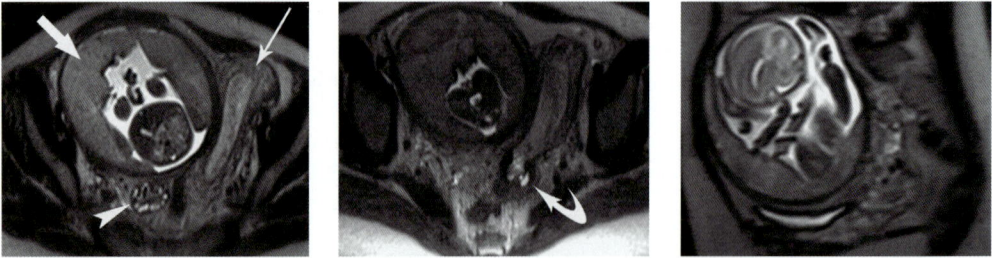

E   F   G

Findings

▶ The left-sided uterus (*skinny arrow* in **E**) is non-gravid with a thickened endometrium representing decidual reaction. The left-sided uterus has a normal cervix (*curved arrow* in **F**).

▶ The separate right-sided uterus (*fat arrow* in **E**) contains a 20-week gestation with a living fetus. No cervix is present on the right (**G**).

▶ The normal right ovary (*arrowhead* in **E**) lies between the two uterine horns.

▶ The mother has two normal kidneys (not shown).

▶ Diagnosis was corneal ectopic pregnancy in a non-communicating rudimentary cavitary horn of a unicornuate uterus.

Differential diagnosis

▶ Bicornuate uterus is excluded because there is no communication with the uterine cavity.

▶ Uterus didelphys is excluded because there is absence of the cervix.

Teaching points

▶ Unicornuate uterus may be simple or have a rudimentary horn on the contralateral side with or without connection to the uterine cavity. It may or may not contain functioning endometrium.

▶ A pregnancy in the rudimentary horn that does not communicate with the uterine cavity results from intraperitoneal migration of sperm.

▶ An interstitial ectopic pregnancy refers to a pregnancy implanted in the interstitial segment of the fallopian tube that lies in the muscular wall of the uterus.

▶ A cornual ectopic pregnancy specifically refers to a pregnancy implanted in the interstitial portion of a unicornuate or bicornuate uterus.

▶ Rupture of a cornual or interstitial ectopic pregnancy often results in catastrophic hemorrhage.

▶ A rudimentary horn may be located remotely from the unicornuate uterus as a result of segmental incomplete arrest of one of the Müllerian ducts.

Management

▶ Because of high risk of rupture with massive hemorrhage, emergency surgery is indicated for a corneal ectopic pregnancy.

Further reading

1. DeAngelis GA. Gynecologic MR. In: Brant WE, de Lange EE. Essentials of Body MR Imaging. New York: Oxford University Press, 2012.
2. Falcone T, Gidwani G, Paraiso M, et al. Anatomical variation in the rudimentary horns of a unicornuate uterus: implications for laparoscopic surgery. Hum Reprod 1997;12:263–265.
3. Goel P, Aggarwal A, Devi K, et al. Unicornuate uterus with non-communicating rudimentary horn—different clinical presentations. J Obstet Gynecol India 2005;55:155–158.

History

▶ 50-year-old woman with history of lung cancer for follow-up

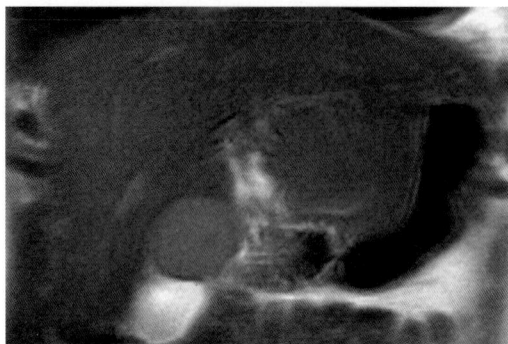

A

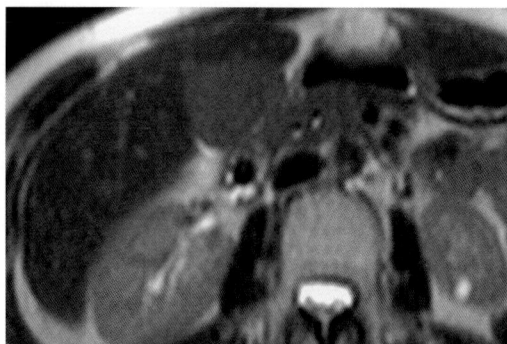

B

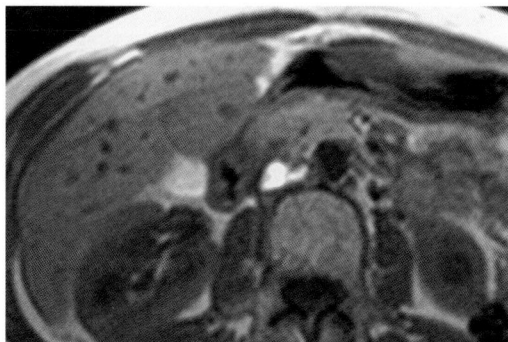

C

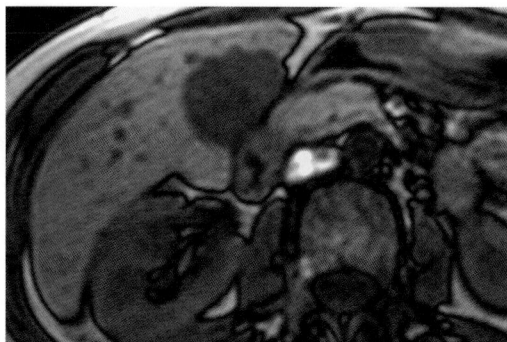

D

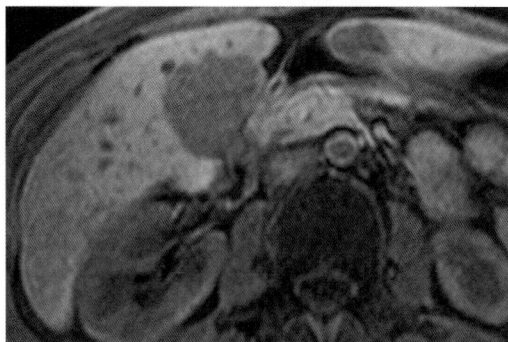

E

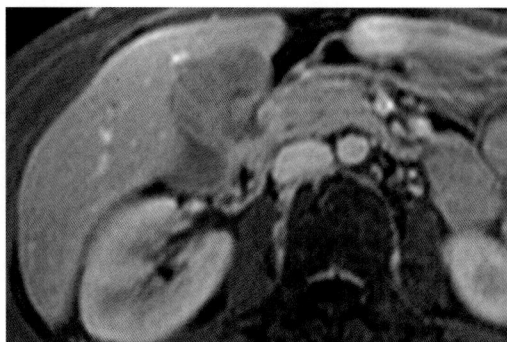

F

A. Coronal and (**B**) axial T2-weighted single-shot FSE/TSE. **C**. Axial in-phase and (**D**) opposed-phase gradient echo. **E**. Axial pre-contrast-enhanced and (**F**) post-gadolinium contrast-enhanced gradient echo with fat saturation.

Case 80 Hepatic Adenoma Containing Intracellular Fat

Findings

- A mass arises exophytically from the inferior aspect of segment 4B of the liver.
- The mass is slightly higher in signal intensity than the liver on T2-weighted images, and is slightly lower in signal intensity than the liver on T1-weighted images.
- The lesion decreases in signal intensity on the out-of-phase images compared with the in-phase images, indicating the presence of intracellular fat within the lesion.
- Enhancement of the lesion is evident on the post-contrast-enhanced sequences; however, the lesion enhances less than the adjacent liver parenchyma.

Differential diagnosis

- Hepatocellular carcinoma
- Hemangioma
- Focal nodular hyperplasia

Teaching points

- Hepatic adenomas are typically found in young women taking oral contraceptives.
- Adenomas tend to be heterogenous in appearance caused by areas of fat and necrosis.
- On T1-weighted images, adenomas can demonstrate increased signal intensity due to fat and recent hemorrhage, or decreased signal due to necrosis, old hemorrhage, or calcification.
- On T2-weighted images, adenomas are heterogenous and predominately hyperintense.
- Many demonstrate signal dropout on out-of-phase imaging due to the presence of intracellular fat. Other hepatic lesions that may contain intracellular fat include hepatocellular carcinoma and focal fatty infiltration.
- Gadolinium contrast-enhanced imaging demonstrates early arterial enhancement due to the presence of capsular feeding vessels.

Management

- Risk of hemorrhage or malignant transformation remains the primary clinical concern.
- Surgical resection if morbidity/mortality is low, versus medical management with cessation of hormone therapy, serial radiological examination, and screening by determining alpha-fetoprotein levels

Further reading

1. Buell JF, Tranchart H, Cannon R, Dagher I. Management of benign hepatic tumors. Surg Clin North Am 2010;90:719–735.
2. Grazioli L, Federle, MP, Brancatelli G, et al. Hepatic adenomas: imaging and pathologic findings. RadioGraphics 2001;21:877–892.
3. Prasad SR, Wang H, Rosas H, et al. Fat-containing lesions of the liver: radiologic-pathologic correlation. RadioGraphics 2005;25:321–331.

History

▶ 60-year-old man with lung cancer undergoing staging workup.

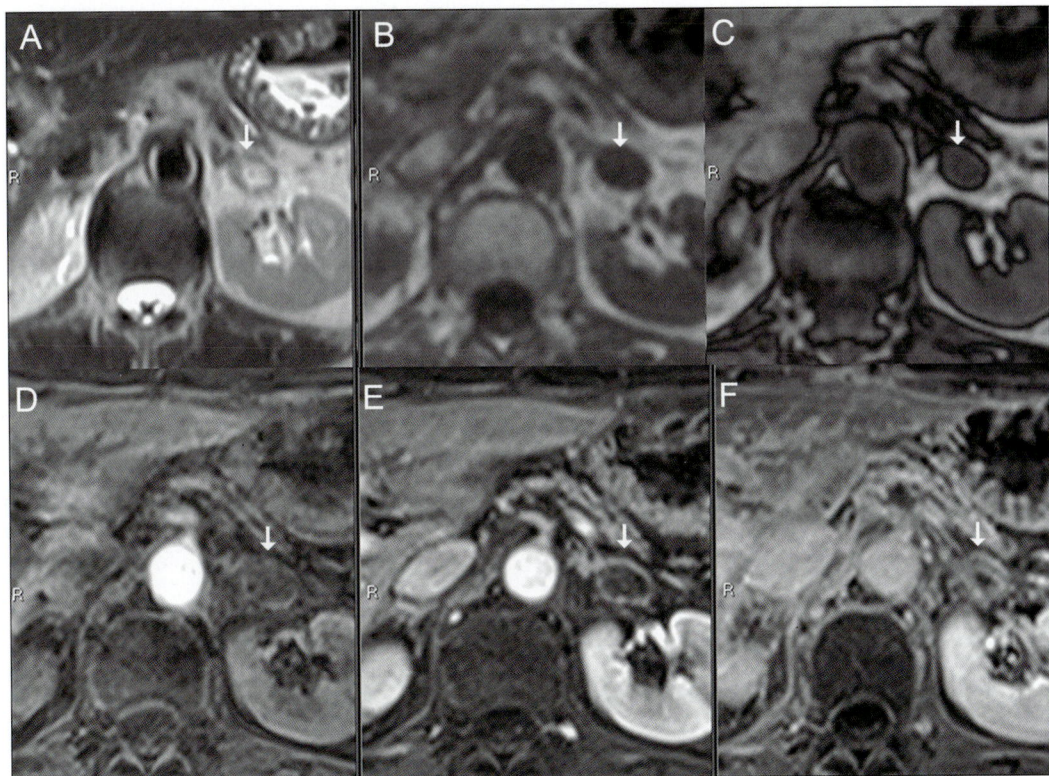

A. Axial T2-weighted single-shot FSE/TSE. **B**. Axial in-phase and (**C**) opposed-phase T1-weighted gradient echo. **D**. Pre-, (**E**) early, and (**F**) delayed axial gadolinium contrast-enhanced T1-weighted gradient echo with fat saturation.

Case 81   Adrenal Metastasis from Lung Carcinoma

Findings

- Left adrenal mass (*arrows*) with central necrosis
- High signal intensity within the mass on T2-weighted image (**A**) is consistent with central fluid.
- The lesion does not decrease in signal intensity on opposed-phase image (**C**) compared with in-phase image (**B**).
- The lesion does not contain macroscopic fat (adipose tissue) as it does not show signal intensity similar to that of the surrounding retroperitoneal fat (**B** and **C**).
- Following gadolinium-based contrast material administration, the central necrotic areas do not enhance (**E** and **F**).

Differential diagnosis

- Atypical or lipid-poor adrenal adenoma
- Pheochromocytoma
- Adrenal cyst or pseudocyst
- Rare entities (ganglioneuroma)
- Adrenal cortical carcinoma

Teaching points

- A specific diagnosis cannot be ascertained in this case, but findings are highly suspicious for necrotic metastasis in a patient with a known primary malignancy.
- Metastasis is the most common malignancy involving the adrenal gland.
- Adrenal metastases are most commonly bilateral but may be unilateral.
- Adrenal metastases most commonly display low signal intensity on T1-weighted images and intermediate high signal intensity on T2-weighted images.
- Enhancement of a metastasis is typically progressive following contrast material administration.
- Metastases do not contain microscopic fat causing signal dropout on opposed-phase images.

Management

- If with MRI a definitive diagnosis cannot be made, a possible metastatic deposit in an adrenal gland needs to be biopsied for definitive diagnosis and accurate staging of the patient's disease.

Further reading

1. Boland GW, Blake MA, Hahn PF, Mayo-Smith WW. Incidental adrenal lesions: principles, techniques, and algorithms for imaging characterization. Radiology 2008;249:756–775.
2. Elsayes KM, Mukundan G, Narra VR, et al. Adrenal masses: MR imaging features with pathologic correlation. RadioGraphics 2004;24:S73–S86.
3. Lam KY, Lo CY. Metastatic tumours of the adrenal glands: a 30-year experience in a teaching hospital. Clin Endocrinol (Oxf) 2002;56:95–101.
4. McNicholas MM, Lee MJ, Mayo-Smith WW, Hahn PF, Boland GW, Mueller PR. An imaging algorithm for the differential diagnosis of adrenal adenomas and metastases. AJR Am J Roentgenol 1995;165:1453–1459.

History

▶ 45-year-old woman with biopsy-proven hepatic sarcoidosis with resultant cirrhosis. MR obtained for pre-liver transplantation evaluation.

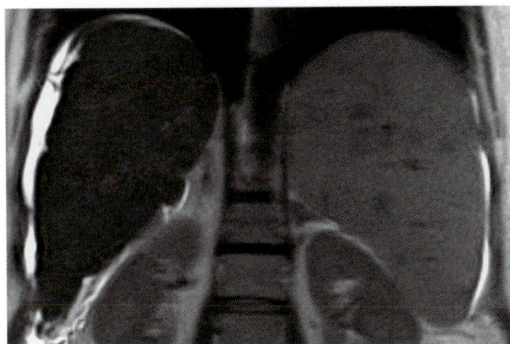

A

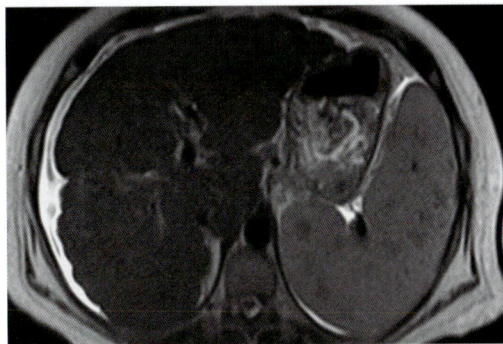

B

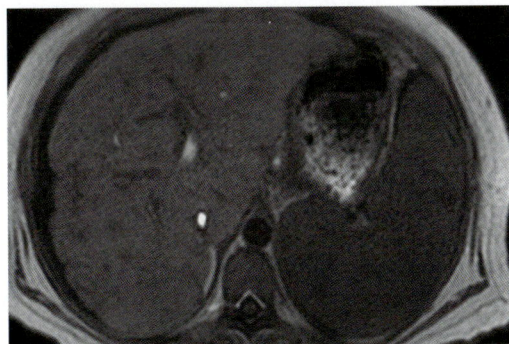

C

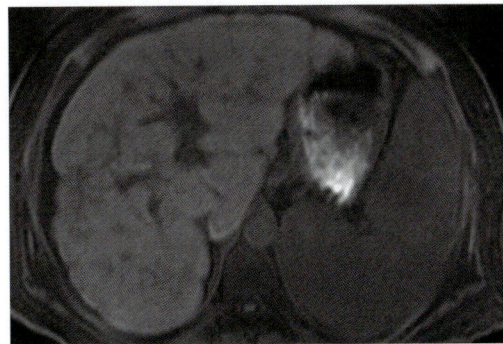

D

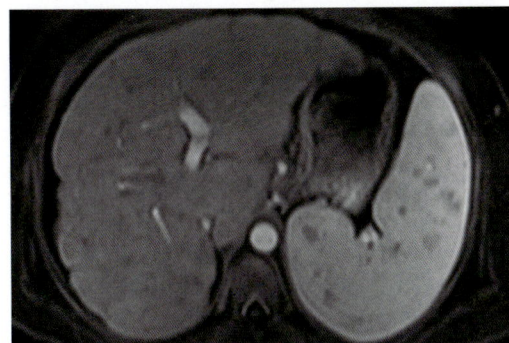

E

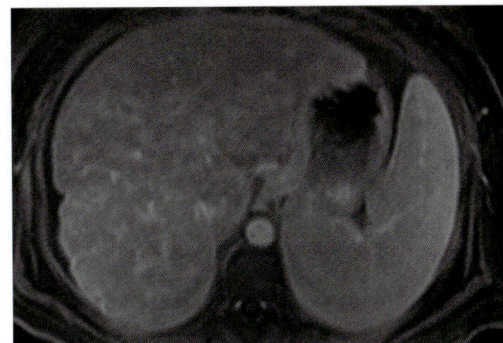

F

A. Coronal and (**B**) axial T2-weighted single-shot FSE/TSE. **C**. Axial in-phase T1-weighted gradient echo. **D**. Axial pre-, (**E**) early, and (**F**) delayed contrast-enhanced T1-weighted gradient echo with fat saturation.

Case 82   Sarcoidosis of the Spleen

Findings

- ▶ The liver is nodular in contour consistent with cirrhosis. Ascites is present.
- ▶ The spleen is enlarged and contains multiple ill-defined nodules.
- ▶ The nodules in the spleen display low signal intensity on both T1- and T2-weighted images.
- ▶ The nodules are best seen on the relatively early post-contrast-enhanced T1-weighted images and show late contrast enhancement, becoming isointense with the splenic parenchyma on delayed contrast-enhanced images.
- ▶ Liver biopsy had shown diffuse infiltration by sarcoidosis. MR shows findings of cirrhosis but no focal hepatic lesions to suggest sarcoidosis.

Differential diagnosis

- ▶ Splenic lymphoma may also appear as multiple low-signal-intensity nodules with little to no contrast enhancement.
- ▶ Metastases to the spleen usually display high signal intensity on T2-weighted images. The nodules show variable enhancement dependent upon the nature of the primary neoplasm.
- ▶ Extramedullary hematopoiesis may present as multiple masslike nodules showing intermediate signal intensity on T1-weighted images and high signal intensity on T2-weighted images. Lesion enhancement is minimal.
- ▶ Multiple splenic abscesses show low signal intensity on T1-weighted and high signal intensity on T2-weighted images. Peripheral enhancement is characteristic.

Teaching points

- ▶ The noncaseous granulomas of sarcoidosis demonstrate low signal intensity on all MR sequences. The lesions are most easily seen on early-phase post-contrast-enhanced T1-weighted images or on T2-weighted fat-suppressed sequences. Enhancement following intravenous gadolinium-based contrast material administration is minimal and is delayed, as shown in this case.

Management

- ▶ Sarcoidosis involving the liver or spleen has no specific treatment. Prednisone is most commonly used. Ursodiol (ursodeoxycholic acid) may be of some benefit.

Further reading

1. Elasyes KM, Narra VR, Mukundan G, et al. MR imaging of the spleen: spectrum of abnormalities. RadioGraphics 2005;25:967–982.
2. Koyama T, Ueda H, Togashi K, et al. Radiologic manifestations of sarcoidosis in various organs. RadioGraphics 2004;24:87–104.

Case 83

History

▶ 38-year-old woman with abdominal pain

A

A. Coronal reconstructed maximum intensity projection MRCP image generated from respiratory gated 3D FSE/TSE

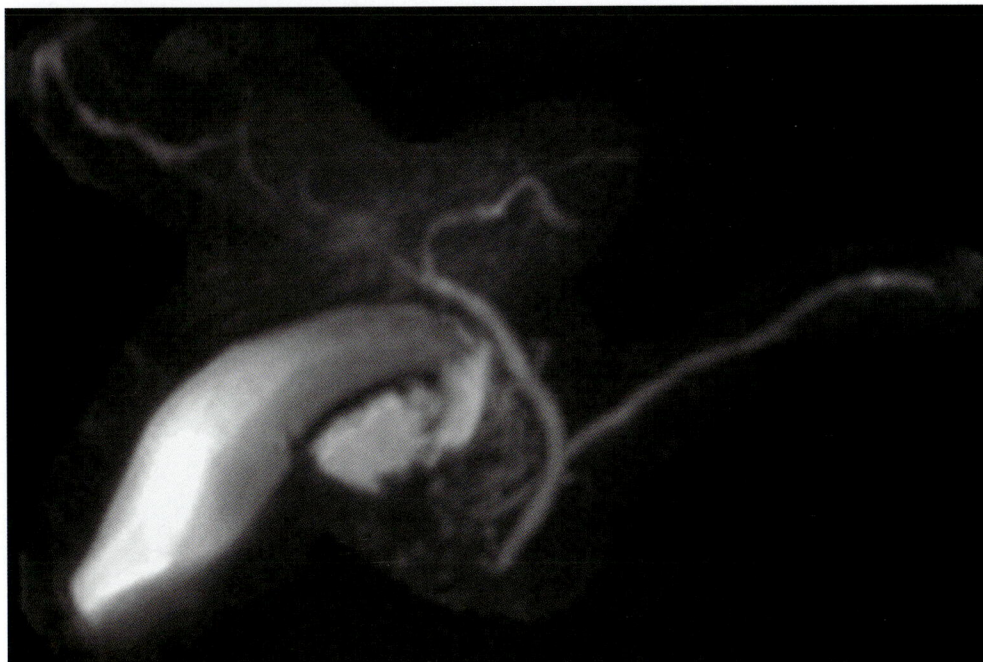

Case 83 Pancreas Divisum

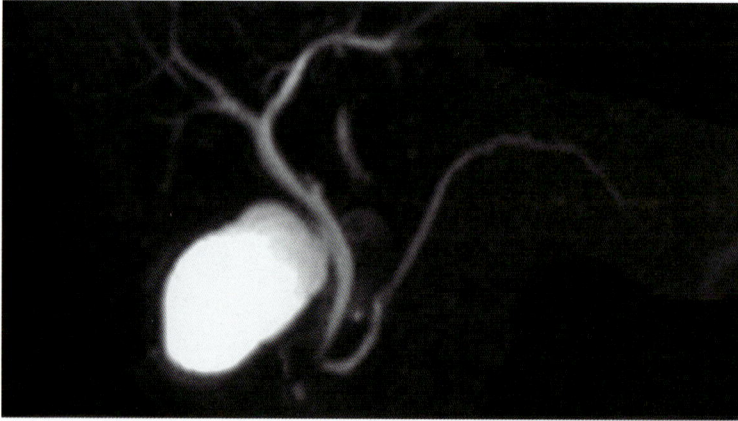

B

Findings

▶ MRCP shows main pancreatic duct entering the minor papilla in the duodenum without joining with common bile duct. Point of entry is cephalad and anterior to major papilla.
▶ Compare this to the finding in **B** obtained in a different individual showing the normal insertion of the pancreatic duct at the major papilla along with the common bile duct.

Differential diagnosis

▶ Agenesis of the dorsal pancreas

Teaching points

▶ Pancreas divisum is the most common congenital pancreatic ductal anatomic variant, found in approximately 4% to 14% of the population at autopsy, 3% to 8% at ERCP, and 9% at MRCP.
▶ The abnormality results from failure of the dorsal and ventral pancreatic anlage to fuse during the sixth to eighth weeks of gestation. In pancreatic divisum, no communication exists between the dorsal and ventral pancreatic ducts, and most pancreatic secretions drain through the minor ampulla.
▶ In some patients, the ventral pancreatic duct may be absent.
▶ Pancreas divisum is usually asymptomatic but is more frequently seen in patients with chronic abdominal pain and idiopathic pancreatitis than in the general population. Approximately 20% of patients with pancreas divisum develop chronic pancreatitis.

Management

▶ In asymptomatic patients, no specific treatment is needed.
▶ Symptomatic patients are treated both medically and surgically. The medical management includes conservative measures or pancreatic enzyme therapy. Patients not responding to medical management may undergo surgical or endoscopic correction, which includes sphincteroplasty of minor papilla.

Further reading

1. Jinxing Y, Turner MA, Fulcher AS, Halvorsen RA. Congenital anomalies and normal variants of the pancreaticobiliary tract and the pancreas in adults: Part 2, pancreatic duct and pancreas. AJR Am J Roentgenol 2006;187:1544–1553.

History

▶ 40-year-old woman with heavy menses, postcoital bleeding and cramping lower pelvic pain

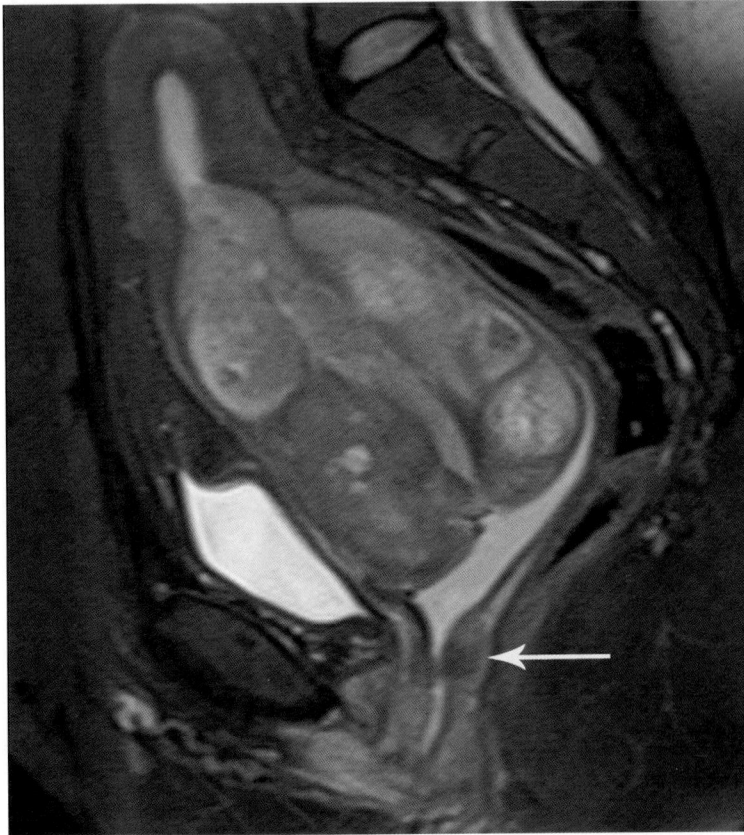

A

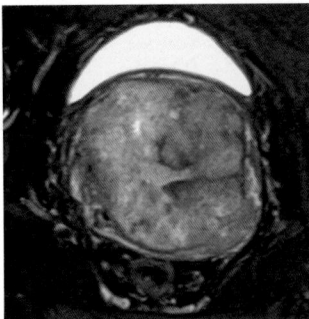

B

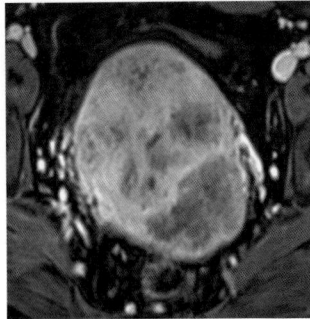

C

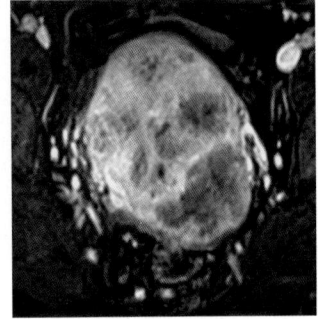

D

A. Sagittal T2-weighted FSE/TSE with fat saturation. **B**. Axial T2-weighted FSE/TSE with fat saturation. **C**. Axial contrast-enhanced T1-weighted gradient echo with fat saturation. **D**. Subtraction image obtained by subtracting the pre-contrast enhanced image from **C**.

Case 84 Undifferentiated Sarcoma of the Cervix with Metastasis to the Posterior Vaginal Wall

Findings

- ▶ Large multilobulated enhancing mass completely replaces the cervical stroma.
- ▶ Poor definition of its peripheral margins suggests parametrial invasion.
- ▶ Its epicenter is mid-cervical, indicating that the tumor origin is in the cervix with extension to the lower uterine segment.
- ▶ No demonstrable invasion of the rectum or bladder
- ▶ Oval nodule (*arrow*) in the posterior wall of the vagina

Differential diagnosis

- ▶ Cervical carcinoma
- ▶ Multiple cervical leiomyoma

Teaching points

- ▶ Primary cervical sarcomas are rare; they constitute less than 1% of all cervical malignancies. Histological subtypes include rhabdomyosarcoma, leiomyosarcoma, liposarcoma, alveolar soft part sarcoma, Ewing sarcoma/primitive neuroectodermal tumor, undifferentiated endocervical sarcoma, and malignant peripheral nerve sheath tumor (MPNST).
- ▶ These neoplasms have an aggressive course and inferior prognosis compared to squamous cell carcinomas and adenocarcinomas matched by stage.
- ▶ Tumors and tumor-like lesions of the cervix may have similar MRI features and it is therefore difficult to make a histological diagnosis based on the imaging findings alone.

Further reading

1. Basal S, Lewin SN, Burke WM, et al. Sarcoma of the cervix: Natural history and outcomes. Gynecol Oncol 2010;118:134–138.
2. Fadare O. Uncommon sarcomas of the uterine cervix: a review of selected entities. Diagn Pathol 2006;18:1–30.
3. Okamoto Y, Tanaka YO, Nishida M, et al. MR imaging of the uterine cervix: imaging–pathologic correlation. RadioGraphics 2003;23:425–445.
4. Sala E, Wakely S, Senior E, Lomas D. MRI of Malignant neoplasms of the uterine corpus and cervix. AJR Am J Roentgenol 2007;188:1577–1587.

History

▶ 63-year-old woman with a history of radiation therapy and abdominoperineal resection of the rectum and sigmoid colon for colon carcinoma presents with increasing pelvic pain.

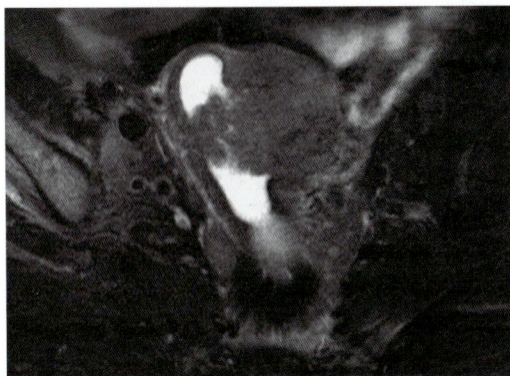
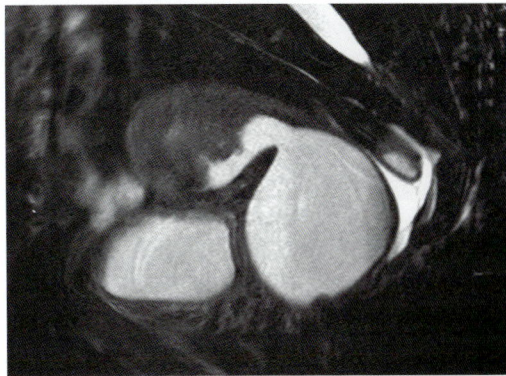

A   B

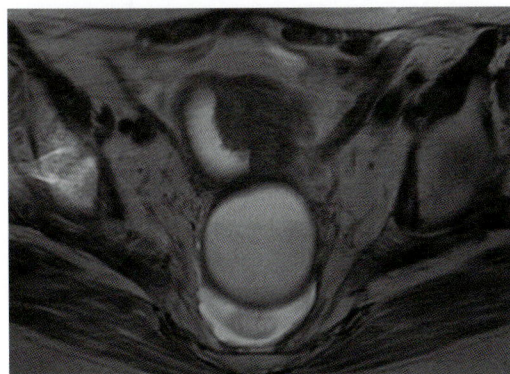
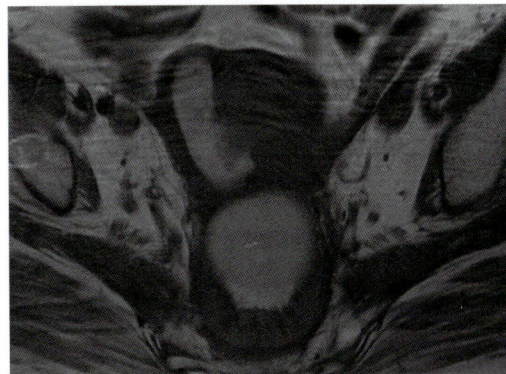

C   D

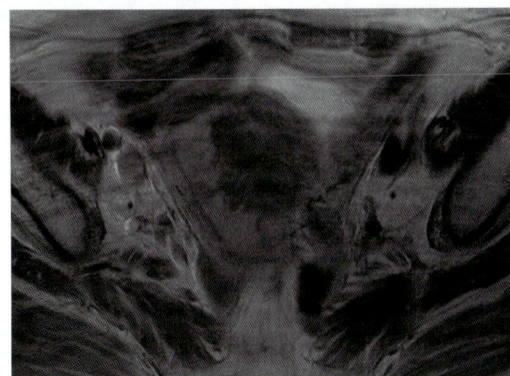
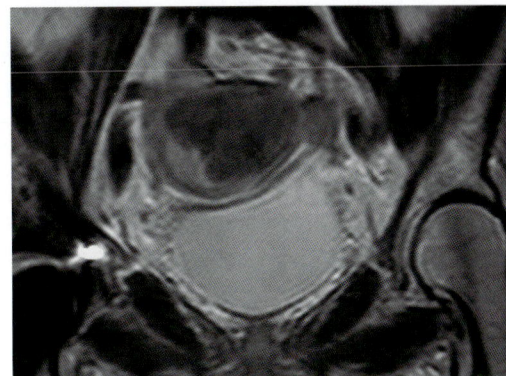

E   F

A. Axial and (**B**) sagittal T2-weighted FSE/TSE with fat saturation. **C**. Axial T2-weighted FSE/TSE without fat saturation. **D**. Axial T1-weighted spin echo without contrast enhancement. **E**. Axial and (**F**) coronal T1-weighted spin echo with gadolinium contrast enhancement.

Case 85 Endometrial Adenocarcinoma

Findings

▶ A large lobulated mass extends from the left fundus of the uterus into the uterine canal. The mass extends nearly through the myometrium.

▶ The uterine canal and the vagina are distended with fluid that shows with high signal intensity on both T1- and T2-weighted images. Findings are consistent with blood (i.e., hematometra and hematocolpos).

▶ The tumor invaded the myometrium to 19 mm of the 20-mm thickness of the myometrial wall. The vagina and uterine cavity were filled with bloody fluid. Hematocolpos was caused by adhesions near the introitus that were thought to be secondary to previous radiation therapy.

Differential diagnosis

▶ Endometrial polyp

▶ leiomyoma

▶ adenomyosis

Teaching points

▶ Transvaginal ultrasound generally provides first-line assessment of the endometrium in patients with postmenopausal bleeding. Endometrial biopsy then confirms the diagnosis of endometrial cancer.

▶ Surgical staging is generally considered necessary and may preclude imaging staging unless the patient is not a surgical candidate due to advanced disease or comorbidities that increase the risk of surgery. MRI is considered by most to be the imaging staging modality of choice.

▶ Determination of myometrial invasion of endometrial carcinoma greater than or less than 50% of the thickness of the myometrium differentiates between stage T1a and T1b. The reported sensitivity, specificity, and accuracy for determining depth of myometrial invasion by MRI are approximately 70%, 85%, and 58% respectively.

▶ Determination of involvement of the cervix by the endometrial tumor differentiates between state T1 and stage T2. The reported sensitivity, specificity, and accuracy of MRI staging of endometrial carcinoma invasion of the cervix are approximately 40%, 97%, and 45% respectively.

▶ Pitfalls in MR tumor staging are related to the tumor being isointense with the myometrium, tumors that are polypoid, abnormal thinning or irregularity of the myometrium, or the presence of adenomyosis or leiomyomas.

Management

▶ Accurate tumor staging assists in the planning of optimal therapy.

Further reading

1 Sanjuan A, Escaramis G, Ayuso JR, et al. Role of magnetic resonance imaging and cause of pitfalls in detecting myometrial invasion and cervical involvement in endometrial cancer. Arch Gynecol Obstet 2008;278:535–539.
2. Shin KE, Park BK, Kim CK, et al. MR staging accuracy for endometrial cancer based on the new FIGO stage. Acta Radiol 2011;52:818–824.
3. Viswanathan AN, Buttin BM, Kennedy AM. Ovarian, cervical, and endometrial cancer. RadioGraphics 2008;28:289–307.

History

► 46-year-old woman underwent ultrasound for abdominal pain. A well-defined hyperechoic lesion was seen in segment 4A.

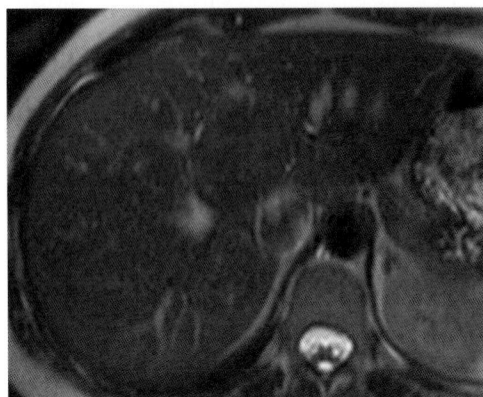

A

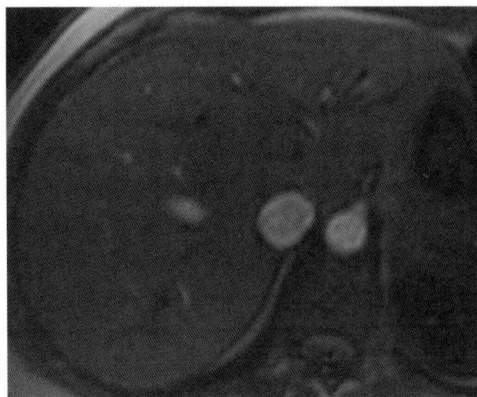

B

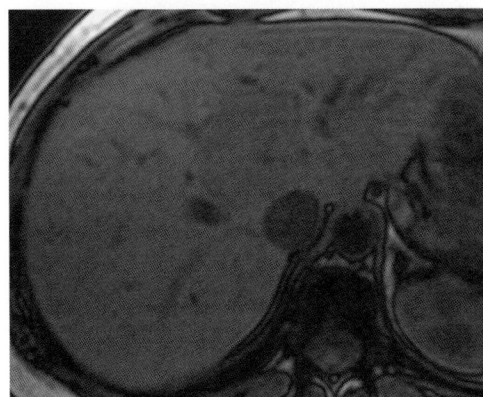

C

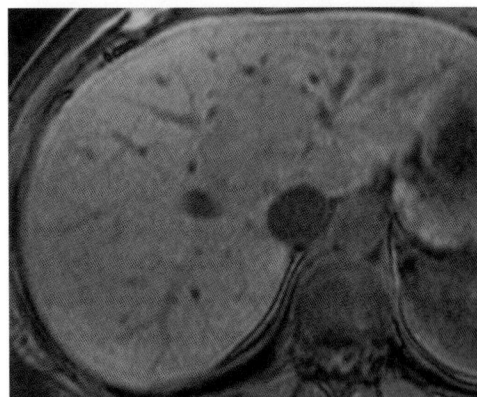

D

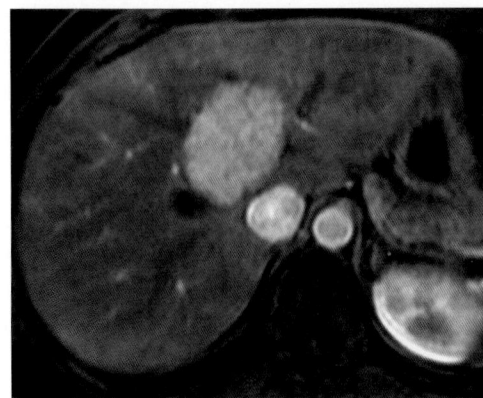

E

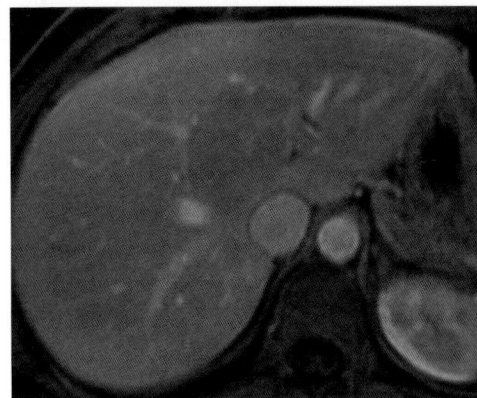

F

A. Axial T2-weighted single-shot FSE/TSE. **B.** Axial magnetization-prepared gradient echo. **C**. Axial T1-weighted opposed-phase gradient echo. **D**. Axial pre-contrast (**E**) early and (**F**) slightly delayed contrast-enhanced T1-weighted gradient echo with fat saturation.

Case 86 Focal Nodular Hyperplasia

Findings

- Mass lesion in segment 4A of the liver shows signal intensity nearly equal to that of liver on T2-weighted and unenhanced T1-weighted sequences.
- Following intravenous gadolinium contrast administration, prominent homogeneous enhancement is evident immediately with rapid washout of contrast agent on the next phase of the dynamic post-contrast sequence.

Differential diagnosis

- Hepatic adenoma
- Cavernous hemangioma
- Hypervascular metastasis
- Fibrolamellar hepatocellular carcinoma

Teaching points

- Focal nodular hyperplasia (FNH) is the second most common benign liver lesion (following hemangioma), with a prevalence of 0.9%.
- FNH occurs much more frequently in women than in men (8:1), and tends to occur in relatively young patients.
- The best diagnostic clues are near iso-intensity on unenhanced T1- and T2-weighted images, marked homogeneous enhancement on arterial phase post-contrast-enhanced images, with delayed enhancement of central scar. Iso-intensity with liver parenchyma on pre-contrast-enhanced sequences is characteristic, representing the components of the lesion that are nearly the same as that of normal liver parenchyma. The lesions are isointense to liver on delayed enhanced images when hepatocyte specific contrast agent is used (not shown).
- In patients with FNH, 20% to 25% will have more than one lesion.
- Some FNHs can have a pseudo-capsule from compression of adjacent hepatic parenchyma. This pseudo-capsule displays high signal intensity on T2-weighted images. The fibrous capsule of hepatocellular carcinoma generally shows low signal intensity on T2-weighted images.

Management

- In asymptomatic patients with classic imaging findings, no treatment or further evaluation is necessary.
- In symptomatic patients, or if the imaging findings are uncertain, biopsy should be considered.
- Oral contraceptives should be discontinued.

Further reading

1. Elsayes KM, Narra VR, Yin Y, et al. Focal hepatic lesions: Diagnostic value of enhancement pattern approach with contrast-enhanced 3D gradient-echo MR imaging. RadioGraphics 2005;25:1299–1320.
2. Hussain SM, Terkivatan T, Zondervan PE, et al. Focal nodular hyperplasia: Findings at state-of-the-art MR imaging, US, CT, and pathologic analysis. RadioGraphics 2004;24:3–17.

History

▶ 6-year-old boy with malignant hypertension

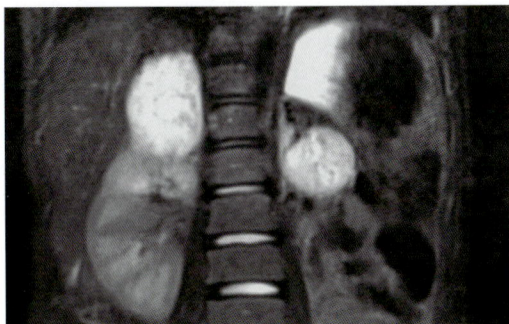
A

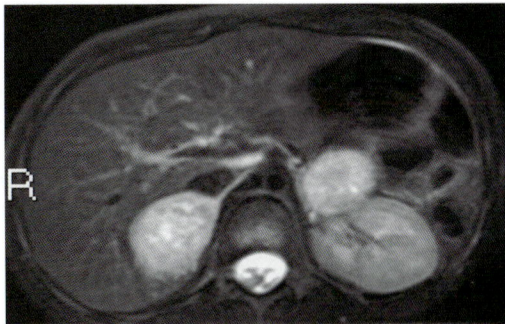
B

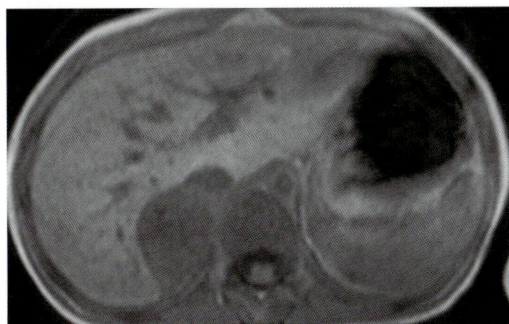
C

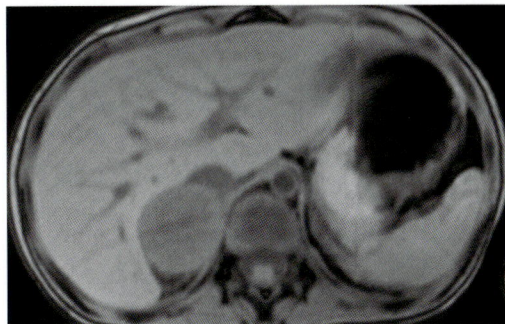
D

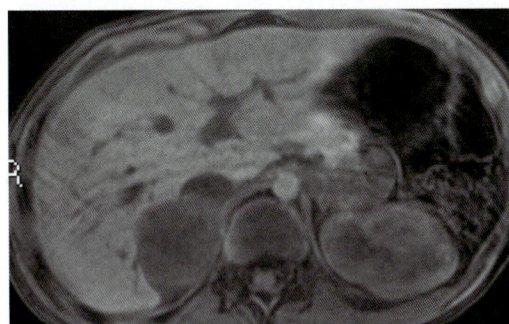
E

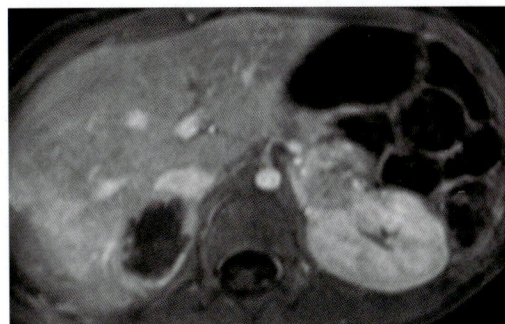
F

A. Coronal T2-weighted inversion-recovery spin echo. **B**. Axial T2-weighted FSE/TSE with fat saturation. **C**. In-phase and (**D**) opposed-phase T1-weighted GRE. **E**. Pre- and (**F**) post-gadolinium contrast-enhanced gradient echo with fat saturation.

Case 87   Bilateral Adrenal Pheochromocytomas in the Setting of Undiagnosed Von Hippel-Lindau (VHL) Disease

Findings

- Bilateral adrenal lesions displaying high signal intensity on T2-weighted inversion-recovery and fat-saturated sequences
- The adrenal lesions do not demonstrate decreased signal intensity on opposed-phase images compared to in-phase images.
- Contrast-enhanced sequences show peripheral enhancement in the right adrenal mass suggestive of a central "outgrowth" of its vascular supply.
- The left adrenal mass enhances heterogeneously in a "salt and pepper" pattern.
- The kidneys are unaffected. There is no lymphadenopathy.

Differential diagnosis

- Adrenal hemorrhage
- Bilateral adrenal adenomas

Teaching points

- Pheochromocytoma has a wide range of prevalence, from 0% in some family groups to 60% in others.
- VHL-associated pheochromocytomas tend to be multiple and ectopic with a low malignant potential compared to sporadic lesions in the general population.
- 50% to 80% of VHL-associated pheochromocytomas are bilateral and 15% to 18% are reported to have ectopic sites.
- Classically, pheochromocytomas manifest as masses displaying high signal intensity on T2-weighted images and low to intermediate signal intensity on T1-weighted images. Additionally, these tumors exemplify marked gadolinium contrast material enhancement with a classic "salt and pepper" appearance secondary to their high vascular nature.
- Patients with VHL disease are highly likely to develop renal cysts (50% to 63% of patients) and eventually renal cell carcinoma (24% to 45%).

Management

- Laparoscopic partial adrenalectomy is often the treatment of choice for bilateral pheochromocytoma.
- A multidisciplinary approach to care of patients with VHL disease is recommended. Periodic imaging screening should include ultrasound of the kidneys after age 10 and MRI of the brain and spine after age 20.

Further reading

1. Leung RS, Biswas SV, Duncan M, Rankin S. Imaging features of von Hippel-Lindau disease. RadioGraphics 2008;28:65–79.

History

▶ 20-year-old Asian man with history of aortic enlargement and aortic insufficiency. The patient had prior aortic valve replacement

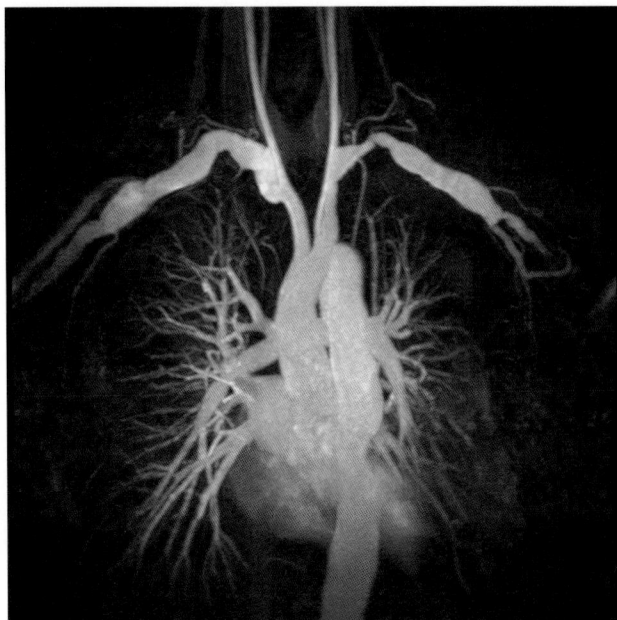

A

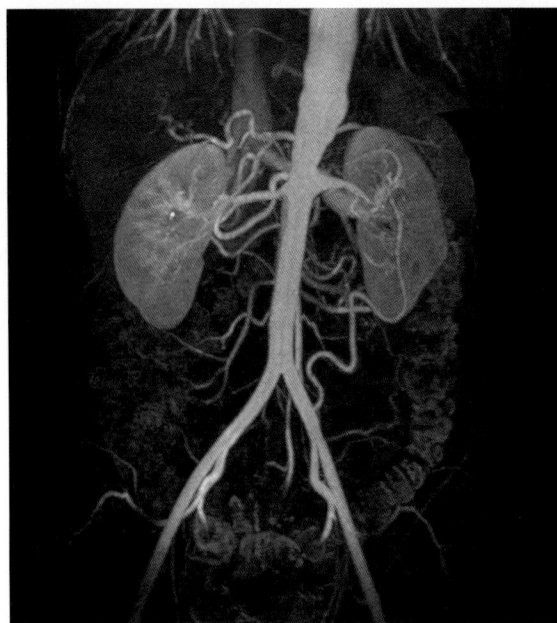

B

A. Coronal maximum intensity projection MRA image of the main vessels of the neck and chest and (**B**) of the abdomen and pelvis. The images were generated from gadolinium-contrast-enhanced 3D gradient echo with fat saturation.

Case 88 Takayasu's Arteritis

Findings

▶ Irregular aneurysmal dilatation of the subclavian arteries
▶ Irregular, undulating dilatation of the descending thoracic and suprarenal abdominal aorta
▶ Normal appearance of the infrarenal aorta and iliac vessels

Differential diagnosis

▶ Giant cell arteritis
▶ Atheromatous disease

Teaching points

▶ Vasculitis affecting the aorta and its branches
▶ Early imaging findings of wall thickening, contrast enhancement, and edema (the latter seen on T2-weighted images)
▶ Late findings include luminal narrowing or occlusion of the aorta (55%) or aortic aneurysm (45%).
▶ Tri-phase disease process: pre-pulseless phase (nonspecific constitutional symptoms), vascular inflammatory phase, late fibrotic stage (stenosis, occlusion, aneurysms)
▶ The clinical presentation due to vascular abnormalities is variable and includes mesenteric angina, claudication, reduced or absent pulses, and hypertension.
▶ Takayasu's arteritis is the most common arteritis to cause mesenteric ischemia.
▶ Rare disease (2.6 cases per 1,000,000 per year), occurs primarily in women (80% to 90%) predominantly from Asian descent, and usually manifests in the second and third decades
▶ Vasculitis of the aorta and main branches in a young person favors Takayasu's arteritis.

Management

▶ High-dose corticosteroid therapy is the mainstay of treatment.
▶ In cases of corticosteroid resistance, cytotoxic agents such as methotrexate, cyclophosphamide, or azathioprine may be required.
▶ Hemodynamically significant stenoses can be treated with percutaneous angioplasty or surgery. Treatment during remission is preferred.

Further reading

1. Nastri MV, Baptista LPS, Baroin RH, et al. Gadolinium-enhanced three-dimensional MR angiography of Takayasu arteritis. RadioGraphics 2004;24:773–786.
2. Restrepo CS, Ocazionez D, Suri R, Vargas D. Aortitis: imaging spectrum of the infectious and inflammatory conditions of the aorta. RadioGraphics 2011;31:435–451.

History

▶ 35-year-old man with symptoms of night sweats, fatigue, and weight loss

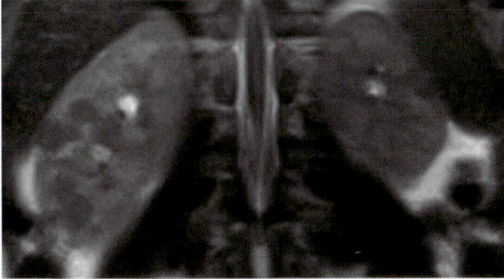
A

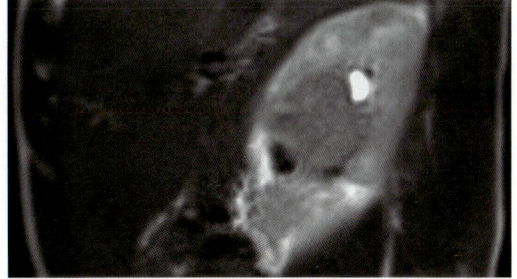
B

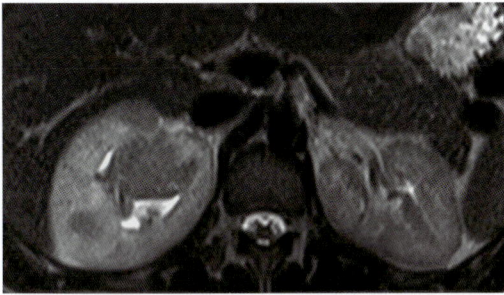
C

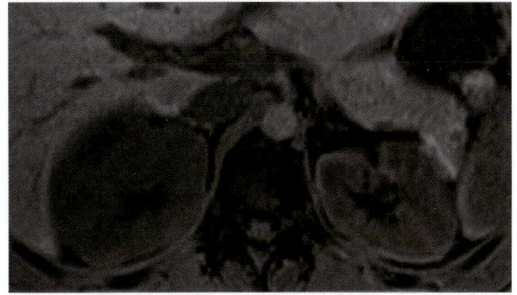
D

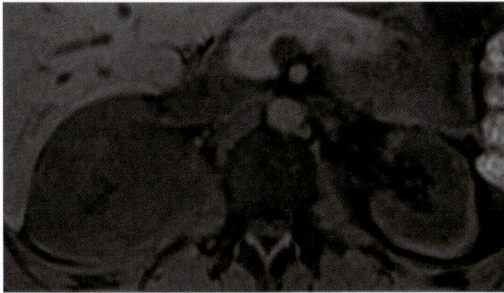
E

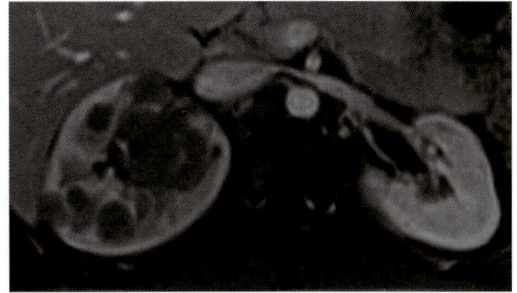
F

A. Coronal, (**B**) sagittal, and (**C**) axial T2-weighted single-shot FSE/TSE. **D** and **E**. Axial pre-contrast-enhanced T1-weighted gradient echo with fat saturation (**E** at slightly lower level than **D**). **F**. Axial post-gadolinium contrast-enhanced T1-weighted gradient echo with fat saturation.

Case 89 Renal Lymphoma (Burkitt Lymphoma)

Findings
- ▶ Multiple nodules of varying size are seen within the parenchyma of both kidneys. The right kidney is more involved than the left.
- ▶ The nodules display low signal intensity on both T1- and T2-weighted images.
- ▶ The nodules show minimal enhancement.

Differential diagnosis
- ▶ Metastases to the kidney
- ▶ Atypical renal infection
- ▶ Multifocal renal cell carcinoma

Teaching points
- ▶ Renal lymphoma occurs most frequently in the presence of widespread non-Hodgkin's B-cell or American Burkitt lymphoma. Hodgkin's lymphoma involves the kidneys in less than 1% of cases. Immuno-compromised patients are at significantly higher risk of developing renal lymphoma.
- ▶ Typical MR findings of renal lymphoma include multiple parenchymal nodules of varying size that are relatively low in signal intensity on T1- and T2-weighted images, and showing poor enhancement. Larger lesions are more heterogeneous.
- ▶ Additional pathologic and imaging patterns of renal lymphoma include:
  - ▪ Solitary mass (10% to 25%), occasionally necrotic or cystic
  - ▪ Direct tumor extension from retroperitoneal lymphadenopathy (25% to 35%)
  - ▪ Perinephric disease with lymphomatous tissue surrounding and compressing the renal parenchyma
  - ▪ Diffuse enlargement of the kidney without distorting the renal contour—most common with Burkitt lymphoma
  - ▪ Renal sinus mass with characteristic minimal hydronephrosis because of the soft nature of lymphomatous tumors

Management
- ▶ Percutaneous biopsy is needed to confirm the diagnosis of lymphoma, unless renal involvement is apparent in the setting of widespread lymphoma to other body areas or organs.

Further reading
1. Sheth S, Ali S, Fishman E. Imaging of renal lymphoma: patterns of disease with pathologic correlation. RadioGraphics 2006;26:1151–1168.
2. Zhang J, Isreal GM, Krinsky GA, Lee VS. Masses and pseudomasses of the kidney: imaging spectrum on MR. J Comput Assist Tomogr 2004;28:588–595.

History

▶ 65-year-old woman with an enlarging pelvic mass and new vaginal bleeding

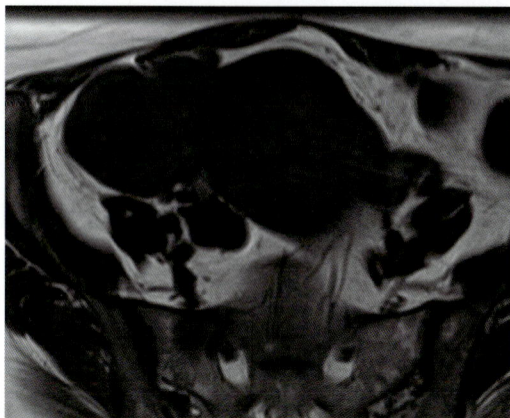

A

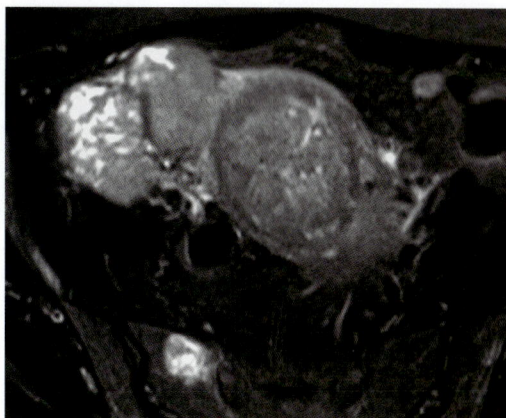

B

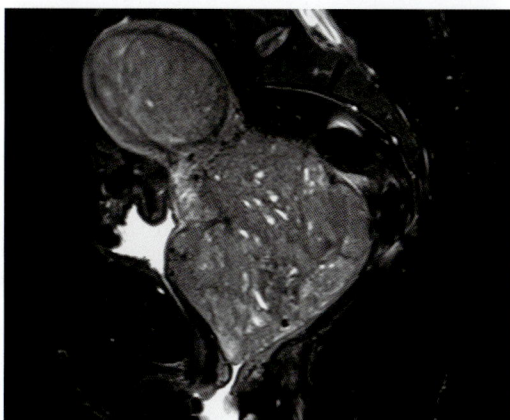

C

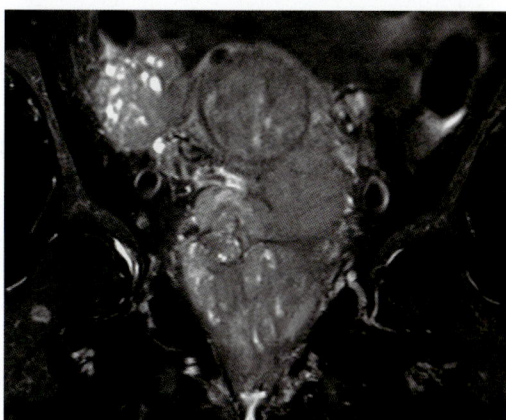

D

A. Axial T1-weighted spin echo. **B**. Axial, (**C**) sagittal, and (**D**) coronal T2-weighted FSE/TSE with fat saturation.

Case 90 Carcinosarcoma of the Uterus (Uterine Malignant Mixed Müllerian Tumor)

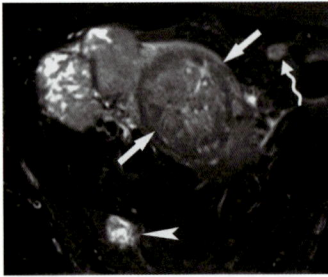

E

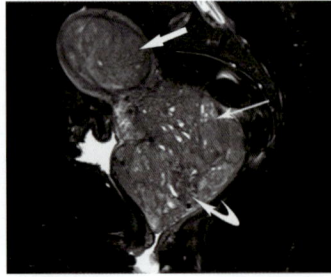

F

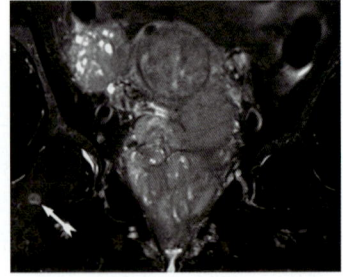

G

Findings

- ▶ The uterus and the mass are indistinguishable from each other on the T1-weighted image.
- ▶ A large solid mass markedly distends the endometrial canal (*fat arrows* in E and F) and cervical canal (*skinny arrow* in F) and extends as an exophytic mass into the upper two thirds of the vagina (*curved arrow* in F).
- ▶ A right sacral metastasis (*arrowhead*, in E), right femoral neck metastasis (*tailed arrow* in G), and peritoneal implant (*squiggly arrow* in E) were present at diagnosis as well as para-aortic lymphadenopathy (not shown).

Differential diagnosis

- ▶ High-grade endometrial malignancy including carcinosarcoma.
- ▶ Papillary serous endometrioid carcinoma.
- ▶ Endometrial stromal sarcoma.

Teaching points

- ▶ High-grade endometrial malignancies are typically large bulky polypoid masses that markedly distend the endometrial cavity, distort the uterus, and often protrude through the external cervical os into the vagina. Hemorrhage and cystic necrosis are common. Extrauterine spread is common at diagnosis.
- ▶ Carcinosarcomas are metaplastic carcinomas with sarcomatous metaplasia that are now classified as high-grade endometrial carcinomas. Prognosis and treatment are similar to those of endometrioid adenocarcinoma.
- ▶ Papillary serous endometrial cancer is likely to have extrauterine spread with superficial or no myometrial invasion. The other high-grade malignancies often deeply invade the myometrium.

Management

- ▶ Early extrauterine spread is common in carcinosarcoma, and therefore imaging plays a greater role in treatment planning than it does for evaluating the lower-grade endometrioid adenocarcinoma.

Further reading

1. Bharwani N, Newland A, Tunariu N, et al. MRI appearance of uterine malignant mixed Müllerian tumors. AJR Am J Roentgenol 2010;195:1268–1275.
2. DeAngelis G. Gynecologic MR imaging. In: Brant WE, de Lange EE (Eds), Essentials of Body MRI. New York: Oxford University Press, 2012.

History

▶ 50-year-old woman presents with progressive abdominal swelling, hematuria, abdominal pain, nausea, and vomiting.

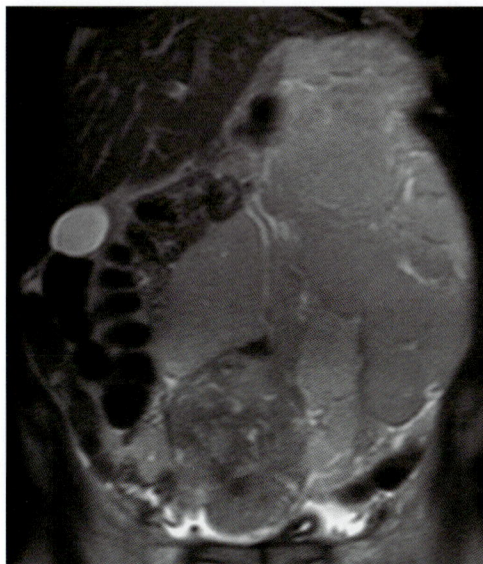

A

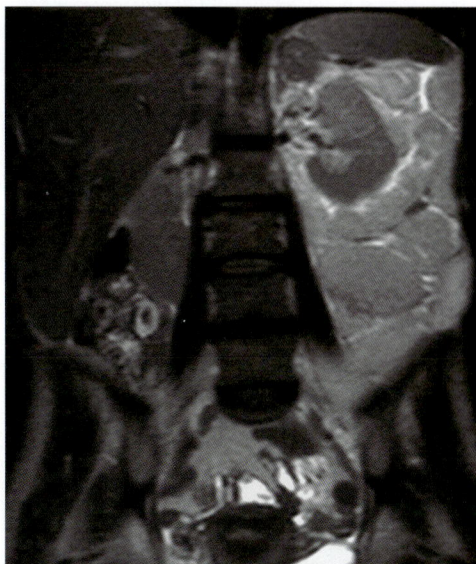

B

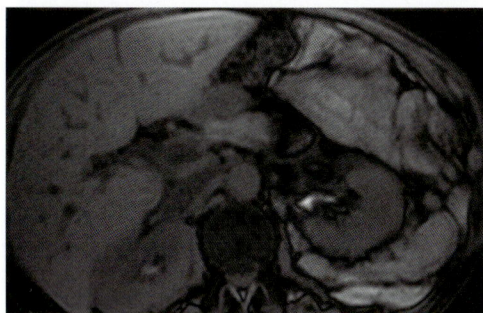

C

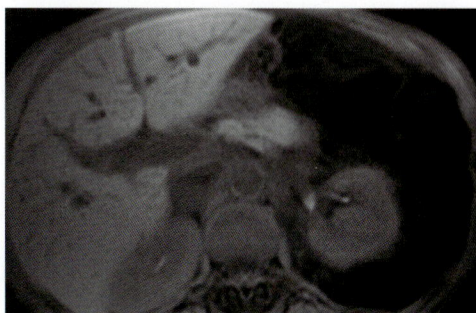

D

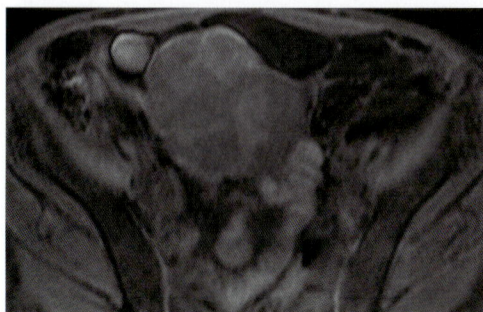

E

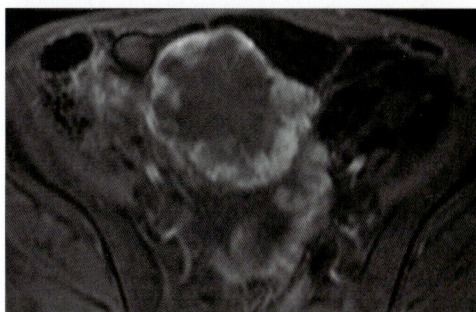

F

A, B. Coronal T2-weighted single-shot FSE/TSE at different levels. **C**. Axial T1-weighted opposed-phase gradient echo. **D**. Axial T1-weighted gradient echo with fat saturation. **E**. Axial pre- and (**F**) post-gadolinium contrast-enhanced T1-weighted gradient echo.

Case 91 Retroperitoneal Sarcoma

Findings

► Large retroperitoneal mass extends from diaphragm to pelvis, crossing the midline. The mass envelops and displaces the left kidney, pancreas, and spleen.
► A large portion of the mass is composed of fatty tissue that demonstrates marked loss of signal intensity on fat-suppressed images.
► A portion of the mass consists of heterogeneous, necrotic tissue that demonstrates contrast enhancement and has no fatty component.
► The mass represented well-differentiated liposarcoma around the left kidney, transverse colon, pancreas, and left adrenal gland, and high-grade non-lipogenic (dedifferentiated) sarcoma in the pelvis.

Differential diagnosis

► Lipoma
► Hibernoma
► Myelolipoma

Teaching points

► Primary retroperitoneal neoplasms arise within the retroperitoneal space but not within any particular organ. Signs that allow identification of a tumor arising in the retroperitoneal space include anterior displacement of the kidneys, adrenal glands, ureters, ascending and descending colon, and other retroperitoneal anatomic structures.
► Liposarcoma is the most common retroperitoneal sarcoma, accounting for 35% of malignant retroperitoneal tumors in adults. Liposarcoma is subclassified into (1) well-differentiated, (2) myxoid/round cell, and (3) pleomorphic types. Dedifferentiated sarcoma is a subgroup of well-differentiated liposarcoma.
► Mature fatty elements of well-differentiated liposarcoma are indistinguishable on imaging from normal fat. Dedifferentiated portions of the tumors are solid lesions that are well demarcated from the fatty components. MR signal and enhancement characteristics of dedifferentiated liposarcoma are variable and nonspecific. Calcification or ossification indicates dedifferentiation and is associated with a poor prognosis.
► Benign lipomas rarely occur in the retroperitoneum. Therefore, fat-containing retroperitoneal tumors should all be considered potentially malignant.

Management

► Surgical resection is indicated for both primary and recurrent retroperitoneal liposarcomas with the goal of complete resection with tumor-free margins.

Further reading

1. Craig WD, Fanburg-Smith JC, Henry LR, et al. Fat-containing lesions of the retroperitoneum: Radiologic-pathologic correlation. RadioGraphics 2009;29:261–290.
2. Nishino M, Hayakawa K, Minami M, et al. Primary retroperitoneal neoplasms: CT and MR imaging findings with anatomic and pathologic diagnostic clues. RadioGraphics 2003;23:45–57.

History

▶ 53-year-old woman with lesion in pancreatic tail

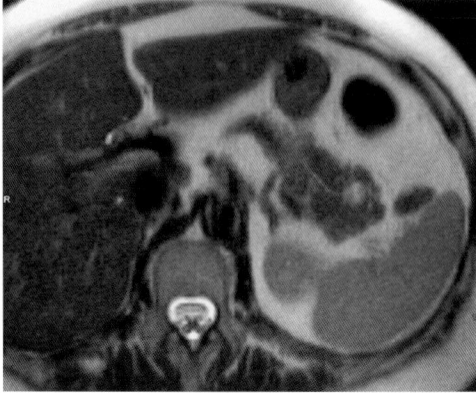

A

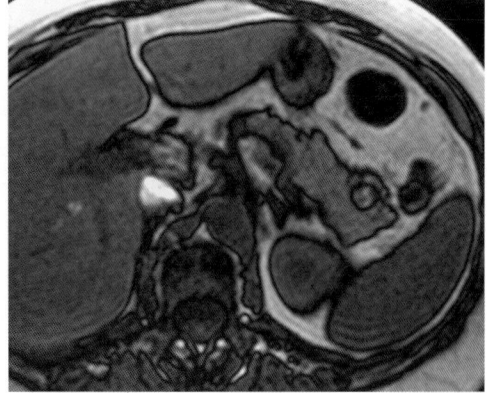

B

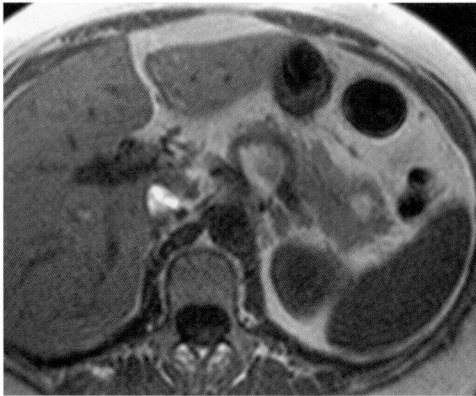

C

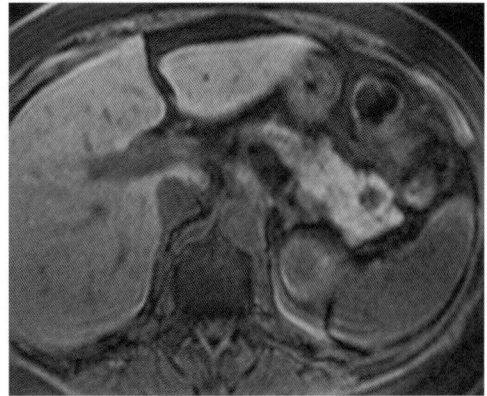

D

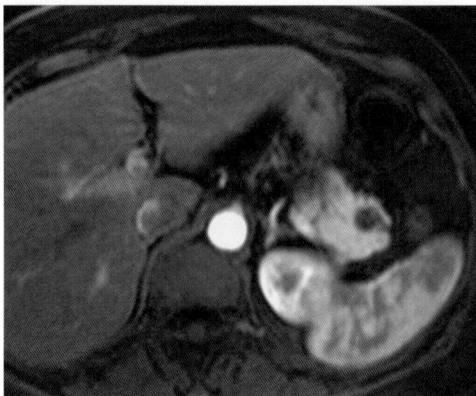

E

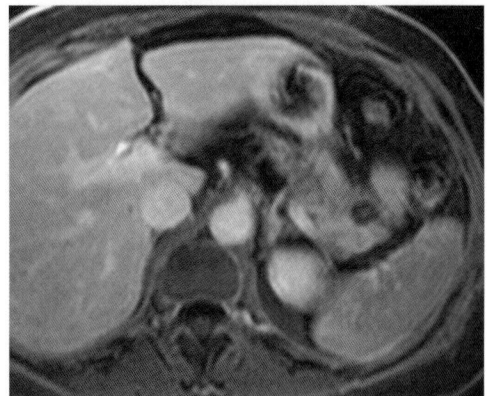

F

A. Axial T2-weighted single-shot FSE/TSE. **B**. Axial opposed-phase and (**C**) in-phase T1-weighted gradient echo. **D**. Axial pre-contrast-enhanced T1-weighted gradient echo. **E**. Axial arterial-phase and (**F**) delayed gadolinium-contrast-enhanced T1-weighted gradient echo.

Case 92 Pancreatic Lipoma

Findings

▶ Well-defined mass in pancreatic tail displaying relatively high signal intensity on non-fat-suppressed T2-weighted (**A**) and T1-weighted images (**B, C**).

▶ The lesion is outlined by a low signal intensity margin on the opposed-phase T1-weighted image (**B**), which is not seen on the in-phase image (**C**).

▶ The lesion displays low signal intensity on the fat-suppressed unenhanced image (**D**), and shows late enhancement of few septa following intravenous administration of gadolinium-based contrast material (**E, F**).

▶ Multiple follow-up imaging studies showed no interval change.

Differential diagnosis

▶ Focal fatty infiltration

▶ Liposarcoma

Teaching points

▶ Pancreatic lipoma is a rare entity with typical findings of a well-defined fat-containing mass that may have few septa.

▶ The fat within the mass consists of adipose (macroscopic) fat. As a result, the signal intensity follows that of adipose fat elsewhere in the body for all pulse sequences and the mass displays low signal intensity on fat-suppressed images.

▶ The low signal intensity at the boundary between the mass and the surrounding normal, water-containing pancreatic parenchyma on the opposed-phase image, in conjunction with the absence of this low-signal-intensity rim on the in-phase image, is diagnostic that the lesion consists of fat.

▶ The low-signal-intensity rim represents an artifact that occurs at the interface between fat and water, and results from the difference in resonant frequency of signal-producing protons in the two tissues. The artifact is caused by cancellation of the fat signal by the water signal because the two signals have opposite (opposed) phases, and occurs in voxels that contain signal from *both* tissues. The low-signal-intensity rim outlining the lesion is not a fibrous capsule; the latter would be visible as a low-intensity structure on both in- and opposed-phase images.

▶ When a mass contains microscopic fat, and hence consists of a mixture of fat and water, such as in a lipid-rich adrenal adenoma or liver adenoma, the entire lesion displays low signal intensity on opposed-phase images from cancellation of the fat and water signals within the lesion. However, if a mass consists largely of adipose fat such as lipoma, the cancellation effect is seen only at the interface between the lesion and the adjacent water-containing tissues.

Further reading

1. de Lange EE, Mugler JP. MR acquisition techniques & practical considerations for abdominal imaging. In: Brant WE, de Lange EE (Eds), Essentials of Body MR Imaging. New York: Oxford University Press, 2012.
2. Temizoz O, Genchellac H, Unlu E, et al. Incidental pancreatic lipomas: Computed tomography imaging findings with emphasis on diagnostic challenges. Can Assoc Radiol J 2010;61:156–161.

History

► 78-year-old woman presents with jaundice.

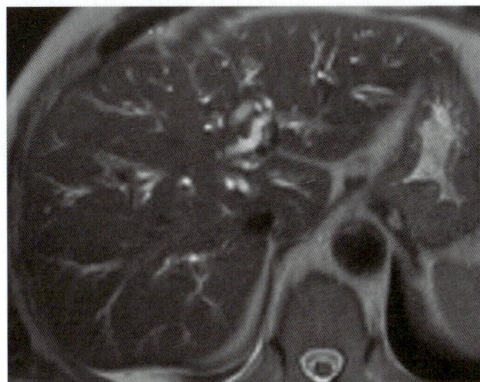

A

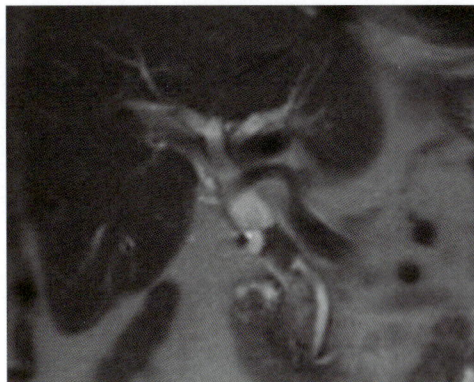

B

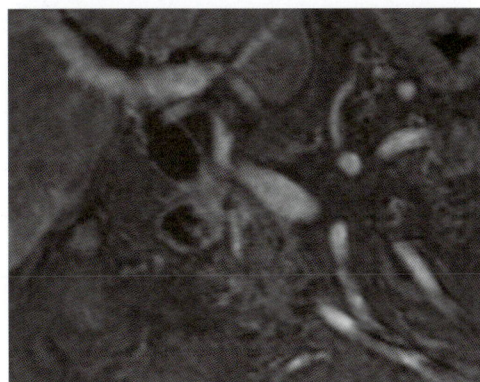

C

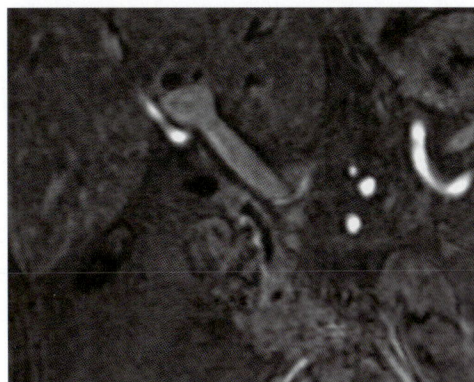

D

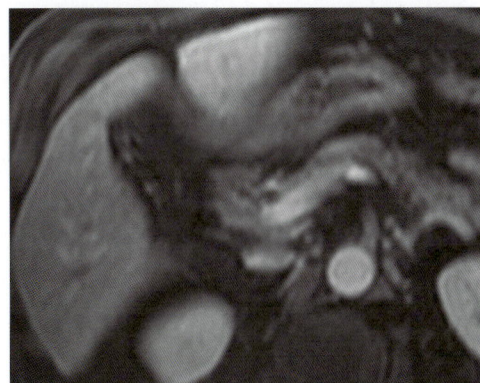

E

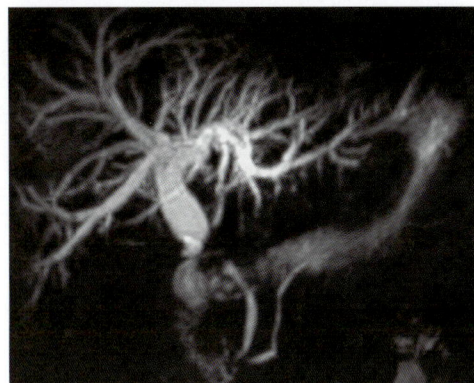

F

A. Axial and (**B**) coronal T2-weighted single-shot FSE/TSE. **C**. Coronal portal venous-phase and (**D**) arterial-phase gadolinium contrast-enhanced T1-weighted gradient echo with fat saturation.(**C** obtained slightly anterior to **D**). **E**. Axial T1-weighted portal venous-phase contrast-enhanced T1-weighted gradient echo with fat saturation. **F**. MRCP (MIP) image generated from respiratory-gated 3D FSE/TSE with fat saturation.

Case 93 Extrahepatic Cholangiocarcinoma Involving the Common Bile Duct

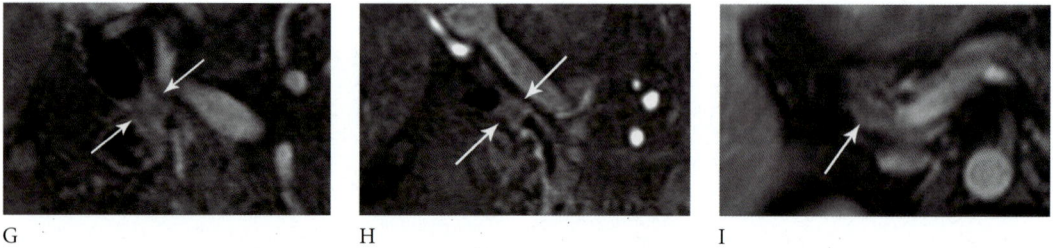

G   H   I

Findings

▶ Diffuse intra- and extrahepatic biliary ductal dilatation
▶ Circumferential wall thickening (*arrows*) with luminal narrowing abruptly terminating the dilated proximal common bile duct (**G, H**)
▶ Tumor enhances (*arrows*) following intravenous gadolinium contrast agent administration (**I**).

Differential diagnosis

▶ Benign stricture
▶ Sclerosing cholangitis
▶ AIDS cholangiopathy

Teaching points

▶ Extrahepatic cholangiocarcinoma may develop in any portion of the extrahepatic bile ducts. Most cases (95%) present with biliary obstruction. Up to 65% of all cholangiocarcinomas are extrahepatic.
▶ The tumors may be mass-forming, producing a small nodule usually 1 to 2 cm in diameter.
▶ Periductal-infiltrating tumors cause circumferential thickening of the wall of the extrahepatic bile duct.
▶ Intraductal tumors spread superficially along the wall of the bile duct or produce a sessile or polypoid tumor nodule within the duct lumen.
▶ Cholangiocarcinoma below the confluence of the left and right hepatic duct is classified as a Bismuth type I tumor and is potentially resectable.

Management

▶ Surgical treatment tailored to the morphology of the tumor

Further reading

1. Chung YE, Kim M-J, Park YN, et al. Varying appearances of cholangiocarcinoma: radiologic pathologic correlation. RadioGraphics 2009;29:683–700.
2. Lim JH. Cholangiocarcinoma: morphologic classification according to growth pattern and imaging findings. AJR Am J Roentgenol 2003;181:819–827.

History

▶ 34-year-old woman complains of pelvic pain. Questionable left adnexal mass was palpated on pelvic examination.

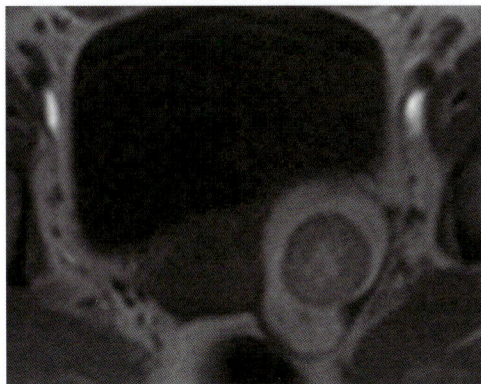

A

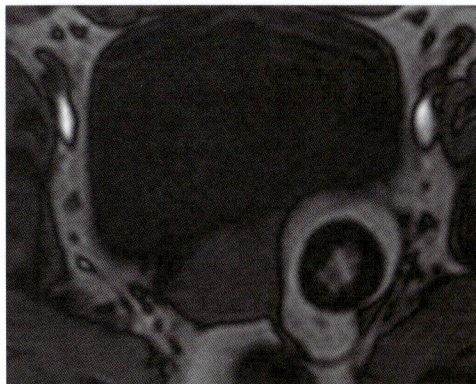

B

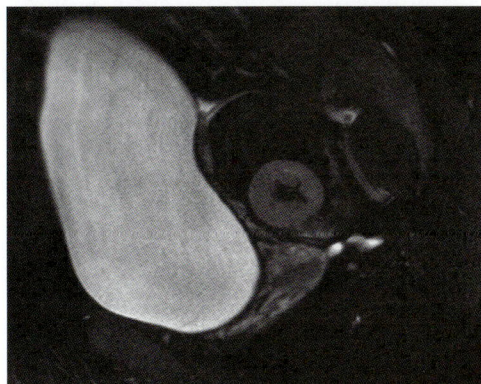

C

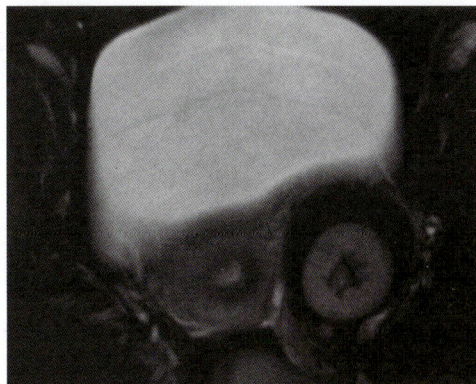

D

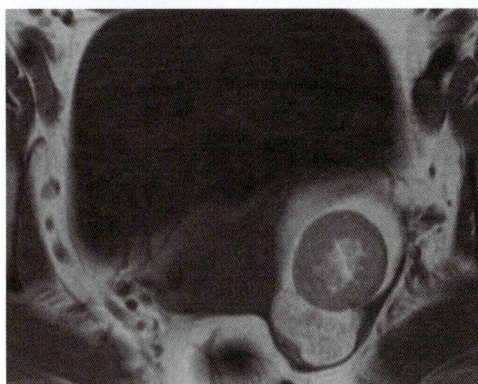

E

A. Axial in-phase and (**B**) opposed-phase T1-weighted gradient echo. **C**. Sagittal and (**D**) axial T2-weighted FSE/TSE with fat saturation. **E**. Axial T1-weighted spin echo.

Case 94 Benign Cystic Teratoma (Mature Teratoma)

Findings

- Complex, predominantly cystic, left adnexal mass with central solid-appearing component
- Cyst fluid shows marked signal decrease on fat-suppressed images.
- Internal solid component shows marked decrease in signal intensity on opposed-phase compared to in-phase images.

Differential diagnosis

- Endometrioma
- Ovarian carcinoma

Teaching points

- Mature cystic teratoma is the most common benign ovarian neoplasm in women less than 45 years of age. This neoplasm accounts for 20% of all ovarian tumors in adults and 50% of ovarian tumors in children. The tumor is composed of well-differentiated components of at least two of three germ-cell layers (endoderm, mesoderm, and ectoderm). When ectodermal elements predominate, the lesion is commonly called a "dermoid" cyst.
- Definitive MR diagnosis of mature cystic teratoma is based on demonstration of intratumoral fat. Adipose tissue displays high signal intensity on T1-weighted images and shows signal-intensity loss on fat-suppressed T1- or T2-weighted images. Chemical shift (in-phase/opposed-phase) imaging is sensitive in demonstrating microscopic fat, showing signal loss on opposed-phase images compared to in-phase images. Additional findings may include fat–fluid levels, floating debris, and calcifications (the latter evidenced by signal void).
- The "dermoid plug," or Rokitansky nodule, consists of a mixture of fat, hair, teeth, bone, skin, muscle, and solid tissue that may enhance.
- Enhancement of the solid portion of mature teratomas is common and is not necessarily evidence of malignancy.
- Tumor growth beyond the capsule of the tumor is evidence of malignant degeneration.

Management

- Mature teratomas are usually surgically removed because of the risk of ovarian torsion and a 1% to 2% risk of malignant transformation.

Further reading

1. Outwater EK, Siegelman ES, Hunt JL. Ovarian teratomas: tumor types and imaging characteristics. RadioGraphics 2001;21:475–490.
2. Park SB, Kim JK, Kim K-R, Cho K-S. Imaging findings of complications and unusual manifestations of ovarian teratomas. RadioGraphics 2008;28:969–983.

History

▶ 50-year-old woman with a history of several months of vague abdominal pain, early satiety, and weight loss

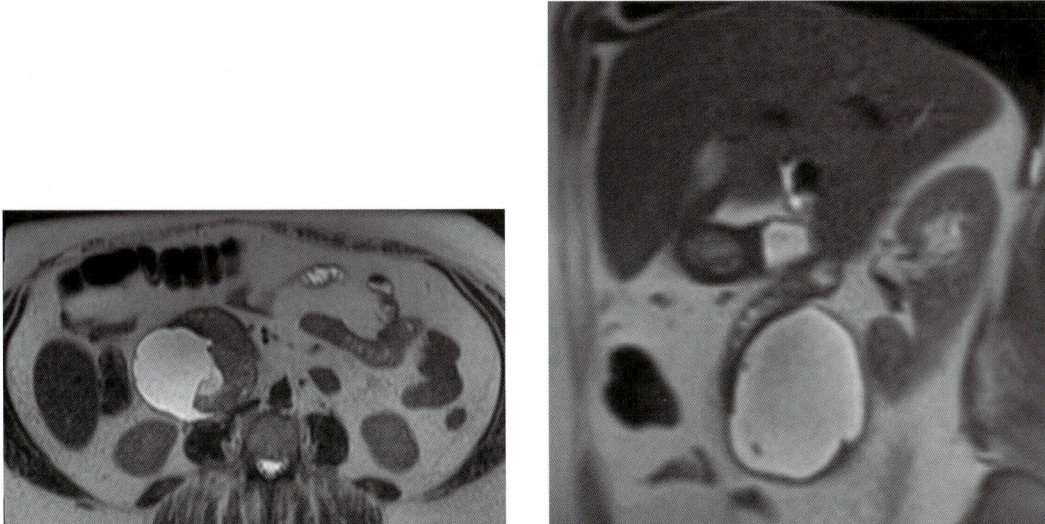

A   B

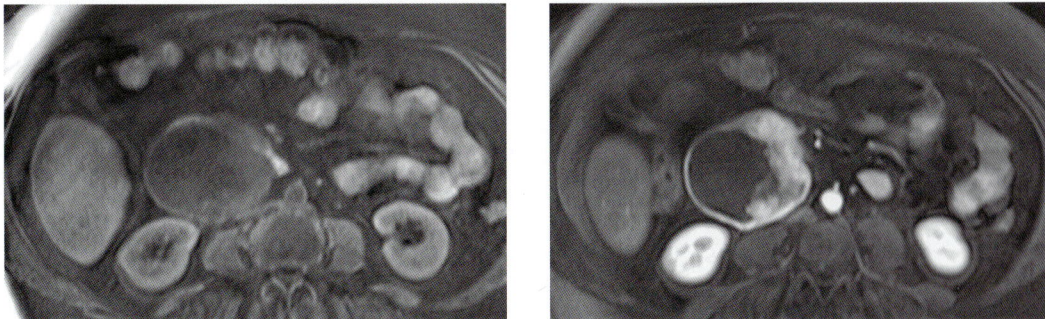

C   D

A. Axial and (**B**) sagittal T2-weighted single-shot FSE/TSE. **C**. Unenhanced and (**D**) gadolinium contrast-enhanced T1-weighted gradient echo with fat saturation.

Case 95 Gastrointestinal Stromal Tumor (GIST) Arising from the Duodenum

Findings

▶ **A** and **B** demonstrate a partially cystic soft-tissue mass originating from the wall of the second portion of the duodenum.

▶ **C** and **D** show that the soft-tissue component of this complex mass demonstrates avid enhancement.

Differential diagnosis

▶ Duodenal adenoma/adenocarcinoma
▶ Lymphoma
▶ Carcinoid
▶ Metastatic disease

Teaching points

▶ GISTs are the most common mesenchymal tumors of the gastrointestinal tract. They are characterized by exophytic growth as opposed to annular growth and luminal narrowing that characterizes adenocarcinoma.

▶ Cross-sectional imaging studies demonstrate a well-circumscribed submucosal mass. Areas of necrosis and ulceration are common. The mucosa is ulcerated in 50% of cases.

▶ GISTs are most common in the stomach (60%), followed by small bowel (20% to 30%) and colon, and they are rare in the esophagus.

▶ Approximately 80% exhibit mutations in the c-KIT gene.

▶ The most common presentation is acute or chronic gastrointestinal bleeding.

▶ Tumors may also present with symptoms related to tumor bulk.

Management

▶ Treatment involves surgical resection and chemotherapy (imatinib mesylate [Gleevec®]) for c-KIT-positive metastatic disease.

▶ Prognosis is related to tumor size, and mortality is increased when lesions are greater than 5 cm.

▶ Positron emission tomography (PET) is helpful in predicting response to imatinib mesylate treatment.

Further reading

1. Horowitz BM, Zamora GE, Gallegos MP. Gastrointestinal stromal tumor of the small bowel. RadioGraphics 2011;31:429–434.
2. King DM. The radiology of gastrointestinal stromal tumors. Cancer Imaging 2005;5:150–156.
3. Miettinen M, Lasota J. Gastrointestinal stromal tumors: Review on morphology, molecular pathology, prognosis and differential diagnosis. Arch Pathol Lab Med 2006;130:1466–1478.

History

▶ 77-year-old woman presents with a lifelong cardiac murmur. An echocardiogram demonstrated a cardiac lesion and MRI was ordered for further evaluation.

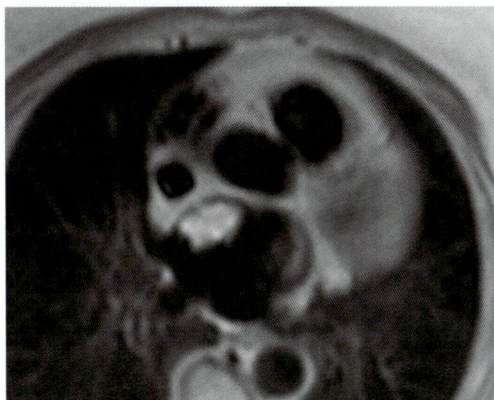

A

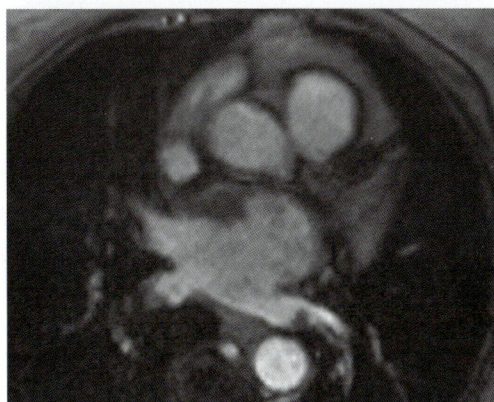

B

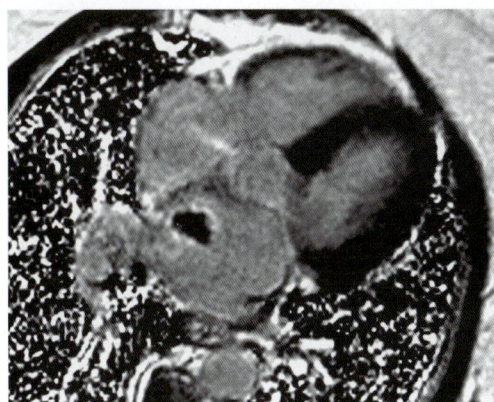

C

A. Axial T2-weighted single-shot FSE/TSE. **B**. Axial balanced steady-state free precession (SSFP). **C**. Axial late gadolinium-enhanced (LGE) phase-sensitive inversion-recovery (PSIR) gradient echo.

Case 96 Atrial Myxoma

Findings

▶ Rounded, pedunculated mass within the left atrium with a narrow stalk of attachment to the interatrial septum (**A**).
▶ The mass is mildly hyperintense to normal myocardium on T2-weighted images, it is iso-intense to normal myocardium on SSFP images, and it demonstrates heterogeneous enhancement on late gadolinium enhanced (LGE) images.

Differential diagnosis

▶ Atrial thrombus
▶ Primary cardiac malignancy
▶ Metastatic malignancy

Teaching points

▶ Myxomas are the most common primary intracavitary cardiac neoplasm.
▶ They may be clinically silent or cause constitutional symptoms (fever, malaise, weight loss), valvular obstruction, or embolic events.
▶ 75% occur in the left atrium, 20% in the right atrium.
▶ Nearly all myxomas are spherical or ovoid in shape with lobular contours.
▶ Myxomas are gelatinous masses with corresponding high signal on T2-weighted images.
▶ Low signal intensity and heterogeneity are present on gradient-echo images due to components of thrombus and calcifications. Myxomas also may be shown to be mobile on cine imaging.
▶ Contrast enhancement of myxomas is typically mildly heterogeneous.
▶ The most important differentiation is between a myxoma and thrombus. Morphology and the demonstration of a stalk connecting to the interatrial septum are useful features to discriminate between the two entities. Myxoma will show some enhancement, whereas thrombus does not.

Management

▶ Surgical resection to prevent obstruction or tumor embolization

Further reading

1. Grebenc ML, Rosado-de-Christenson ML, Green CE, et al. Cardiac myxoma: imaging features in 83 Patients. RadioGraphics 2002;22:673–689.
2. Sparrow PJ, Kurian JB, Jones TR, Sivananthan MU. MR imaging of cardiac tumors. RadioGraphics 2005;25:1255–1276.

History

▶ 48-year-man with a cystic mass discovered in the abdomen on a CT scan performed for trauma

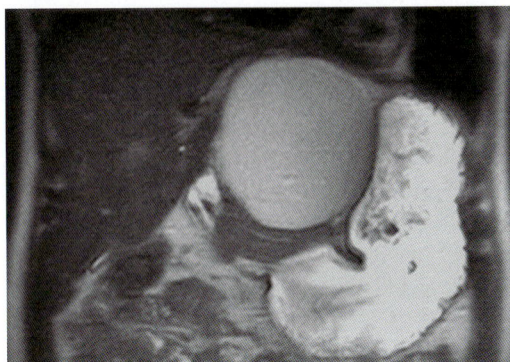

A

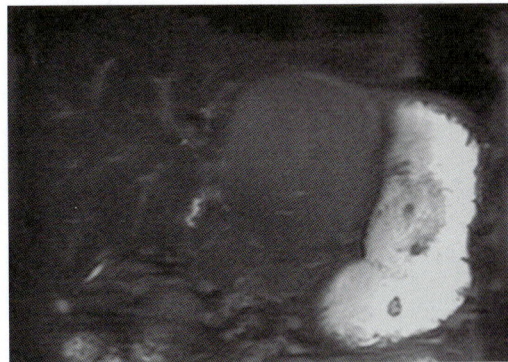

B

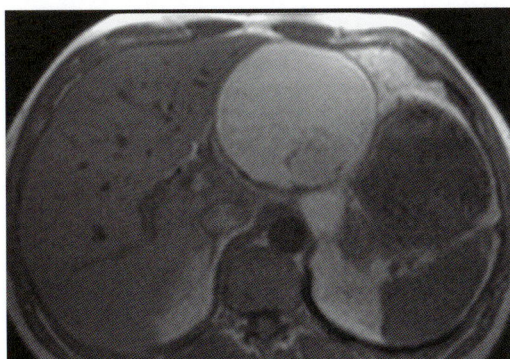

C

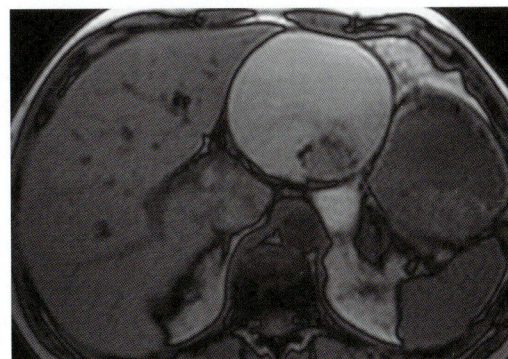

D

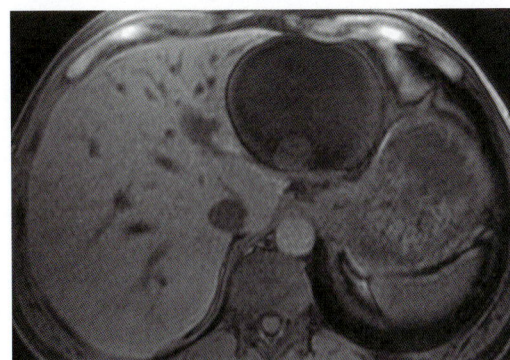

E

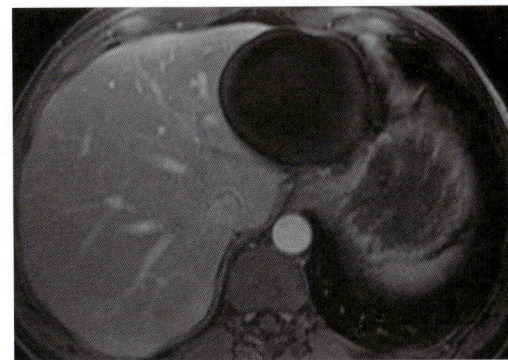

F

A. Coronal T2-weighted single-shot FSE/TSE without and (**B**) with fat saturation. **C**. Axial in-phase and (**D**) opposed-phase T1-weighted gradient echo. **E**. Axial pre-contrast-enhanced and (**F**) post-gadolinium contrast-enhanced T1-weighted gradient echo with fat saturation.

Case 97 Mature Cystic Teratoma

Findings

- A well-defined thin-walled cystic mass displaces the stomach and pancreas inferiorly and laterally.
- The contents of the mass displays high signal intensity on both T1- and T2-weighted images.
- With fat suppression there is marked decrease in signal intensity of the mass contents which is not seen on the non-fat-suppressed images.
- Debris within the mass, seen best on the in-phase and opposed-phase gradient-echo images, shows no evidence of gadolinium contrast enhancement. There are also several small low intensity foci on the opposed-phase image compared with in-phase image indicating the presence of fat.
- At surgery the mass did not involve the liver and stomach but was adherent to the pancreas and the celiac artery and its branches.

Differential diagnosis

- Pancreatic pseudocyst
- Cystic neoplasm of the pancreas, liver, or stomach

Teaching points

- Mature cystic teratomas are composed of mature tissue elements derived from at least two germ-cell layers (endoderm, mesoderm, or ectoderm). Most tumors are unilocular and filled with fatty, sebaceous material. Other mature tissue types within the lesion include mesodermal (fat, bone, cartilage, muscle), ectodermal (skin, neural tissue), or endodermal (thyroid tissue, gastrointestinal or bronchial epithelium) tissues. Teratomas occur commonly in the ovary and are rare in the testis. The most common extragonadal location is sacrococcygeal. Other locations are mediastinal, retroperitoneal, cervical, and intracranial.
- MR demonstration of fat content is the key to definitive diagnosis. Mature fat or fatty sebum displays high signal intensity on T1-weighted images and variable but usually relatively high signal intensity on T2-weighted images. Fat-saturated sequences are optimal for differentiating fat from hemorrhage.

Management

- Surgical excision is needed to confirm the diagnosis.

Further reading

1. Khan A, Khosa F, Eisenberg RL. Cystic lesions of the pancreas. AJR Am J Roentgenol 2011;196:W668–W677.
2. Pereira JM, Sirlin CB, Pinto PS, Casola G. CT and MR imaging of extrahepatic fatty masses of the abdomen and pelvis: techniques, diagnosis, differential diagnosis, and pitfalls. RadioGraphics 2005;25:69–85.
3. Yang DM, Jung DH, Kim H, et al. Retroperitoneal cystic masses: CT, clinical and pathologic findings and literature review. RadioGraphics 2004;24:1353–1365.

History

▶ 49-year-old man with history of recurrent pancreatitis

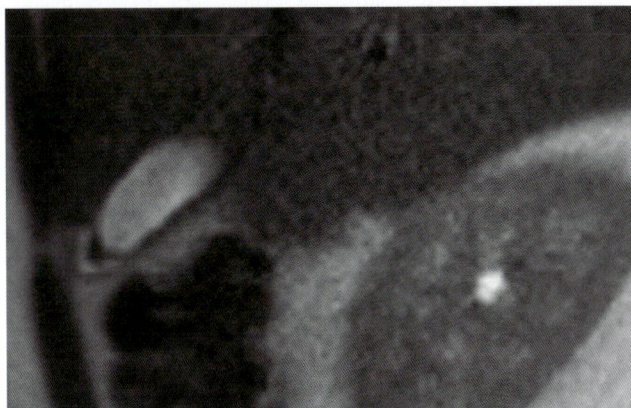

A

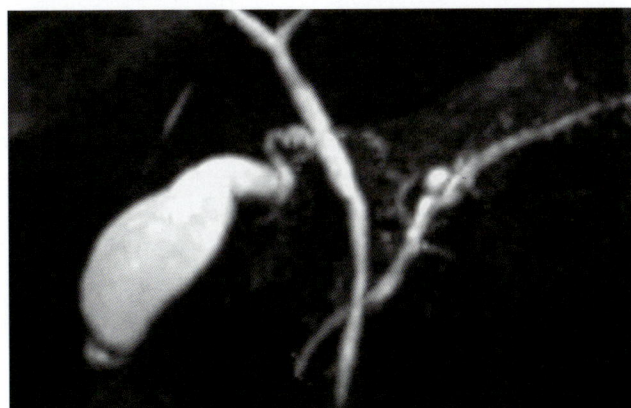

B

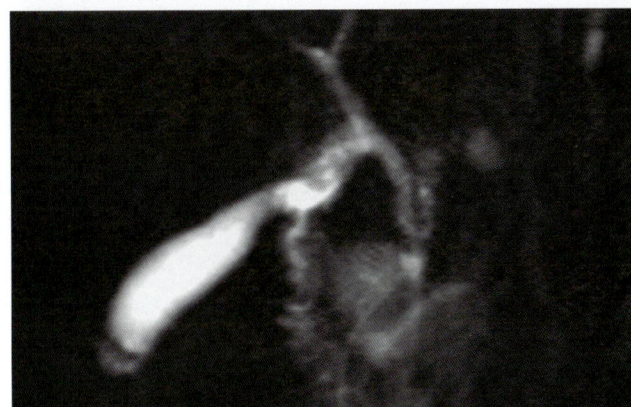

C

A. Sagittal T2-weighted single-shot FSE/TSE. **B**. Maximum intensity reconstruction MRCP frontal view image created from 3D FSE/TSE. **C**. MRCP oblique view, thick-slab single-shot FSE/TSE.

Case 98 Adenomyomatosis of the Gallbladder

Findings

▶ Focal thickening of the wall of the gallbladder is confined to the fundus. The wall thickening is associated with narrowing and segmentation of the gallbladder lumen.
▶ Pancreas divisum is present with associated changes of chronic pancreatitis affecting the pancreatic duct.

Differential diagnosis

▶ Gallbladder carcinoma
▶ Gallbladder polyp
▶ Chronic cholecystitis
▶ Gallbladder diverticulum

Teaching points

▶ Adenomyomatosis is relatively common benign hyperplasia of the gallbladder wall identified in 5% of cholecystectomy specimens.
▶ Wall thickening is associated with the development of intramural diverticula lined with mucosa termed Rokitansky-Aschoff sinuses. The diverticula trap bile, causing stasis, which may result in the formation of cholesterol crystals, sludge, and calculi.
▶ Wall thickening may be focal, most commonly involving the fundus, or diffuse.
▶ T2-weighted MR images show low-signal-intensity wall thickening with the Rokitansky-Aschoff sinuses appearing hyperintense and resembling a "string of pearls." Intravenous gadolinium-based contrast material administration shows little to no enhancement, differentiating this condition from gallbladder carcinoma. PET-CT shows no abnormal uptake in adenomyomatosis.
▶ The gallbladder lumen is often narrowed focally or diffusely by the wall thickening.

Management

▶ Adenomyomatosis has no malignant potential and requires no specific treatment.

Further reading

1. Boscak AR, Mahmoud A-H, Ramsburgh SR. Adenomyomatosis of the gallbladder. RadioGraphics 2006;26:941–946.
2. Levy AD, Murakata LA, Abbott RM, Rohrmann CA. Benign tumors and tumorlike lesions of the gallbladder and extrahepatic bile ducts: Radiologic-pathologic correlation. RadioGraphics 2002;22:387–413.

History

▶ 31-year-old woman with a reported "liver mass" was referred for further characterization.

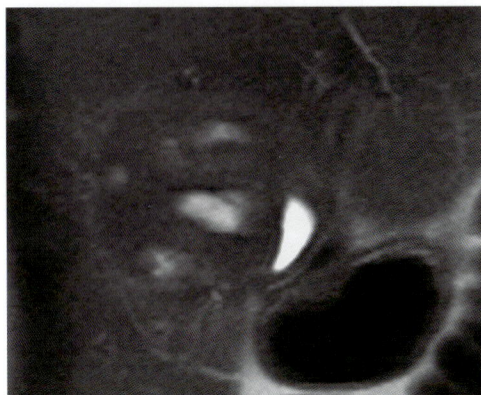

A

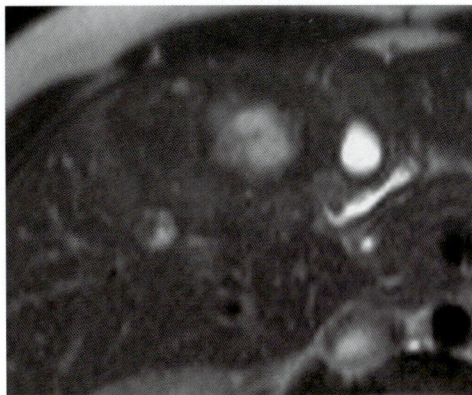

B

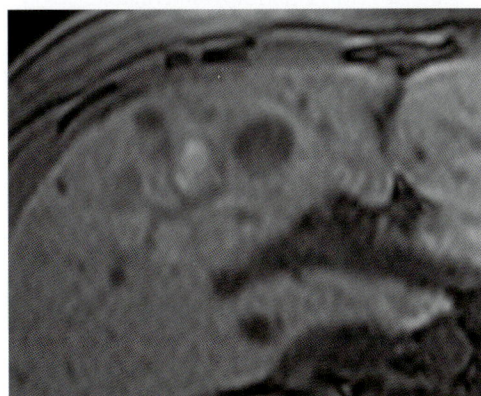

C

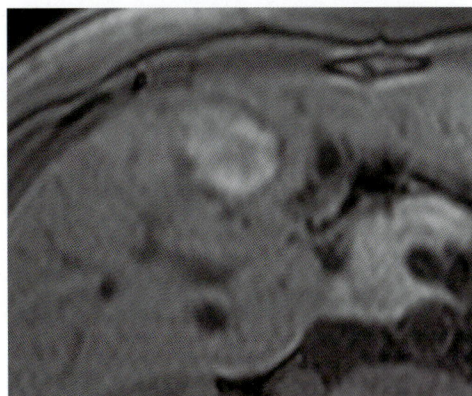

D

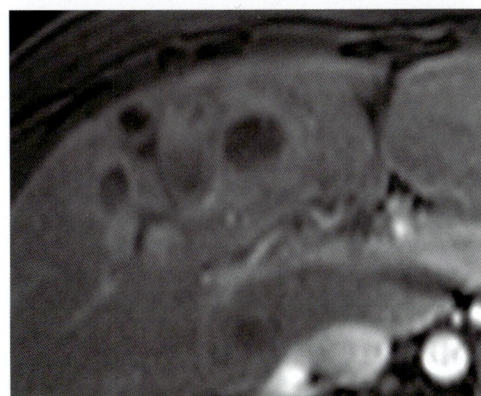

E

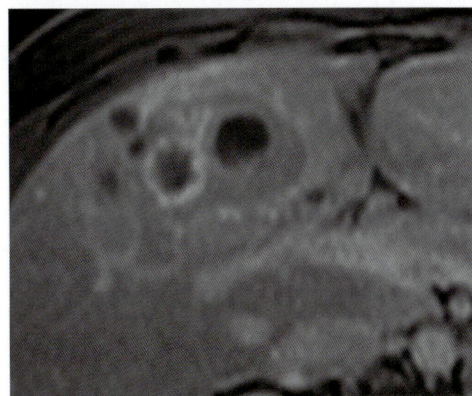

F

A. Coronal and (**B**) axial T2-weighted single-shot FSE/TSE. **C, D**. Axial pre-contrast-enhanced (**D** at lower level than **C**), (**E**) portal venous-phase gadolinium contrast-enhanced and (**F**) delayed-phase contrast-enhanced T1-weighted gradient echo with fat saturation.

Case 99 Hepatic Adenoma with Internal Hemorrhage

Findings

▶ There is a heterogeneous mass in the liver that is slightly hyperintense on T1- and T2-weighted images. Internal regions of low signal intensity on T1-weighted images are seen, some of which correspond with focal, increased signal intensity on T2 weighted images. Post-gadolinium contrast-enhanced images demonstrate early and delayed hyper-enhancement.

Differential diagnosis

▶ Hepatocellular carcinoma, especially fibrolamellar subtype
▶ Hypervascular metastasis
▶ Focal nodular hyperplasia

Teaching points

▶ Hepatic adenoma is a rare benign neoplasm. The reported incidence in the general population is 1 per million, and in women using oral contraceptives it is 30 to 40 per million. Another risk factor is glycogen storage disease, which is often associated with multiple adenomas. The risk of malignant degeneration is up to 10% and increases with size. These lesions are usually problematic due to pain, hemorrhage, and rupture. The lesions have abnormal hepatocytes and Kupffer cells, and may contain fat, mucin, glycogen, and blood products.

▶ Not surprisingly, their imaging appearance is variable and heterogeneous. Usually hepatic adenomas are hyperintense to parenchyma on both T1- and T2-weighted images, but this varies. One third demonstrate a peripheral rim corresponding to a capsule. Early arterial enhancement is typical and is due to the presence of subcapsular feeding vessels. Evidence of blood products and fat is often seen.

▶ The major differential considerations in young patients without cirrhosis are fibrolamellar hepatocellular carcinoma, focal nodular hyperplasia (FNH), and hypervascular metastasis. Clues pointing to fibrolamellar HCC are abdominal lympadenopathy (65%), calcifications (40% to 68%), radiating fibrous septa, and local invasion of the bile ducts or blood vessels. FNH tends to have a central scar and is usually homogeneously isointense to liver on unenhanced, portal venous-phase, and delayed-phase images in contradistinction to adenoma. Adenomas have abnormally functioning Kupffer cells and do not take up iron oxide particles (or sulfur colloid), unlike FNH. Hypervascular metastases tend to be low in signal intensity on T1-weighted images and high in signal on T2-weighted images, and are usually multiple.

Management

▶ Hormone cessation often results in stability or regression of the lesions, and many physicians feel comfortable managing these with serial imaging. Symptomatic, large, and growing lesions are considered at risk for rupture and bleeding, and are treated with resection or occasionally with hepatic arterial embolization. Prophylactic resection on the basis of risk for malignant degeneration can be performed, especially in the case of large lesions.

Further reading

1. Gore RM, Newmark GM, Thakrar KH, et al. Hepatic incidentalomas. Radiol Clin North Am 2011;49:291–322.
2. Grazioli L, Federle MP, Brancatelli G, et al. Hepatic adenomas: imaging and pathologic findings. RadioGraphics 2001;21:877–894.

History

▶ 49-year-old man with cirrhosis presents with failure to thrive.

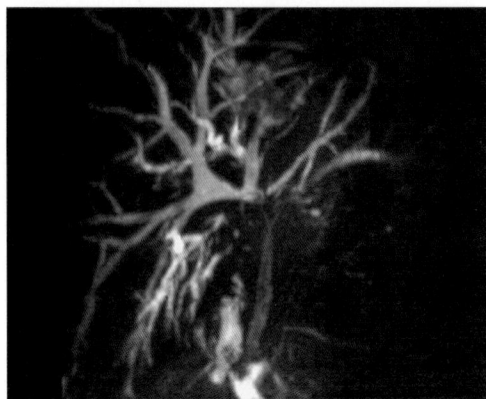
A

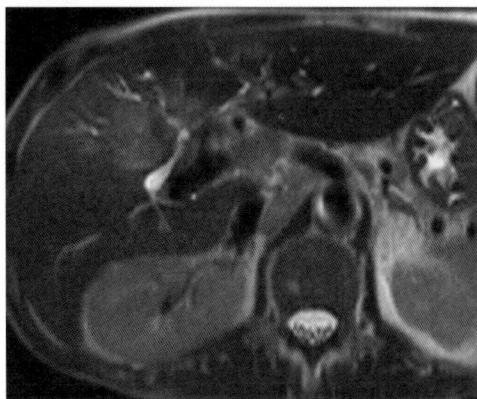
B

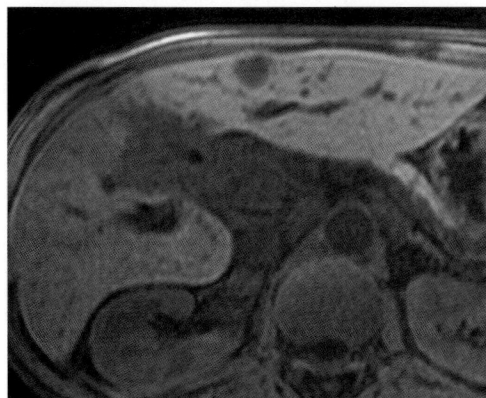
C

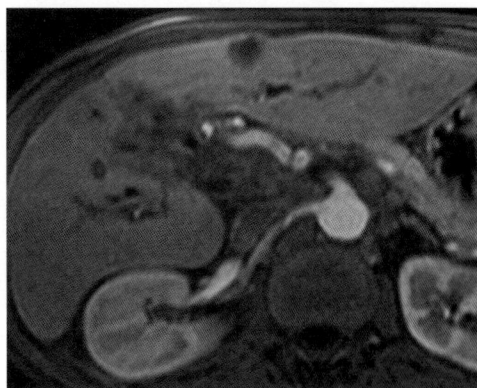
D

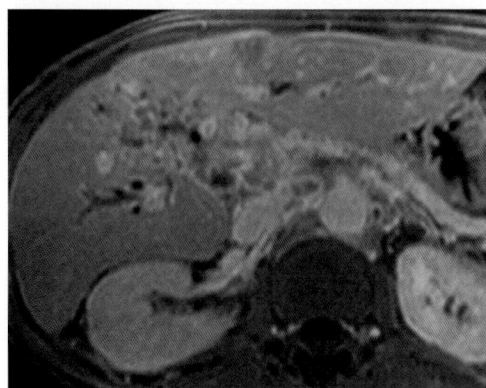
E

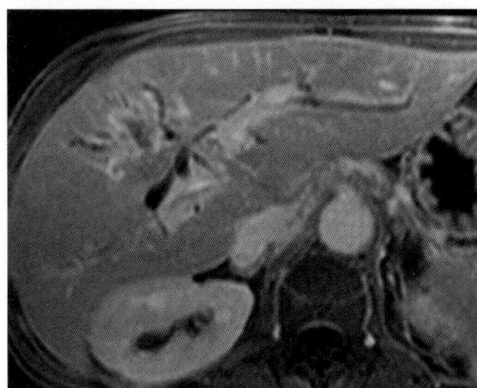
F

A. Coronal maximum intensity projection MRCP image generated from respiratory-gated 3D FSE/TSE. **B**. Axial T2-weighted single-shot FSE/TSE. **C**. Pre-contrast-enhanced, (**D**) arterial-phase, and (**E**) delayed-phase gadolinium-based contrast-enhanced T1-weighted gradient echo at same level, and (**F**) delayed-phase contrast-enhanced image at slightly higher level.

Case 100 Cholangiocarcinoma of the Liver Hilum (Klatskin Tumor)

Findings

▶ MRCP shows dilated intrahepatic ducts converging to a stricture at the liver hilum.
▶ T2-weighted image shows a mass with moderately high signal intensity enveloping the bile duct at the liver hilum.
▶ Post-gadolinium contrast-enhanced images show the hilar mass to have minimal enhancement early. Delayed enhanced images show avid enhancement of the tumor extending along the bile ducts toward the liver periphery.
▶ A metastatic deposit is evident in the left lobe.

Differential diagnosis

▶ Sclerosing cholangitis
▶ Hepatocellular carcinoma
▶ Metastatic disease

Teaching points

▶ Hilar cholangiocarcinomas or Klatskin tumors arise at the junction of the right and left hepatic ducts within the porta hepatis. This type of tumors represent 25% of cholangiocarcinomas.
▶ MR is used to determine the extent of bile duct involvement, involvement of the portal vein and hepatic arteries, presence of liver atrophy, and nodal or hepatic metastatic disease.
▶ Patients with extension into the second-order intrahepatic biliary radicles, vascular involvement with encasement or occlusion of the portal vein, or concomitant involvement of the contralateral hepatic artery and portal vein are poor candidates for surgery.
▶ Mass-forming cholangiocarcinomas show with hypointense to iso-intense signal intensity compared to hepatic parenchyma on T1-weighted images and show variable mild hyperintensity on T2-weighted images. Delayed post-gadolinium contrast-enhanced MR shows progressive enhancement in the active peripheral portion of the lesion and little to no enhancement in the central desmoplastic portion of the lesion. MRCP documents ductal stricture and upstream dilatation.

Management

▶ Surgical resection is the only effective cure for a Klatskin tumor. Palliation includes biliary stenting, biliary bypass procedures, and radiation therapy.

Further reading

1. Choi J-Y, Kim M-J, Lee JM, et al. Hilar cholangiocarcinoma: role of preoperative imaging with sonography, MDCT, MRI, and direct cholangiography. AJR Am J Roentgenol 2008;191:1448–1457.
2. Menias CO, Surabhi VR, Prasad SR, et al. Mimics of cholangiocarcinoma: Spectrum of disease. RadioGraphics 2008;28:1115–1129.
3. Sainani NI, Catalano OA, Holalkere N-S, et al. Cholangiocarcinoma: current and novel imaging techniques. RadioGraphics 2008;28:1263–1287.

History

▶ 31-year-old man with pain and discoloration of the right arm during weight lifting. He has a history of prior right upper extremity deep venous thrombosis that underwent successful lysis.

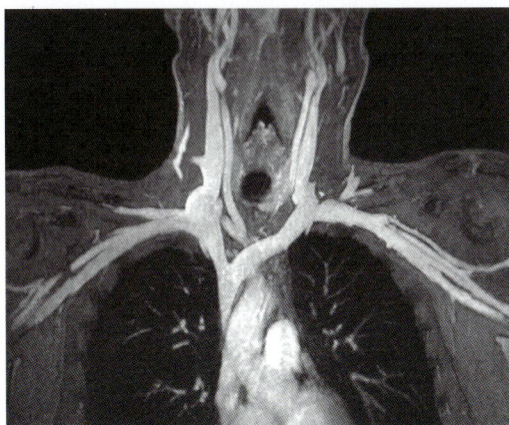

A

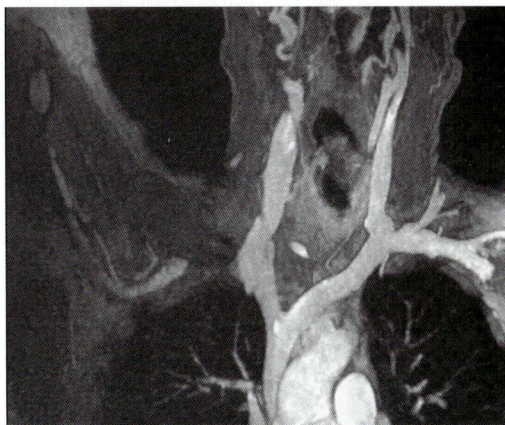

B

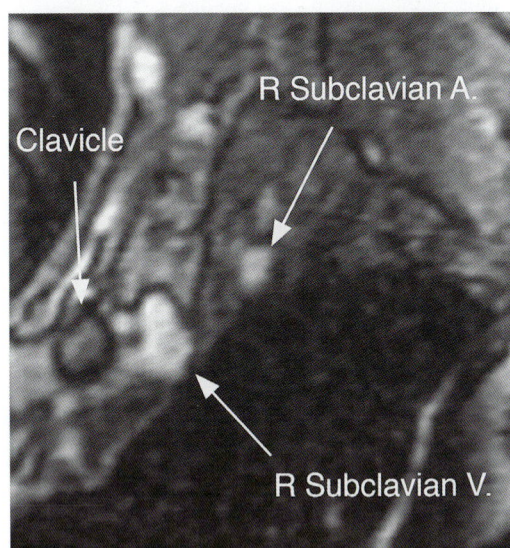

C

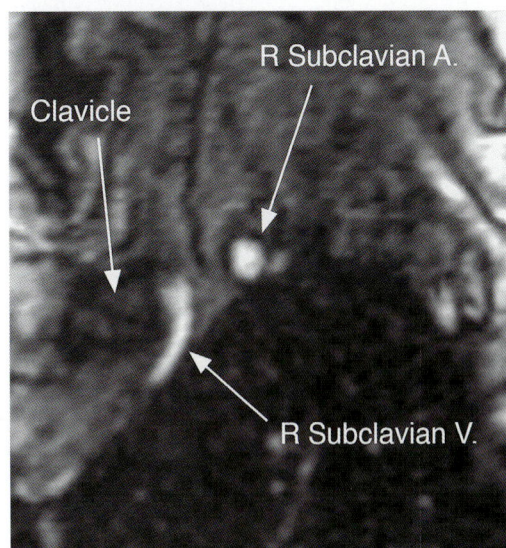

D

A. MR venogram of the chest with the patient holding the arms in neutral position at the sides, using gadolinium contrast-enhanced 3D gradient echo. **B**. MR venogram obtained with the right arm in hyperabducted position. **C**. MR venogram reconstructed in sagittal plane with the patient holding the arms in neutral and (**D**) in hyperabducted position.

Case 101 Venous Thoracic Outlet Syndrome (TOS)

Findings

- Normal appearance of the bilateral subclavian veins with the right upper extremity in the neutral position (**A**).
- Stenosis of the distal right subclavian vein as it passes over the first rib with hyperabduction of the extremity (**B**).
- Sagittal view (**C**) demonstrates relationship of the clavicle with the right subclavian vein and artery in neutral position.
- With hyperabduction of the extremity the clavicle moves posteriorly relative to the first rib, pinching the vein (**D**) and compressing it between the clavicle and first rib (rib not shown).

Differential diagnosis

- Neurogenic or arterial TOS
- History of prior ipsilateral central venous catheter placement
- Trauma
- Malignant involvement of subclavian vein (Pancoast tumor)

Teaching points

- Venous TOS refers to compression of one or more of the neurovascular bundles crossing the thoracic outlet resulting in pain, tingling, weakness, or other symptoms of the upper extremity.
- The syndrome is most frequent in women (F:M, 4:1) between 20 and 40 years of age, and is most commonly caused by compression of the subclavian vein by a skeletal or soft-tissue abnormality (cervical rib, prominent C7 transverse process, hypertrophied subclavius or anterior scalene muscle), or by repetitive trauma (baseball/softball pitching, swimming, etc.).
- There are three distinct syndromes depending on the injured component: neurogenic (most common), arterial, and venous syndrome.
- Compression of the subclavian vein is often present with hyperabduction in asymptomatic patients, complicating diagnosis. The presence of collateral veins supports the diagnosis of venous TOS.
- Venous compression is best seen on sagittal, reconstructed MR venography images.
- Paget-von Schroetter disease (also known as effort-induced thrombosis) refers to acute subclavian-axillary vein thrombosis occurring after vigorous activity. It may develop as a sequela of TOS.

Management

- Surgical: first-rib resection and scalenectomy
- In case of thrombosis: thrombolysis and anticoagulation

Further reading

1. Charon JP, Milne W, Sheppard DG, Houston JG. Evaluation of MR angiographic technique in the assessment of thoracic outlet syndrome. Clin Radiol 2004;59:588–595.
2. Demondion X, Herbinet P, Jan SVS, et al. Imaging assessment of thoracic outlet syndrome. RadioGraphics 2006;26:1735–1750.
3. Hagspiel KD, Spinosa DJ, Angle JF, Matsumoto AH. Diagnosis of vascular compression at the thoracic outlet using gadolinium-enhanced high-resolution MR angiography in abduction and adduction. Cardiovasc Intervent Radiol 2000;23:152–164.

Case 102

History

► 33-year-old woman complaining of right pelvic pain. Outside ultrasound examination was reported as showing a complex right adnexal mass.

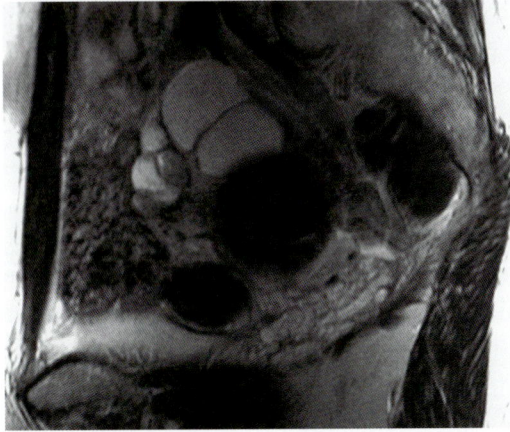

A

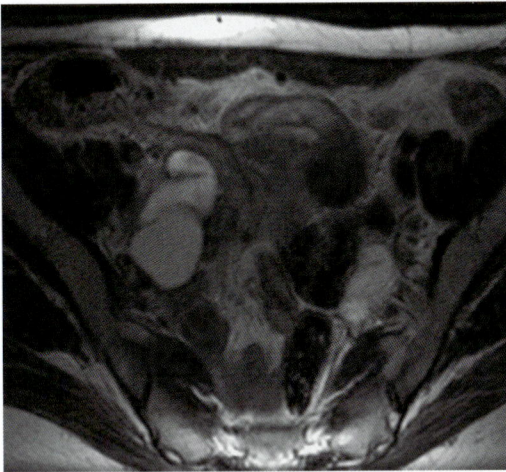

B

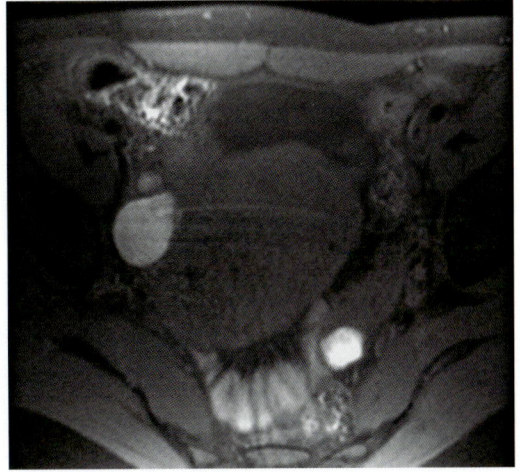

C

A. Sagittal and (**B**) axial T2-weighted FSE/TSE. **C**. Axial T1-weighted spin echo with fat saturation.

Case 102 Hydrosalpinx

Findings

- A cystic mass in the right adnexa has the configuration of a dilated twisted tube.
- Fluid within the cyst displays high signal intensity on both T1- and T2-weighted images, consistent with bloody or proteinaceous material.
- No solid component is evident within the lesion to indicate the presence of tumor.

Differential diagnosis

- Complex ovarian cyst, possibly ovarian tumor
- Endometrioma

Teaching points

- A distended fallopian tube filled with serous fluid is termed a hydrosalpinx. A blood-filled dilated tube is a hematosalpinx. A pus-filled dilated tube is a pyosalpinx. Dilation of the fallopian tube occurs with obstruction of the distal fimbriated end of the tube. This may occur as an isolated event or as a component of complex pelvic disease including pelvic infection, endometriosis, or tumor.
- Hydrosalpinx is usually confidently diagnosed by transvaginal pelvic ultrasound examination. MR may be indicated for problem solving in patients with complex pelvic findings.
- As an isolated finding MR shows a fluid-filled tubular structure arising from the lateral margin of the uterine fundus. The dilated tube frequently folds or twists on itself to produce a C-shaped, S-shaped, or sausage-shaped cystic structure. Tubal diameter may reach 10 cm. The tube is shown to be separate from the ovary. The wall may be thickened as a result of inflammation. A solid enhancing mass or enhancing polypoid projections suggest fallopian tube carcinoma.
- The dilated tube may be a component of a complex adnexal lesion that includes the ovary, bowel, lymph nodes, and peritoneal fluid collections. These complex adnexal masses most commonly represent endometriosis, pelvic inflammatory disease, or complicated malignancy. Tubo-ovarian abscess may be chronic with indolent symptoms.
- Sterile hydrosalpinx is associated with risk of developing pyosalpinx. Hydrosalpinx has an adverse effect on fertility, including a 50% decreased chance of implantation and pregnancy after in vitro fertilization.

Management

- Pelvic inflammatory disease and acute tubo-ovarian abscess are treated with antibiotics, and with catheter or surgical drainage as needed.
- Laparoscopic salpingectomy is usually recommended for symptomatic hydrosalpinx.

Further reading

1. Kim MY, Rha SE, Oh SN, et al. MR imaging findings of hydrosalpinx: a comprehensive review. RadioGraphics 2009;29:495–507.

History

▶ 73-year-old man with remote history of right nephrectomy for benign cause presents for MR with recurrent episodes of gross hematuria.

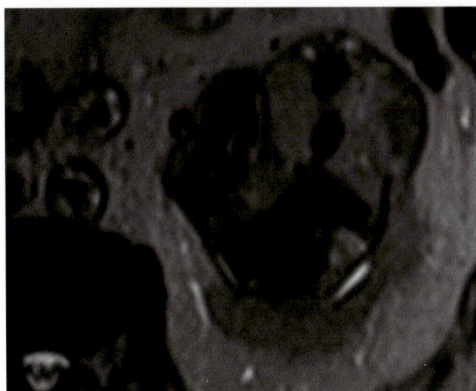

A

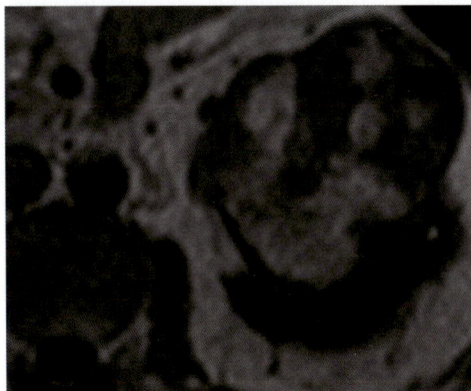

B

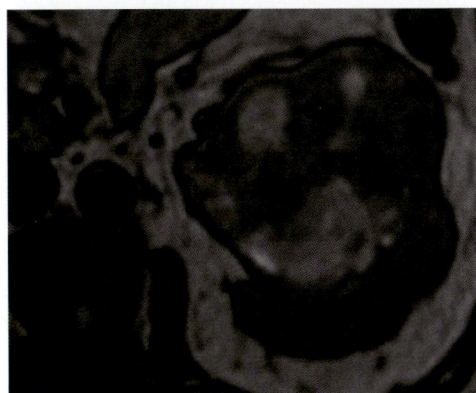

C

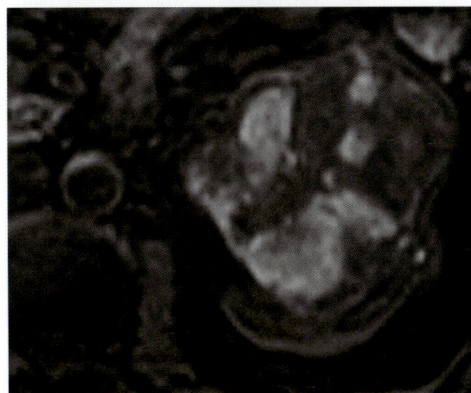

D

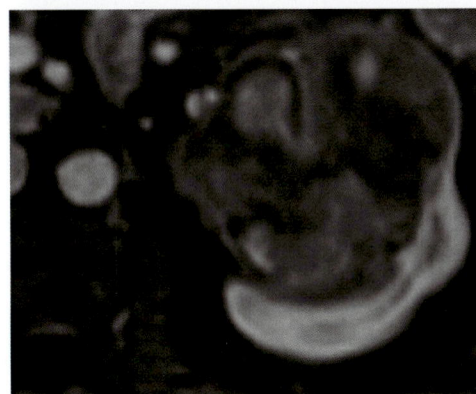

E

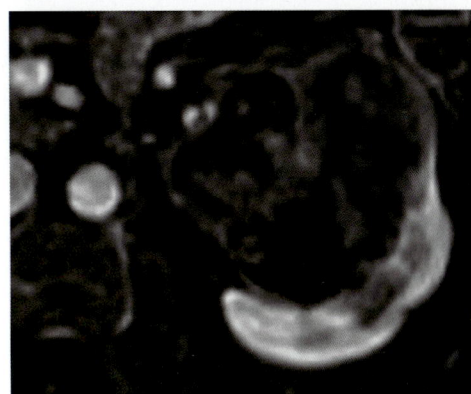

F

A. Axial T2-weighted single-shot FSE/TSE. **B**. Axial in-phase and (**C**) opposed-phase T1-weighted gradient echo. **D**. Axial pre-contrast-enhanced (**E**) and post-gadolinium contrast-enhanced T1-weighted gradient echo with fat saturation. **F**. Subtraction image of **D** and **E**.

Case 103 Hemorrhagic Renal Cyst

Findings

▶ A 9-cm hemorrhagic mass with mildly enhancing thick nodular septations is present within the left renal hilum.

▶ No lymphadenopathy or vascular invasion is identified.

Differential diagnosis

▶ Malignant tumor (renal cell carcinoma, uroepithelial carcinoma, Wilms' tumor)

▶ Benign tumors (multilocular cystic nephroma, angiomyolipoma)

▶ Renal trauma

Teaching points

▶ Renal cysts may be complicated by hemorrhage, infection, inflammation, ischemia, or trauma, and may mimic renal tumors, especially renal cell carcinoma.

▶ Hemorrhagic cysts contain blood products at varying stages of breakdown and can have septations; however, any nodularity within the wall or septations or any enhancement should raise suspicion of renal cell cancer.

▶ Traumatic injury to the kidney can have a variety of appearances and is usually known from the clinical history. However, any hemorrhagic renal lesion not typical for renal trauma should receive a short-interval follow-up imaging examination to confirm resolution.

▶ Hemorrhagic renal cysts show a variety of signal-intensity changes on T1- and T2-weighted images depending on the amount of hemorrhage and the stage of the evolution of the hematoma—that is, the degree of red blood cell lysis, the type of blood breakdown products, and the protein content. Paramagnetic effects of blood-breakdown deoxyhemoglobin, methemoglobin and hemosiderin variably shorten T1 and T2. Hemorrhagic cysts are usually shown with intermediate to high signal intensity on T1-weighted images caused by methemoglobin. On T2-weighted images signal intensity varies and may be high or low depending on the stage of the blood cell breakdown.

▶ The presence of contrast-enhancing nodules in the wall of a hemorrhagic cyst or septations or solid components is highly indicative of cystic tumor rather than benign hemorrhagic cyst.

Management

▶ Imaging follow-up of hemorrhagic renal lesions is generally recommended to confirm expected evolution of hemorrhage and to exclude an underlying malignancy.

Further reading

1. Hilpert PL, Friedman AC, Radecki PD, et al. MRI of hemorrhagic renal cysts in polycystic kidney disease. AJR Am J Roentgenol 1986;1167–1172.
2. Pedrosa I, Sun MR, Spencer M, et al. MR Imaging of renal masses: correlation with findings at surgery and pathologic analysis. RadioGraphics 2008;28:985–1003.
3. Roubidoux MA. MR imaging of hemorrhage and iron deposition in the kidney. RadioGraphics 1994;14:1033–1044.

History

▶ 82-year-old man with new-onset abdominal pain

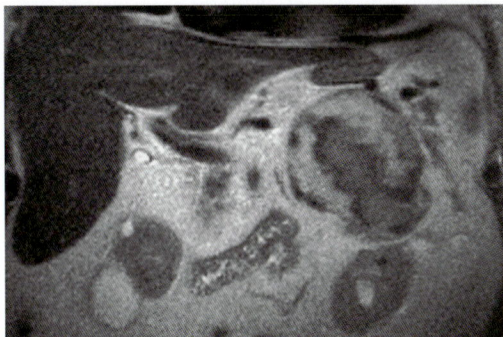 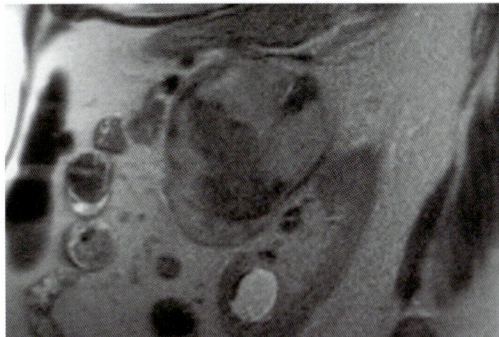

A   B

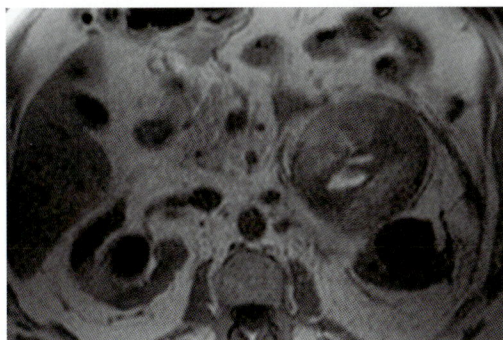 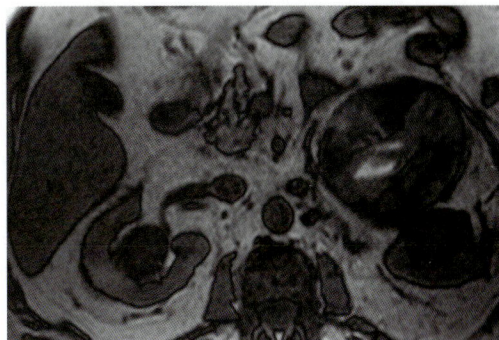

C   D

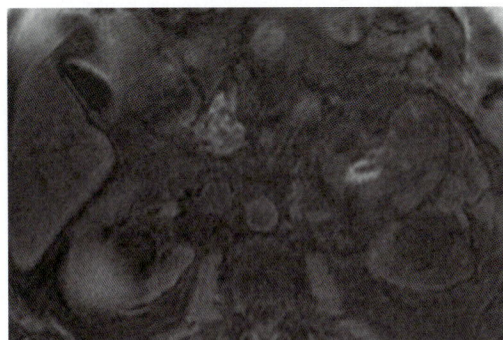 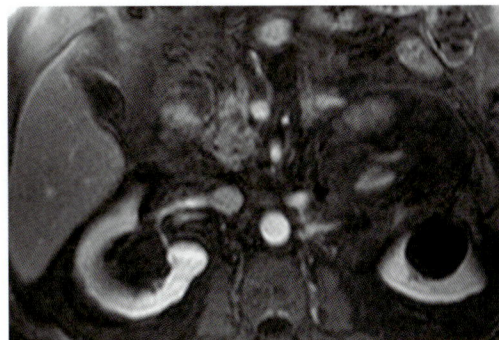

E   F

A. Coronal and (**B**) sagittal T2-weighted single-shot FSE/TSE. **C**. Axial in-phase and (**D**) opposed-phase T1-weighted gradient-echo images. **E**. Axial pre-contrast-enhanced and (**F**) axial post-gadolinium contrast-enhanced T1-weighted gradient echo with fat saturation.

Case 104 Adrenal Myelolipoma Complicated by Hemorrhage

Findings

▶ Heterogeneous well-defined mass in the left suprarenal space with internal central foci of marked hyperintensity on T1-weighted imaging, indicating hemorrhage
▶ Mass shows decreased signal intensity on fat-suppressed images, indicating macroscopic fat.
▶ A portion of the mass shows signal dropout on out-of-phase imaging, indicating a component of the tissue containing microscopic fat. In other areas characteristic dark margins ("India ink artifact") are seen at the interfaces between bulk (adipose) fat and the water-containing tumor tissue.
▶ A portion of the mass shows contrast enhancement consistent with the hematopoietic elements.
▶ The diagnosis was confirmed by surgical resection.

Differential diagnosis

▶ Liposarcoma
▶ Renal angiomyolipoma
▶ Lipoma
▶ Hibernoma

Teaching points

▶ An encapsulated mixed fatty and soft-tissue suprarenal mass can confidently be diagnosed as a myelolipoma.
▶ MRI can identify the separate components of bulk (adipose) fat, hematopoietic tissue, and occasional hemorrhage of myelolipomas with T1- and T2-weighted imaging with and without fat saturation, and in-phase/opposed-phase T1-weighted gradient-echo imaging.
▶ Myelolipoma is an uncommon benign lesion typically discovered incidentally within the adrenal gland in older asymptomatic patients.
▶ Myelolipomas are characterized histologically by the presence of hematopoietic elements (*myelo*) and adipocytes (*lipoma*).

Management

▶ Surgical resection is rarely needed but may be indicated in larger (>7 cm) symptomatic myelolipomas because of complications due to hemorrhage or mass effect.

Further reading

1. Bassignani MJ. Adrenal and retroperitoneal MR imaging. In: Brant WE, de Lange EE (Eds), Essential of Body MRI. New York: Oxford University Press, 2012.
2. Craig WD, Fanburg-Smith JC, Henry LR, et al. Fat containing lesions of the retroperitoneum: radiologic-pathologic correlation. RadioGraphics 2009;29:261–290.
3. Kenney PJ, Wagner BJ, Rao P, Heffess CS. Myelolipoma: CT and pathologic features. Radiology 1998;208:87–95.
4. Routhier JR, Woodfield CA, Mayo-Smith WW. Fat-containing retroperitoneal mass presenting with acute flank pain. AJR Am J Roentgenol 2009;192:S122–S124.

History

▶ 56-year-old man with abdominal pain

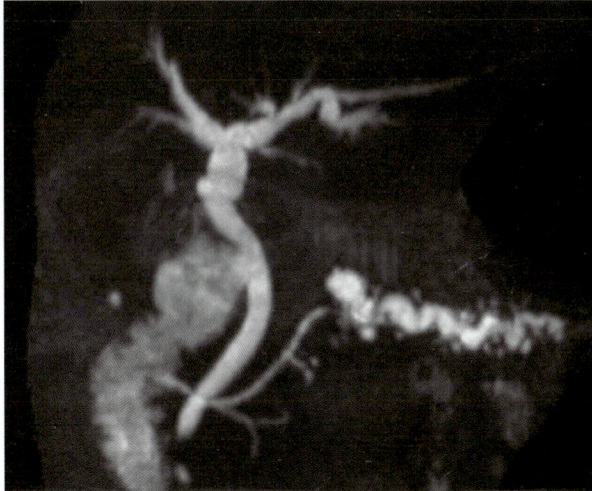

A

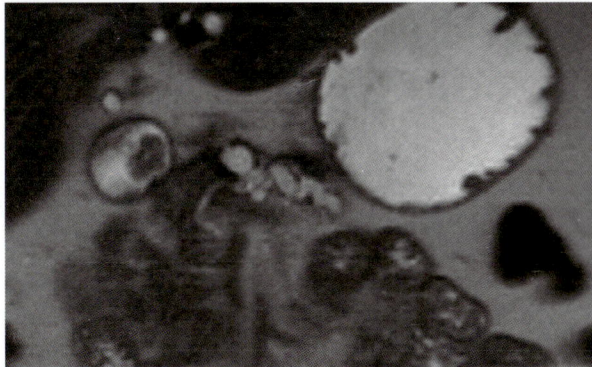

B

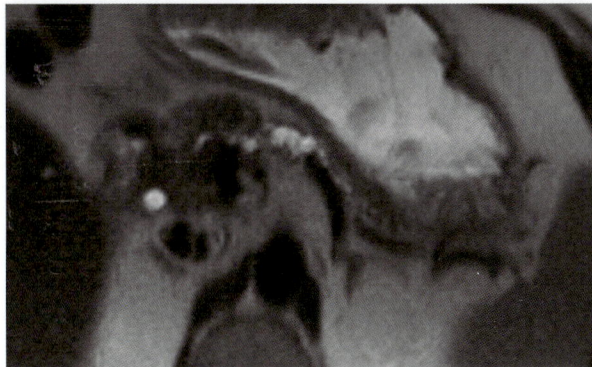

C

A. Coronal maximum intensity projection MRCP image reconstructed from 3D FSE/TSE. **B**. Coronal and (**C**) axial T2-weighted single-shot FSE/TSE.

Case 105 Intraductal Papillary Mucinous Neoplasm (IPMN) or Tumor (IPMT)—Main Duct Type

Findings

► Significant (>7 mm) dilatation of the main pancreatic duct as well as its side branches, only involving the left lateral half of the pancreatic duct
► The dilated portion of the duct is continuous with the main pancreatic duct
► There is atrophy of the pancreatic parenchyma surrounding the dilated duct
► There is pancreas divisum anatomy

Differential diagnosis

► Chronic pancreatitis
► Pancreatic ductal carcinoma
► Pancreatic pseudocyst
► Mucinous cystic neoplasm (MCN) of the pancreas

Teaching points

► Subdivision of IPMNs
► Classified into three subtypes:
  ■ Side branch pancreatic duct type: focal lobulated cystic dilatation of branch ducts
  ■ Main pancreatic duct type: diffuse dilatation of main pancreatic duct
  ■ Combined type: dilatation of both branch ducts and main duct
► Main duct type can be focal or involve the entire duct.
► The risk of developing malignancy (adenocarcinoma) in main duct IPMN is substantially higher than in isolated side branch IPMN.
► A main pancreatic ductal diameter greater than 7 mm should be considered main duct IPMN.
► In contrast to MCN, IPMNs lack an associated ovarian-type stroma. Further, IPMN originates from the ductal mucosa causing the pancreatic duct to dilate from mucin secretion, whereas MCN is not a ductal tumor but orginates in the pancreatic parenchyma and may cause ductal dilatation when the tumor compresses the duct.

Management

► Surgical resection is the treatment of choice for main duct IPMNs because of their malignant potential, and IPMNs resected before the development of invasive carcinoma are highly curable.
► Some surgeons recommend surgical resection as soon as main duct IPMN is suspected because of lack of reliable markers of malignancy; however, for a patient with an asymptomatic small side branch duct type lesion without evidence of malignancy (no mural nodule, absence of main pancreatic duct dilatation), close follow-up with meticulous serial imaging studies should be done.
► Current surgical consensus is that side branch IPMNs more than 3 cm in greatest dimension require surgery because of increased risk for malignancy.

Further reading

1. Kawamoto S, Horton KM, Lawler LP, et al. Intraductal papillary mucinous neoplasm of the pancreas: Can benign lesions be differentiated from malignant lesions with multidetector CT? RadioGraphics 2005;25:1451–1468.
2. Sohn TA, Yeo CJ, Cameron JL, et al. Intraductal papillary mucinous neoplasms of the pancreas: an updated experience. Ann Surg 2004; 239:788–797; discussion 797–799.

History

▶ 63-year-old man who had Whipple procedure for acinar carcinoma of the pancreas

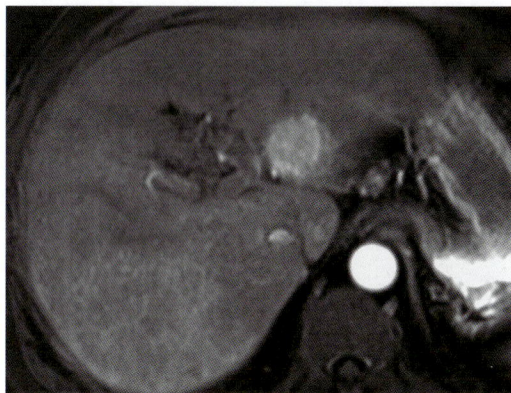

A

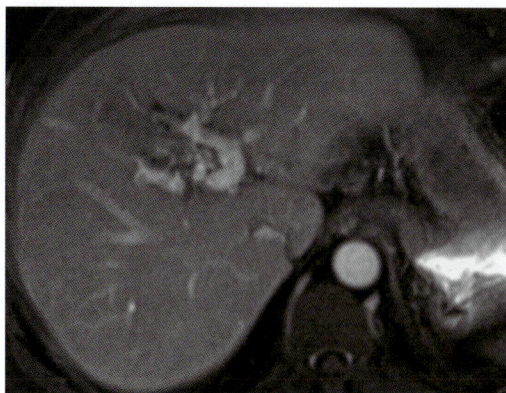

B

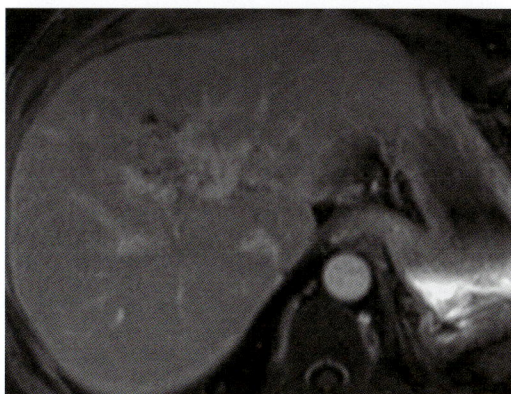

C

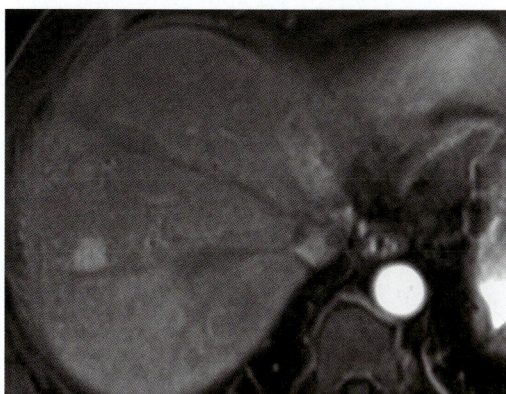

D

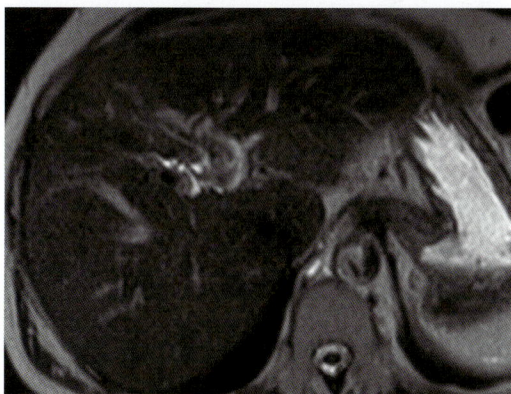

E

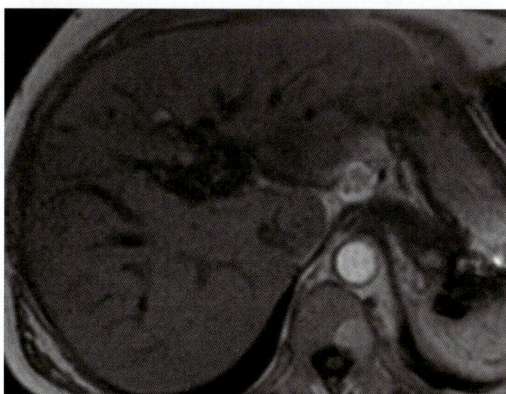

F

A. Axial early arterial-phase, (**B**) portal venous-phase, and (**C**) 10-minute delayed post-gadoliniuim contrast-enhanced gradient echo with fat saturation. **D**. Early arterial-phase contrast-enhanced image at a more cranial level than **A**. **E**. Axial T2-weighted single-shot FSE/TSE. **F**. Axial non-contrast-enhanced T1-weighted gradient echo.

Case 106 Hypervascular Metastases from an Exocrine Gland Carcinoma of the Pancreas

Findings

▶ Mass lesion in segment 4B of the liver shows marked arterial phase enhancement (**A**) with rapid washout of the contrast agent (**B, C**).

▶ The mass shows only slightly increased signal intensity on the T2-weighted image compared with normal liver (**E**) and slightly decreased signal on the T1-weighted image (**F**).

▶ A second arterial-phase hyper-enhancing lesion is seen at a more cranial level in the right lobe (**D**). On other sequences this lesion had similar signal intensity characteristics (not shown) as the segment 4B lesion. Only the arterial-phase image is shown in this example.

Differential diagnosis

▶ Hypervascular liver lesions occurring in the normal liver include focal nodular hyperplasia, hepatic adenoma, some metastases, and hemangioma.

▶ Hypervascular liver lesions occurring in cirrhosis include vascular shunts, regenerative nodules, dysplastic nodules, hepatocellular carcinoma, and vascular fistulas.

Teaching points

▶ Metastases to the liver are most commonly discrete, focal, and multiple, though they may present as a solitary or confluent mass. The margins are typically irregular and indistinct. The blood supply to all hepatic tumors is predominantly from the hepatic artery. The enhancement pattern depends on the vascularity of the tumor.

▶ Hypervascular metastases enhance early and are best seen on arterial-phase post-intravenous contrast-enhanced images. Washout of the contrast agent on delayed images is typical.

▶ The most common hypervascular metastases are primary pancreatic neuroendocrine (islet cell) tumors, carcinoid, pheochromocytoma, renal cell carcinoma, choriocarcinoma, melanoma, and thyroid carcinoma.

▶ Most hypervascular liver metastases display decreased signal intensity on T1-weighted images compared to normal liver and increased signal intensity on T2-weighted images.

▶ The presence of hemorrhage, necrosis, or cystic change within the lesion changes its signal-intensity characteristics. Hemorrhagic lesions and melanoma may show with high signal intensity on T1-weighted images. Perilesional fat deposition is characteristic of metastases from insulinoma.

▶ Treated hypervascular metastases may show non-uniform nodular enhancement. A continuous peripheral rim of enhancement distinguishes these lesions from the discontinuous nodular enhancement of hemangioma.

Management

▶ Percutaneous image-guided biopsy is usually required for pathologic confirmation.

Further reading

1. Khosa F, Khan AN, Eisenberg RL. Hypervascular liver lesions on MRI. AJR Am J Roentgenol 2011;197:W204-W220, Web exclusive article.
2. Silva AC, Evans JM, McCullough AE, et al. MR imaging of hypervascular liver masses: a review of current techniques. RadioGraphics 2009;29:385–402.

History

▶ 73-year-old woman with vague lower abdominal pain

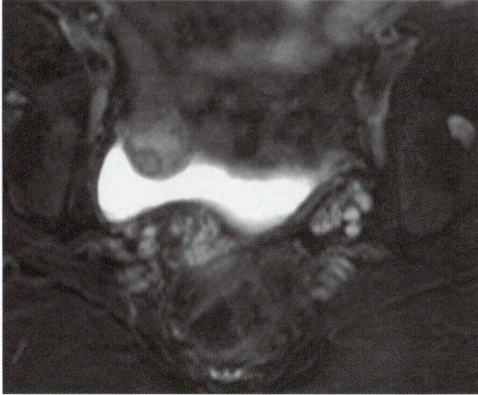

A

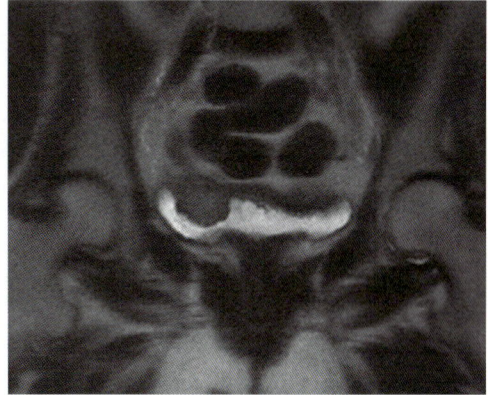

B

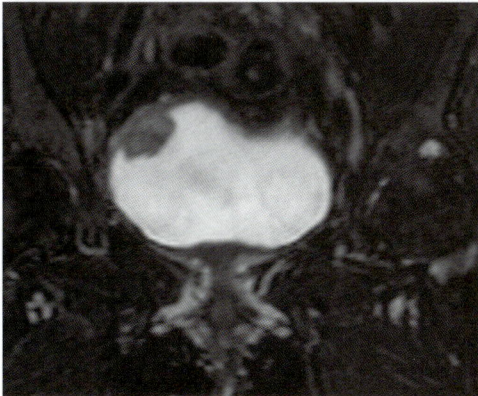

C

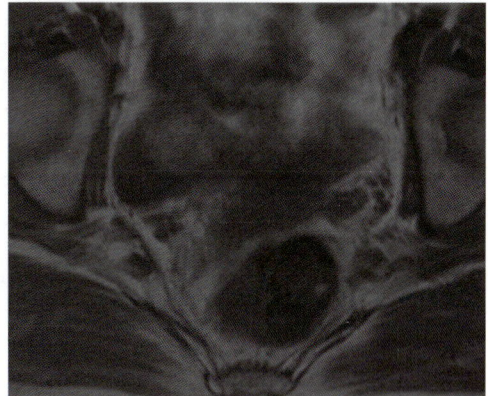

D

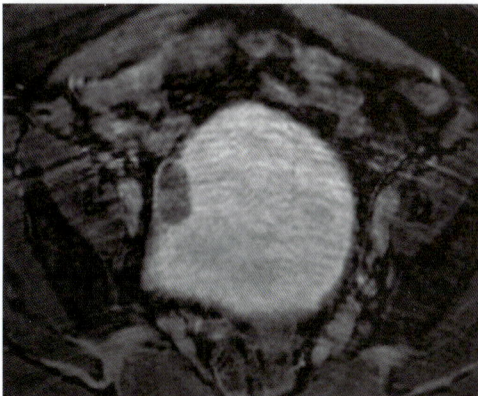

E

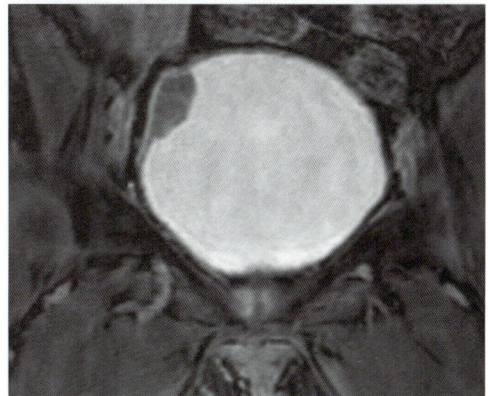

F

A. Axial T2-weighted FSE/TSE with fat saturation. **B**. Coronal T2-weighted single-shot FSE/TSE. **C**. Coronal T2-weighted FSE/TSE with fat saturation. **D**. Axial T1-weighted spin echo. **E**. Axial and (**F**) coronal T1-weighted post-gadolinium contrast-enhanced T1-weighted gradient echo with fat saturation.

Case 107   Paraganglioma, Wall of the Urinary Bladder

Findings

▶ A well-defined small solid mass arising in the bladder wall demonstrates increased signal intensity on T2-weighted images compared to the adjacent normal bladder wall.

▶ The mass demonstrates heterogenous contrast enhancement.

Differential diagnosis

▶ Bladder carcinoma
▶ Endometriosis

Teaching points

▶ Extra-adrenal pheochromocytomas are also called paragangliomas. They are rare neuroendocrine neoplasms arising from chromaffin cells. They account for the 15% of pheochromocytomas that do not arise in the adrenal glands.

▶ Approximately 10% of extra-adrenal paragangliomas arise in the bladder wall. Many of these have no hormonal activity. Hormonally active tumors secrete norepinephrine and rarely dopamine which is in distinction to adrenal pheochromocytomas that secrete epinephrine as well as norepinephrine.

▶ Paragangliomas may be multicentric and are more often malignant (40%) than adrenal pheochromocytomas (2% to 11%).

▶ Paragangliomas are associated with multiple endocrine neoplasia types 2A and 2B, neurofibromatosis type 1 (von Recklinghausen disease), and von Hippel-Lindau disease.

▶ Paragangliomas classically demonstrate increased signal intensity on T2-weighted images compared to the normal bladder wall and show avid contrast enhancement. Contrast-enhanced images are essential to evaluate for additional lesions.

▶ This case is atypical in that the tumor shows weak heterogeneous contrast enhancement rather than the avid homogeneous enhancement more characteristic of bladder pheochromocytoma.

▶ Considerable overlap exists between benign and malignant causes of a bladder mass; therefore, the role of imaging is to evaluate for local extent of disease and for metastasis once a malignant diagnosis has been established.

Management

▶ Surgical excision

Further reading

1. Elsayes KM, Narra VR, Leyendecker JR, et al. MRI of adrenal and extraadrenal pheochromocytoma. AJR Am J Roentgenol 2005;184:860–867.
2. Sahdev A, Sohaib A, Monson JP, Grossman AB, Chew SL, Reznek RH. CT and MR imaging of unusual locations of extra-adrenal paragangliomas (pheochromocytomas). Eur Radiol 2005;15:85–92.

History

▶ 12-year-old girl with primary amenorrhea and pelvic pain

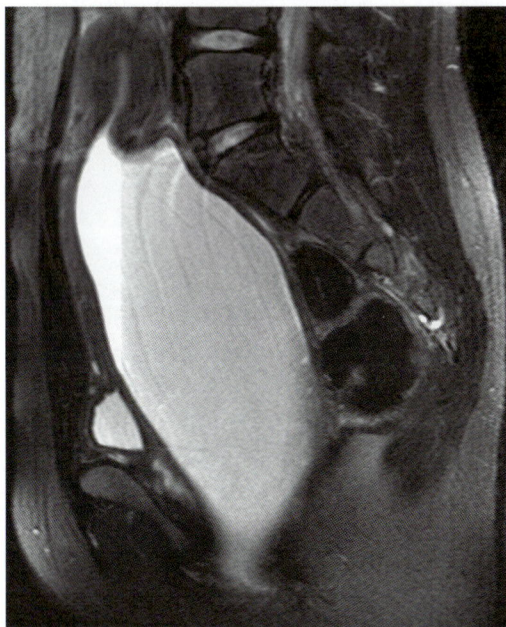

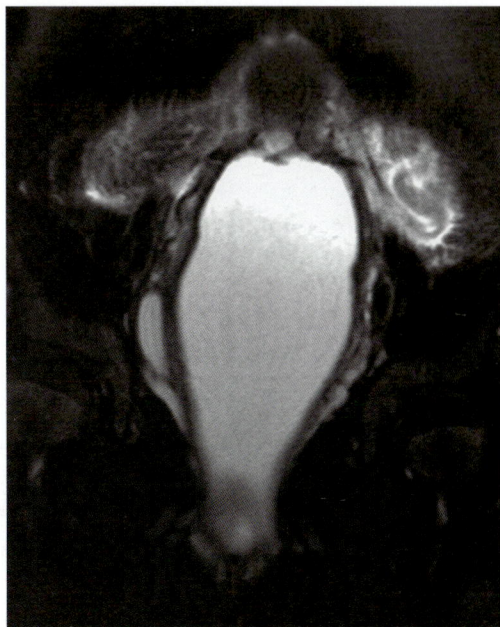

A

B

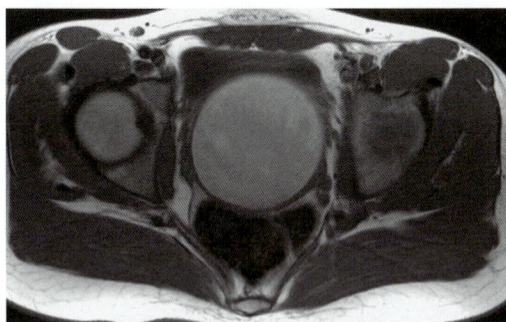

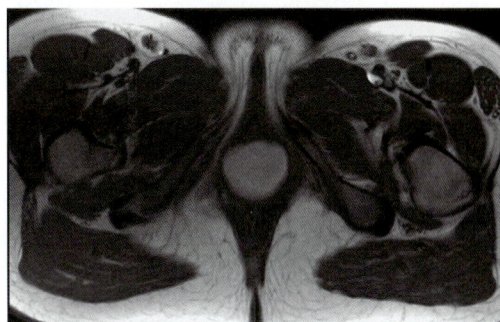

C

D

A. Sagittal T2-weighted FSE/TSE. **B**. Coronal T2-weighted FSE/TSE with fat saturation. **C**, **D**. Axial T1-weighted spin echo (**D** obtained at level inferior to **C**).

Case 108 Hematocolpos Caused by Imperforate Hymen

Findings

▶ Marked distention of the vagina with fluid that displays high signal intensity on both T1- and T2-weighted images consistent with hemorrhagic material. The fluid shows no signal loss with fat suppression. The fluid bulges at the introitus.
▶ The normal-appearing uterus is displaced far superiorly.
▶ Normal-appearing ovaries were confirmed on other images (not shown).

Differential diagnosis

▶ Vaginal septum
▶ Vaginal hypoplasia

Teaching points

▶ Imperforate hymen is a rare but easily curable cause of primary amenorrhea. It is the most common genital outflow anomaly.
▶ Patients typically present with cyclical abdominal and pelvic pain and swelling when menstruating, with menstrual fluid trapped within the closed-off vagina.
▶ Normal onset of puberty and development of secondary sex characteristics are evidence of normal ovarian function.
▶ The lower third of the uterus develops from the urogenital sinus while the upper two thirds of the vagina, the uterus, fallopian tubes and ovaries develop from the müllerian duct system. Failure of fusion of the two systems, or failure of canalization of the vagina, may result in vaginal atresia, or longitudinal or transverse vaginal septa. The hymen may also be imperforate. Any of these conditions affecting the vagina but with normal development of the uterus and ovaries may result in distention of the vagina and/or uterus from filling with blood products from menstruation (hematocolpos or hematometrocolpos).

Management

▶ Hymenectomy is curative. Vaginal hypoplasia or atresia requires reconstructive surgery.

Further reading

1. Junqueira BLP, Allen LM, Spitzer RF, et al. Müllerian duct anomalies and mimics in children and adolescents: correlative intra-operative assessment with clinical imaging. RadioGraphics 2009;29:1085–1103.
2. Oppelt P, von Have M, Paulsen M, et al. Female genital malformations and their associated anomalies. Fertil Steril 2007;87:335–342.

History

▶ 32-year-old woman with of recurrent spontaneous first-trimester abortions

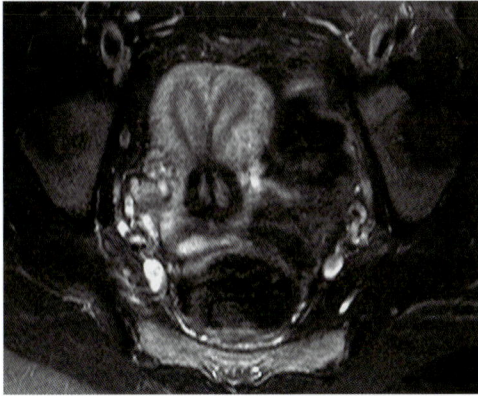

A

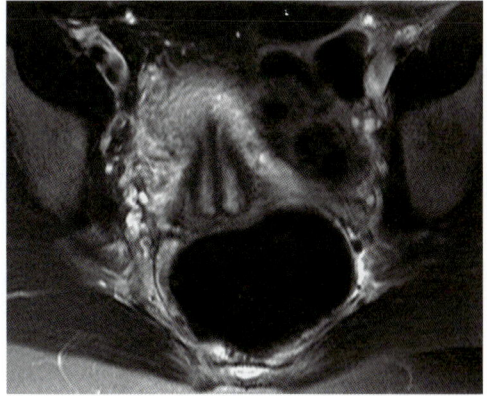

B

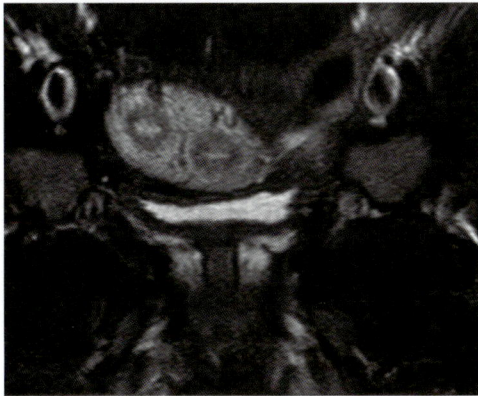

C

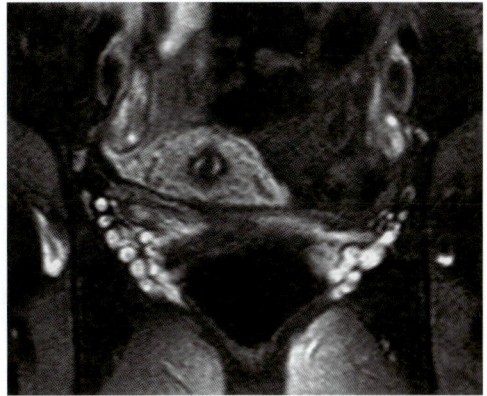

D

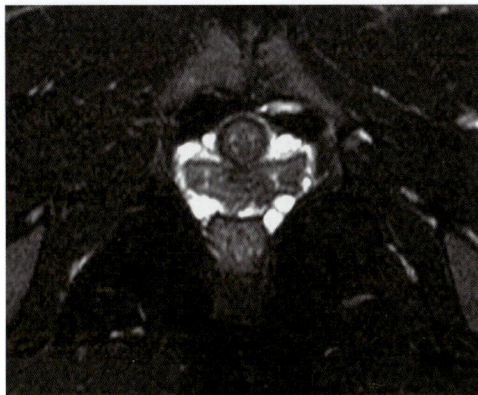

E

A, **B**. Axial oblique T2-weighted FSE/TSE with fat saturation. Image **B** was obtained a few slices inferior to **A**. **C**, **D**. Coronal oblique T2-weighted FSE/TSE with fat saturation. Image **D** was obtained a few slices posterior to **C**. **E.** Axial T2-weighted FSE/TSE with fat saturation.

Case 109 Septate Uterus

Findings

▶ The uterus is normal in size and has a normal external contour (**A**).
▶ On T2-weighted images a low-signal-intensity vertical septum extends through the uterine body, cervix and upper two thirds of the vagina.
▶ The ovaries and kidneys are normal.
▶ The lower vagina and urethra are normal (**E**).

Differential diagnosis

▶ The normal size and external contour with a midline vertical band is diagnostic of a septate uterus.

Teaching points

▶ The normal external contour excludes bicornuate or didelphys uterus.
▶ The septum may variably extend through the uterine body, cervix and vagina. In a septate uterus, the low-signal vertical band through the uterine body and cervix is fibrous tissue, not myometrium.
▶ Bicornuate and septated uterus are not associated with urinary tract anomalies.
▶ Surgical repair of a bicornuate or didelphys uterus involves transabdominal metroplasty.

Management

▶ A septate uterus is treated by transvaginal hysteroscopic resection of the septum to avoid subsequent spontaneous abortions.

Further reading

1. DeAngelis GA. Gynecologic MR imaging. In: Brant WE, de Lange EE (Eds), Essentials of Body MRI. New York: Oxford University Press, 2012.
2. Imaoka I, Wada A, Matsuo M, et al. MR imaging of disorders associated with female infertility: Use in diagnosis, treatment, and management. RadioGraphics 2003;23:1401–1421.

History

▸ 12-year-old boy with impaired renal function

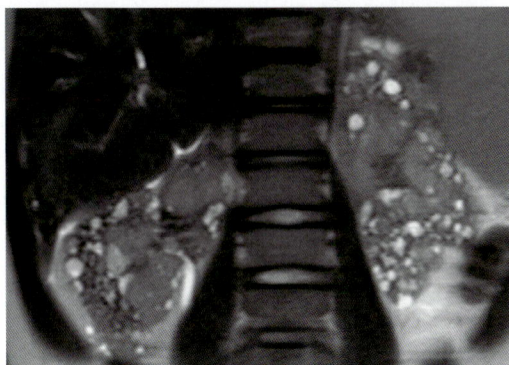

A

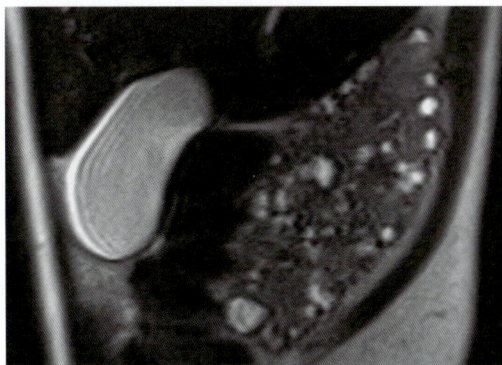

B

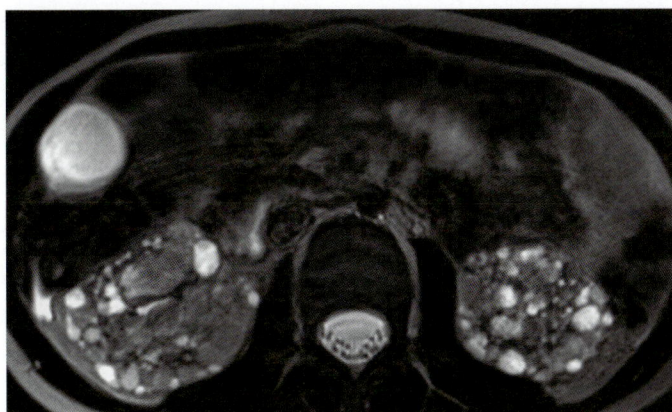

C

A. Coronal and (**B**) sagittal T2-weighted single-shot FSE/TSE. **C**. Axial T2-weighted FSE/TSE.

Case 110   Autosomal Recessive Polycystic Kidney Disease (ARPKD)

Findings

- ▶ Innumerable small cysts within enlarged bilateral kidneys
- ▶ Cysts demonstrate high signal intensity on T2-weighted images and the cyst walls are thin.
- ▶ The cyst walls did not enhance on gadolinium contrast-enhanced images (not shown).

Differential diagnosis

- ▶ Autosomal dominant polycystic kidney disease (ADPKD)
- ▶ Bilateral multicystic dysplastic kidney (MCDK)
- ▶ Tuberous sclerosis
- ▶ Beckwith-Wiedemann syndrome
- ▶ Trisomy 13
- ▶ Meckel-Gruber syndrome

Teaching points

- ▶ ARPKD is caused by a mutation in polycystic kidney and hepatic disease 1 (PKHD1) that results in dilatation of the distal collecting tubules.
- ▶ The majority of patients are identified in utero or at birth. Patients present with enlarged echogenic kidneys and oligohydramnios, which may result in pulmonary hypoplasia.
- ▶ ARPKD can typically be differentiated from other polycystic kidney diseases on the basis of extrarenal manifestations of disease.
- ▶ Perinatal, neonatal, infantile and juvenile forms

Management

- ▶ Initial treatment focuses on optimizing the respiratory status, including the use of mechanical ventilation.
- ▶ Oliguric or anuric neonates may need peritoneal dialysis.
- ▶ Occasionally unilateral or bilateral nephrectomy may be required.

Further reading

1. Guay-Woodford LM, Desmond RA. Autosomal recessive polycystic kidney disease: the clinical experience in North America. Pediatrics 2003;111:1072–1080.
2. Lonergan GJ, Rice RR, Suarez ES. Autosomal recessive polycystic kidney disease: radiologic-pathologic correlation. RadioGraphics 2000;20:837–855.
3. Sweeney WE Jr, Avner ED. Diagnosis and management of childhood polycystic kidney disease. Pediatr Nephrol 2011;26:675–692.

History

▶ 56-year-old woman presents with worsening shortness of breath and chest pain.

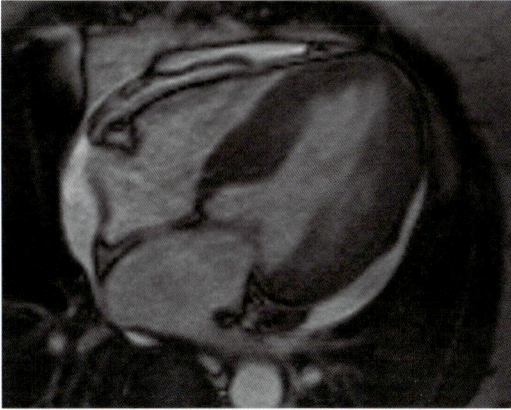

A

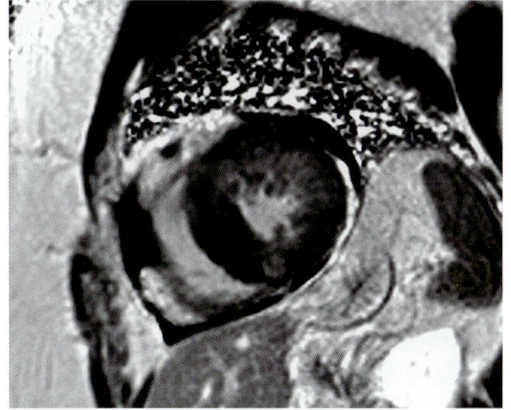

B

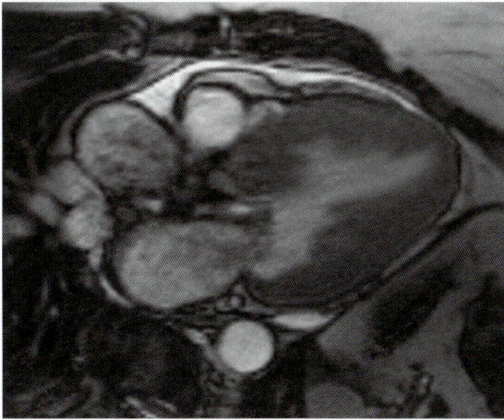

C

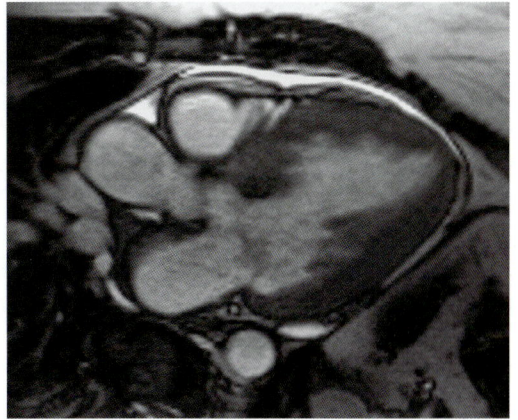

D

A. Horizontal long-axis (4-chamber) steady-state free precession (SSFP). **B**. Short-axis late gadolinium enhancement phase-sensitive inversion recovery (PSIR) gradient echo. **C**. Left ventricular outflow tract (3-chamber) SSFP in systole and (**D**) diastole.

Case 111   Hypertrophic Obstructive Cardiomyopathy

Findings:

- Asymmetric septal hypertrophy
- Left ventricular outflow tract (LVOT) turbulence
- Systolic anterior motion (SAM) of the anterior leaflet of the mitral valve
- Late gadolinium enhancement in a classic pattern at the insertion of the right ventricle on the left ventricle

Differential diagnosis

- Cardiac amyloidosis
- Concentric hypertrophy associated with hypertension or aortic stenosis
- Athlete's heart

Teaching points

- Hypertrophic cardiomyopathy (HCM) is the most common cause of cardiac death in young people. It is inherited as a Mendelian autosomal dominant trait.
- The key physiologic feature is diastolic dysfunction with impaired left ventricular filling and preserved systolic function. Systolic dysfunction is a late manifestation.
- Asymmetric septal hypertrophy is the most common phenotype of HCM. Left ventricular wall thickness >15 mm at end-diastole, or a >1.5 ratio of the septal thickness to inferior wall thickness at the mid-ventricle, is diagnostic of HCM.
- HCM can be classified as obstructive (HOCM) or nonobstructive based on whether there is a pressure gradient between the LVOT and the aorta at rest. Systolic anterior motion (SAM) of the mitral leaflet is a consequence of LVOT flow acceleration, often associated with mitral regurgitation.
- Predictors of sudden death include left ventricular (LV) wall thickness, LVOT obstruction, LV dilatation with depressed ejection fraction (burned-out phase), and the presence of fibrosis and perfusion defects.
- Subepicardial LV enhancement involving the anteroseptum and inferoseptum, at the insertion of the right ventricle, is the classic pattern of late gadolinium enhancement in septal HCM.

Management

- The goal of treatment is to control symptoms and prevent complications. Treatment includes medications and often an implantable cardioverter defibrillator.

Further reading

1. Chun EJ, Choi SI, Jin KN, et al. Hypertrophic cardiomyopathy: assessment with MR imaging and multidetector CT. RadioGraphics 2010;30:1309–1328.
2. Norton P. Cardiac MR imaging. In: Brant WE, de Lange EE (Eds), Essentials of body MR Imaging. New York: Oxford University Press, 2012.

History

▶ 71-year-old woman presents with right upper quadrant pain and dark urine.

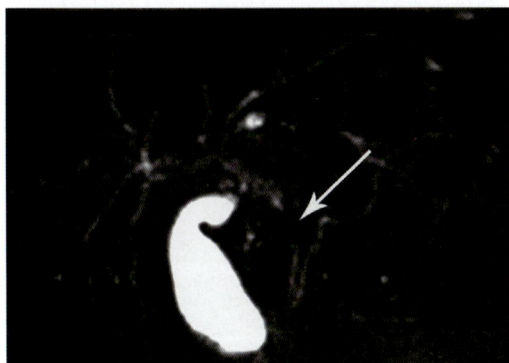

A

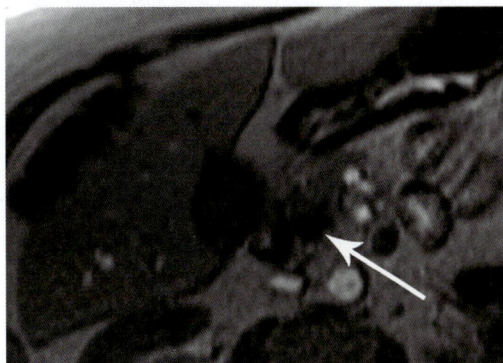

B

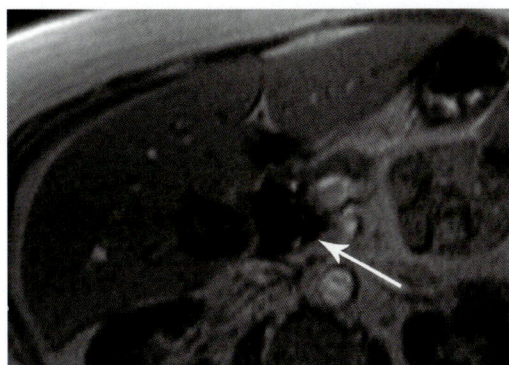

C

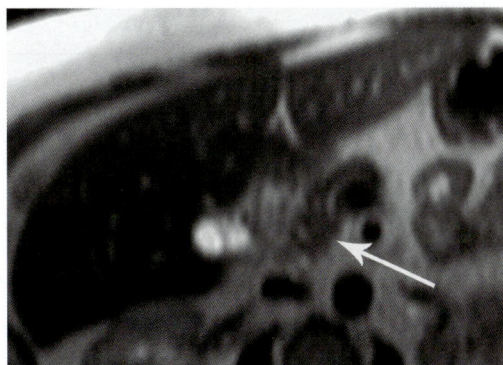

D

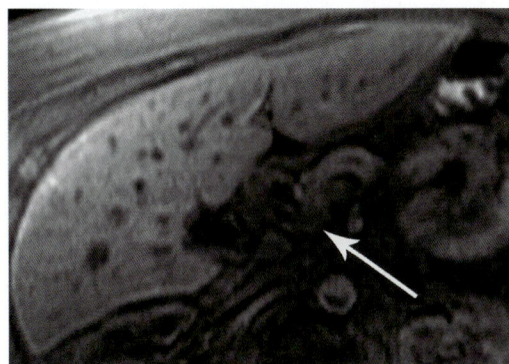

E

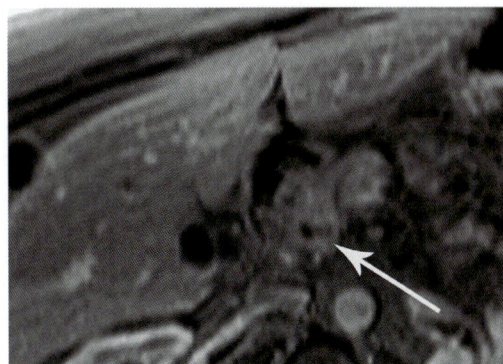

F

A. MRCP using thick-slab single-shot FSE/TSE with fat suppression. **B, C**. Axial magnetization-prepared T1-weighted gradient echo (**B** was obtained slightly lower than **C**). **D**. Axial T2-weighted single-shot FSE/TSE. **E**. Axial T1-weighted pre-enhanced and (**F**) post-gadolinium contrast-enhanced T1-weighted gradient echo with fat saturation.

Case 112 Cholangiocarcinoma Involving the Distal Common Bile Duct within the Pancreatic Head

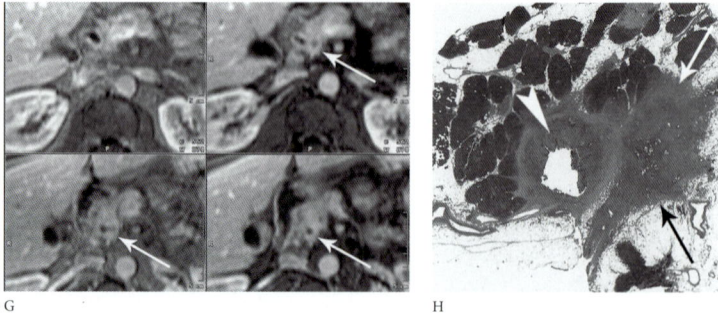

G

H

Findings

- ▶ MRCP (**A**) shows an abrupt stricture (*arrow*) in the common bile duct (CBD).
- ▶ T1–weighted images (**B, C**) show low signal intensity around the distal biliary duct stricture, indicating both tumor (*arrows*). T2-weighted image (**D**) shows iso-intensity in the region of the tumor (*arrow*).
- ▶ Pre-contrast-enhanced T1-weighted image (**E**) shows low signal intensity of the tumor (*arrow*). Post-contrast-enhanced images (**F**) show enhancement of the tumor around the CBD (*arrows*) within the pancreatic head with increasing enhancement on delayed image (**G**)..
- ▶ Pathologic specimen (**H**) matched to axial images shows the tumor (*arrowhead*) surrounding the common bile duct and extension into adjacent pancreatic tissue (*arrows*).
- ▶ Histologic diagnosis was poorly differentiated adenocarcinoma. When poorly differentiated, distinction between pancreatic and cholangiocarcinoma cannot be made histologically and final diagnosis of tumor type is based on imaging features.

Differential diagnosis

- ▶ Pancreatic adenocarcinoma
- ▶ Benign, inflammatory, stricture

Teaching points

- ▶ Cholangiocarcinoma arises in the extrahepatic bile duct in 20% to 25% of cases. The majority (65%) of patients are over age 65. Most (95%) cholangiocarcinomas are adenocarcinomas classified and graded according to the percentage of tumor that is composed of glandular tissue. Histologic grade and stage of disease are critical prognostic factors.
- ▶ MR imaging with MR cholangiography and dynamic gadolinium contrast-enhanced images provides comprehensive evaluation. Intraductal tumors are hypo- to iso-intense compared to normal liver parenchyma on T1-weighted images with variable but often slightly hyperintense signal intensity on T2-weighted images. Enhancement of cholangiocarcinoma on dynamic post-gadolinium contrast-enhanced images is mild on early-phase images with peak enhancement on delayed-phase images.

Management

- ▶ Surgery is the only curative treatment. The patient's suitability for surgery is determined by the tumor extent, the presence of distant metastases and medical risk factors.

Further reading

1. Khan SA, Davidson BR, Goldin R, et al. Guidelines for the diagnosis and treatment of cholangiocarcinoma: consensus document. Gut 2002;1:1–9.
2. Sainani NI, Catalano OA, Holalkere N-S, et al. Cholangiocarcinoma: current and novel imaging techniques. RadioGraphics 2008;28:1263–1287.

History

▶ 39-year-old woman with painful menses

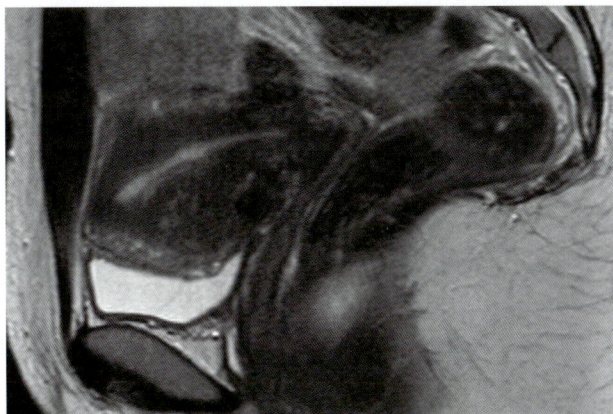

A

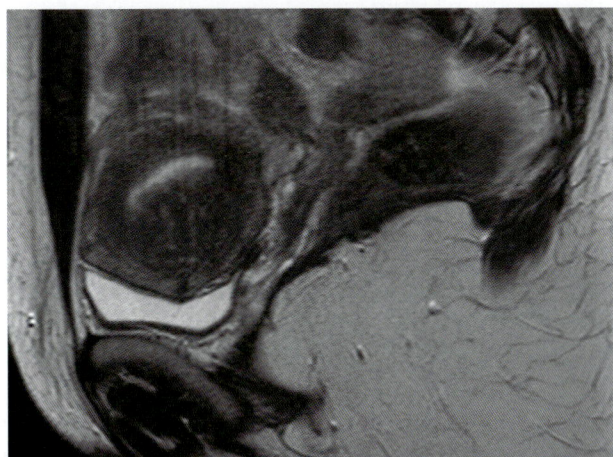

B

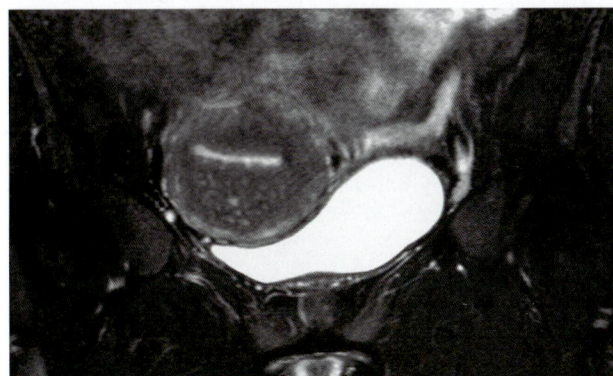

C

A, **B**. Consecutive sagittal T2-weighted FSE/TSE. **C**. Coronal T2-weighted FSE/TSE with fat saturation.

Case 113 Adenomyosis of the Uterus

Findings

- ▶ T2-weighted MR images show a bulky uterus with asymmetric and irregular thickening of the low-signal-intensity junctional-zone myometrium.
- ▶ There is an ill-defined low-signal-intensity mass causing asymmetric thickening of the posterior wall of the uterus. Within the mass are multiple small round and oval high-signal-intensity foci.
- ▶ Adenomyosis of the uterus was confirmed at hysterectomy.

Differential diagnosis

- ▶ Leiomyoma
- ▶ Leiomyosarcoma
- ▶ Stromal sarcoma

Teaching points

- ▶ Adenomyosis of the uterus is characterized by invasion of benign endometrium into the adjacent junctional-zone myometrium. The inflammation induced by periodic bleeding results in myometrial hypertrophy and fibrosis.
- ▶ Associated symptoms include dysmenorrhea, menorrhagia, pelvic pain, and abnormal uterine bleeding. The typical patient is multiparous, over the age of 30, and premenopausal.
- ▶ Adenomyosis may be diffuse or focal. Myometrial hyperplasia enlarges the uterus focally or diffusely. Islands of ectopic endometrium with associated blood products are irregularly distributed within the thickened fibrotic muscle. Malignant transformation of the ectopic endometrium may occur but is rare.
- ▶ MR has high sensitivity and specificity for diagnosis of adenomyosis. T2-weighted images show characteristic findings of ill-defined low-signal-intensity areas bordering the uterine cavity representing hypertrophied fibrotic myometrium with numerous small foci of high signal intensity representing the ectopic endometrium. Hemorrhagic foci associated with the ectopic endometrium show as high-signal-intensity, 1- to 3-mm lesions on T1-weighted images owing to the presence of methemoglobin. Hemosiderin content typically shows the lesions with low signal intensity on T2-weighted images. Gadolinium contrast enhancement of adenomyosis is variable and does not add to the diagnosis.

Management

- ▶ Treatment options include anti-inflammatory drugs, hormones, and hysterectomy.

Further reading

1. Takeuchi M, Matsuzaki K. Adenomyosis: usual and unusual imaging manifestations, pitfalls, and problem-solving MR imaging techniques. RadioGraphics 2011;31:99–115.
2. Tamai K, Togashi K, Ito T, et al. MR imaging findings of adenomyosis: correlation with histopathologic features and diagnostic pitfalls. RadioGraphics 2005;25:21–40.

History

▶ 65-year-old man with history of liver and kidney transplant and bilateral nephrectomies

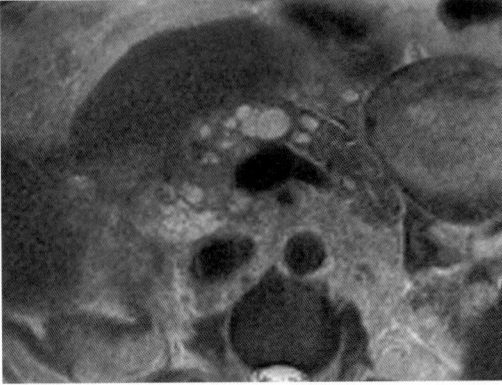
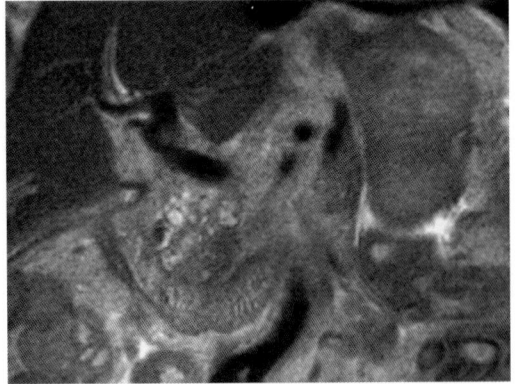

A

B

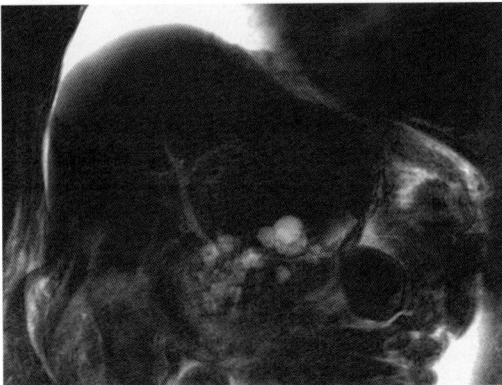
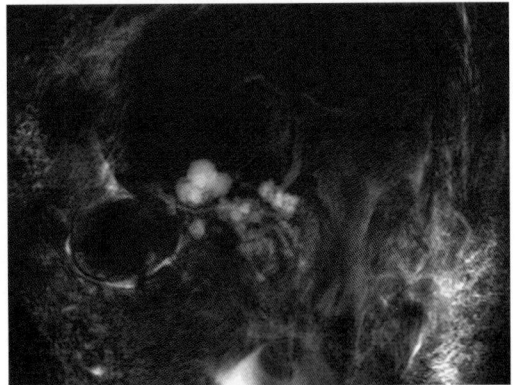

C

D

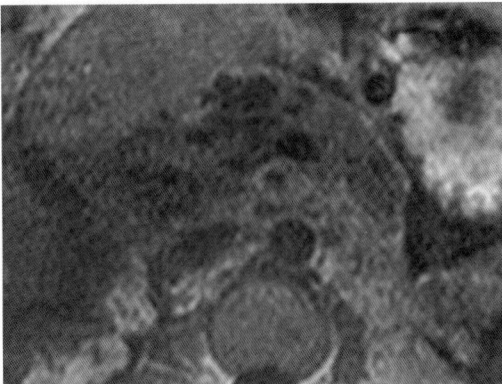
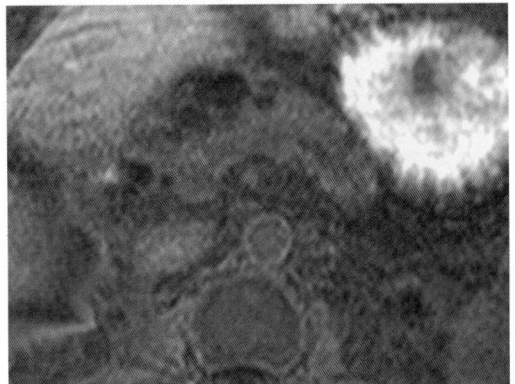

E

F

A. Axial and (**B**) coronal T2-weighted single-shot FSE/TSE. **C**. Coronal and (**D**) oblique coronal MRCP using thick-slab single-shot FSE/TSE with fat saturation. **E**. Axial T1-weighted gradient echo. **F**. Axial 20-minute-delayed post-gadolinium contrast-enhanced T1-weighted gradient echo with fat saturation.

Case 114 Autosomal Dominant Polycystic Disease (ADPCD) Affecting the Pancreas

Findings

▶ Multiple simple-appearing pancreatic cysts of varying size are seen throughout the pancreas.

▶ The cysts contain simple fluid, displaying high signal intensity on T2-weighted images and low signal intensity on T1-weighted images.

▶ The cysts show no significant enhancement.

▶ The patient has undergone liver transplant for liver failure resulting from extensive polycystic liver disease and had a renal transplant for kidney failure. The polycystic kidneys were removed because of their large size.

Differential diagnosis

▶ von Hippel-Lindau syndrome

Teaching points

▶ With the increasing life expectancy of patients with autosomal dominant polycystic kidney disease, the extrarenal manifestations become more clinically relevant. Approximately 10% of patients develop cysts in their pancreas. Other organs affected with cysts include the liver, seminal vesicles, and arachnoid membrane. Additional abnormalities include intracranial aneurysms, dilatation of the aortic root, dissection of the thoracic aorta, mitral valve prolapse, and abdominal wall hernias.

▶ The pancreatic cysts associated with autosomal dominant polycystic disease are simple congenital cysts with thin walls lined by benign epithelium. Internal fluid is simple. Similar cysts may also be present in association with von Hippel-Lindau disease. These cysts are generally classified as "true pancreatic cysts."

▶ The presence of pancreatic cysts in ADPCD seldom affects pancreatic exocrine or endocrine function. Complications are rare, with isolated reports of pancreatic duct obstruction and recurrent pancreatitis, and there is an association with intraductal papillary mucinous neoplasms.

Management

▶ No specific treatment is generally indicated.

Further reading

1. Mosetti MA, Leonardou P, Motohara T, et al. Autosomal dominant polycystic kidney disease: MR imaging evaluation using current techniques. J Magn Reson Imag 2003;18:210–215.
2. Perrone RD, Ruthazer R, Terrin NC. Survival after end-stage renal disease in autosomal dominant polycystic kidney disease: contribution of extrarenal complications to mortality. Am J Kidney Dis 2001;38:777–784.
3. Pirson Y. Extrarenal manifestations of autosomal dominant polycystic kidney disease. Adv Chronic Kidney Dis 2010;17:173–180.

History

▶ 76-year-old man with gross hematuria

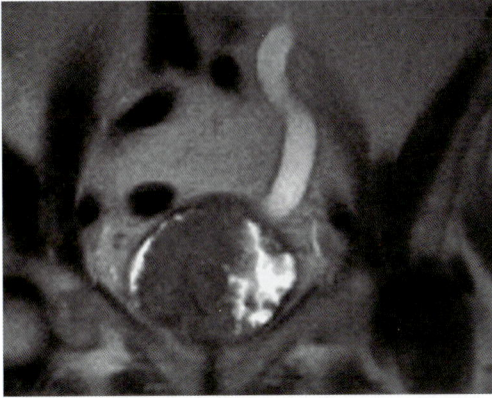

A

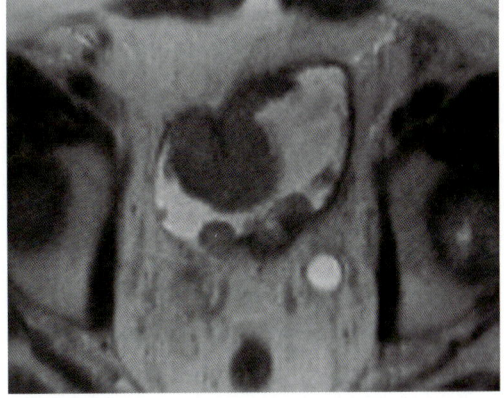

B

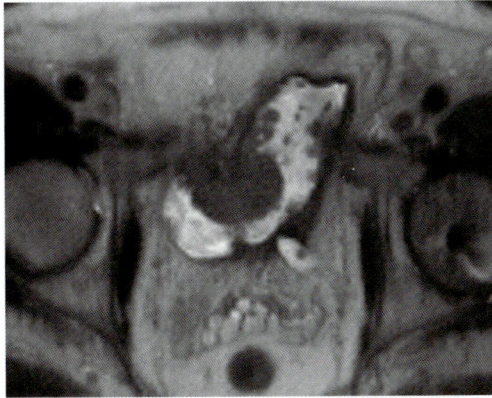

C

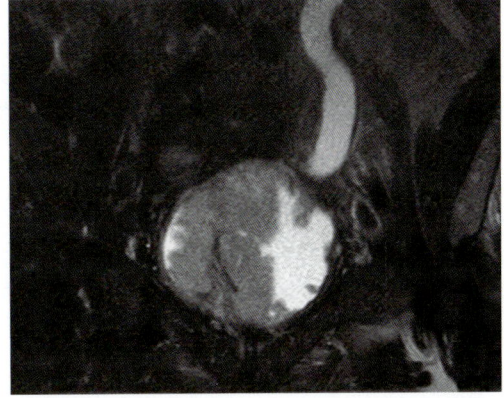

D

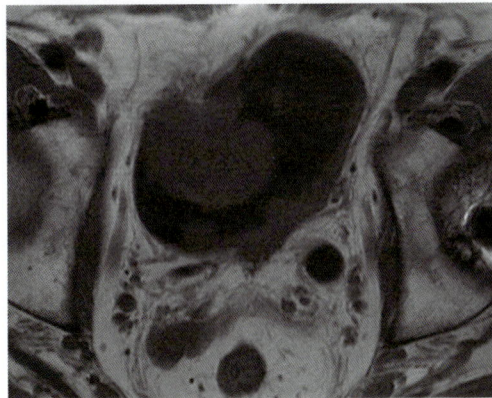

E

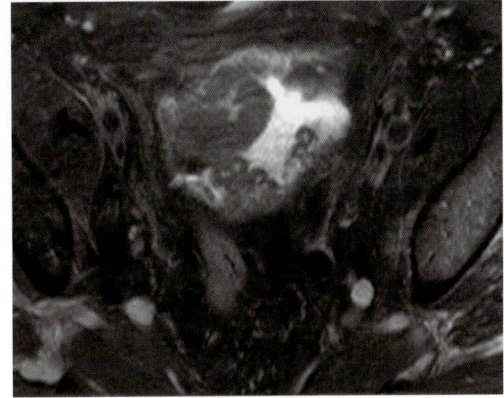

F

A. Coronal, and (**B**, **C**) axial T2-weighted single-shot FSE/TSE. (image **D** is at level slightly caudad to **B**). **D**. Coronal T2-weighted FSE/TSE with fat saturation. **E**. Axial T1-weighted spin echo. **F**. Axial post-gadolinium contrast-enhanced T1-weighted spin echo with fat saturation.

Case 115 Multifocal Papillary Transitional Cell Carcinoma of the Bladder, Grade II–IV

Findings

▶ Numerous polypoid soft-tissue nodules of varying size are seen carpeting the bladder wall.
▶ The tumor involves the left ureterovesicular junction, causing obstruction and hydronephrosis of the left ureter.
▶ The tumor extends through the bladder wall.
▶ The tumor displays intermediate low signal intensity on T1- and T2-weighted images and shows little gadolinium contrast enhancement.

Differential diagnosis

▶ Mesenchymal tumors: leiomyoma, leiomyosarcoma, rhabdomyoma
▶ Lymphoma
▶ Paraganglioma

Teaching points

▶ Bladder cancers most frequently present with gross or microscopic hematuria, urinary urgency and frequency, or, rarely, symptoms of metastatic disease. At presentation 75% of patients have localized disease, 20% have regionally advanced disease, and 5% have distant metastatic disease. Types of urothelial carcinomas include transitional cell (95%), squamous cell (4%), and adenocarcinoma (1%).
▶ Imaging is vital in determining the extent of disease, which determines the appropriate treatment. Examination of the renal collecting system, pelvis, and entire ureter is important because 2% to 3% of patients with bladder cancer have a concomitant urothelial cancer of the upper tracts.
▶ The treating urologist needs to know the location and extent of the primary tumor, and whether there is hydronephrosis, lymph node involvement, or tumor invasion into contiguous organs.

Management

▶ Diagnosis of bladder cancer is made by cystoscopy and biopsy. Imaging is important in the detection, staging, and surveillance of urothelial cancers.

Further reading

1. Bharwani N, Stephens NJ, Heenan SD. Imaging of bladder cancer. Imaging 2008;20:97–111.
2. Lee EK, Dickstein RJ, Kamat AM. Imaging of urothelial cancers: What the urologist needs to know. AJR Am J Roentgenol 2011;196:1249–1254.
3. Wong-You-Cheung JJ, Woodward PJ, Manning MA, Sesterhenn IA. Neoplasms of the urinary bladder: radiologic-pathologic correlation. RadioGraphics 2006;26:553–580.

History

► 47-year-old woman with abdominal pain

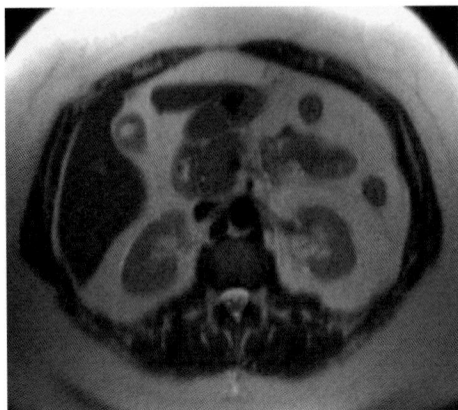

A

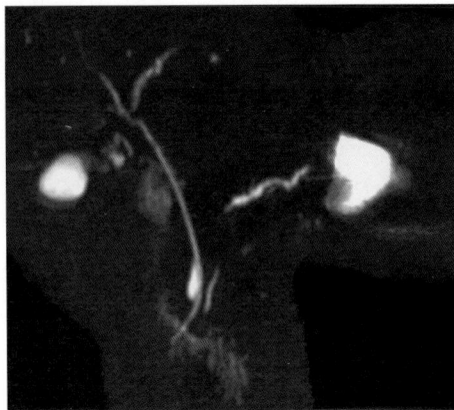

B

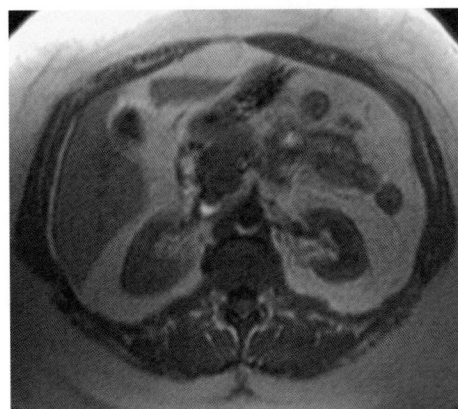

C

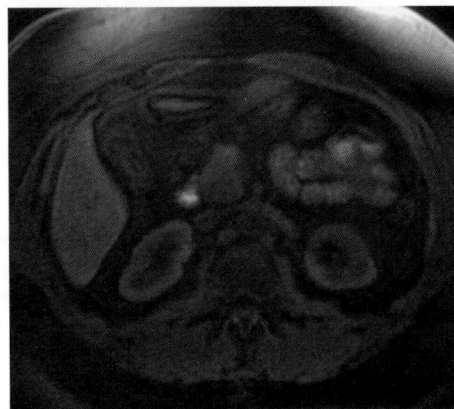

D

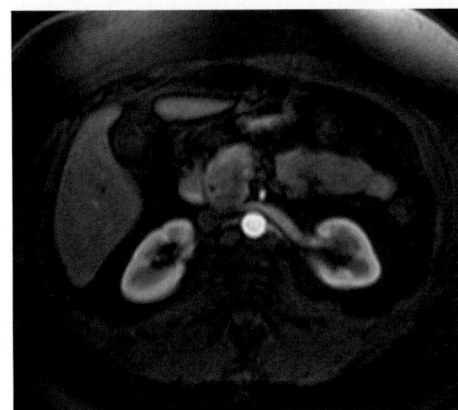

E

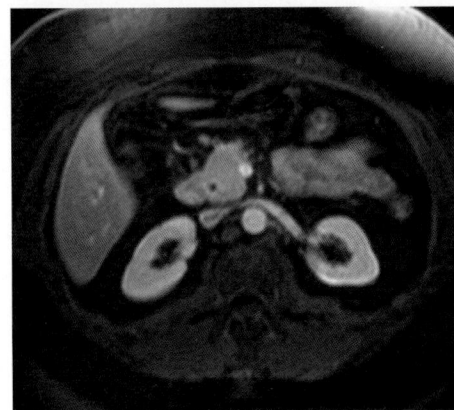

F

A. Axial T2-weighted single-shot FSE/TSE. **B**. MRCP using single-shot FSE/TSE with fat suppression. **C**. Axial T1-weighted gradient echo.
D. Pre-contrast-enhanced and (**E**) early- and (**F**) late-phase gadolinium contrast-enhanced T1-weighted gradient echo with fat saturation.

Case 116   Autoimmune Pancreatitis (AIP), Focal Type

Findings

▶ Solid pancreatic head mass showing decreased signal intensity on T1-weighted images compared to normal pancreas, slightly increased signal on T2-weighted images, hypo-enhancement on early-phase and homogenous enhancement on delayed-phase contrast enhancement.

▶ Narrowing of the common bile duct (CBD) and pancreatic duct (CBD stent is in place).

Differential diagnosis

▶ Ductal adenocarcinoma

Teaching points

▶ AIP is a distinct type of chronic pancreatitis, accounting for 2% to 11% of cases, characterized by an autoimmune inflammatory process, with lymphoplasmacytic infiltration and fibrosis.

▶ Is more than twice as common in men than in women; mean age is approximately 60 years.

▶ Extrapancreatic manifestations include sclerosing cholangitis, primary biliary cirrhosis, inflammatory bowel disease, Sjögren syndrome, sialadenitis, and retroperitoneal fibrosis.

▶ Clinical presentation includes jaundice, abdominal pain, weight loss, and diabetes mellitus. The classic acute attack of pancreatitis or severe abdominal pain is unusual.

▶ Serum amylase and lipase levels are usually normal or mildly elevated.

▶ Gamma globulin, total IgG, and IgG4 are often elevated; IgG4 is most sensitive and specific.

▶ There are three patterns of AIP:
  - *Diffuse*: most common, diffusely enlarged sausage-like pancreas with narrowing and irregularity of the main pancreatic duct, presence of a capsule-like rim believed to represent fluid, phlegmon, or fibrous tissue. Calcifications and pseudocysts are rare.
  - Focal: usually in the head, may mimic malignancy, is relatively well demarcated, may cause obstruction of the pancreatic and CBD.
  - Multifocal (rare)

▶ MRI features that may help differentiate AIP from cancer: slightly decreased early enhancement compared to the adjacent normal pancreatic tissue, homogeneous delayed enhancement, hypointense capsule-like rim, absence of upstream parenchymal atrophy, main pancreatic duct upstream dilatation ≤4 mm

Management

▶ Biopsy if imaging and laboratory criteria are nonconclusive.

▶ Corticosteroid therapy is usually highly effective.

Further readings

1. Law R, Bronner M, Vogt D, Stevens T. Autoimmune pancreatitis: a mimic of pancreatic cancer. Cleve Clin J Med 2009;76:607–615.
2. Shanbhogue AK, Fasih, N, Sarabhi VR, et al. A clinical and radiologic review of uncommon types and causes of pancreatitis. RadioGraphics 2009;29:1003–1026.
3. Vlachou PA, Khalili K, Jang H-J, et al. IgG4-related sclerosing disease: autoimmune pancreatitis and extrapancreatic manifestations. RadioGraphics 2011;31:1379–1402.

History

► 82-year-old woman with recent onset of vaginal bleeding

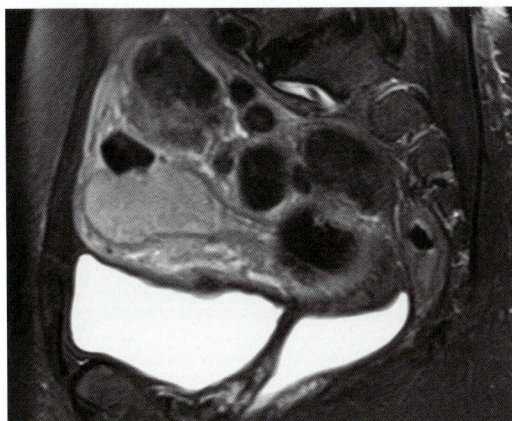

A

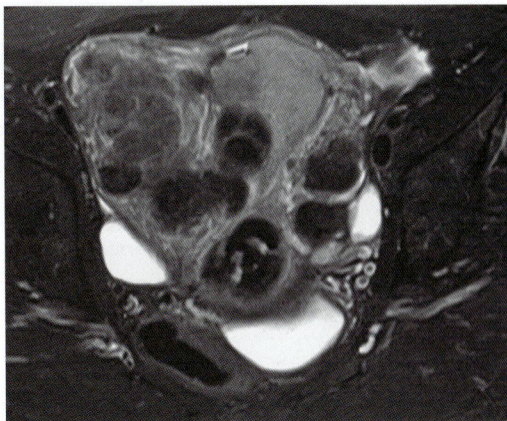

B

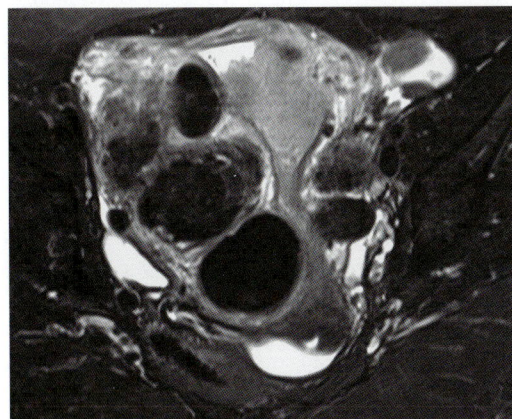

C

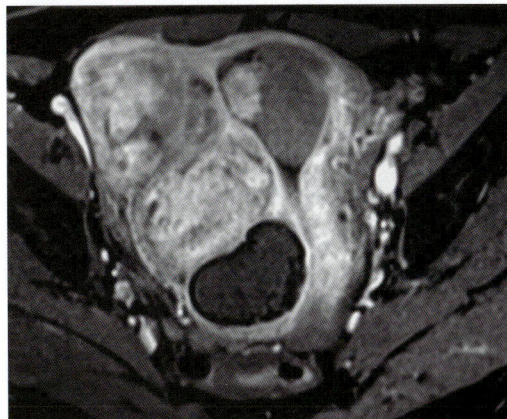

D

A. Sagittal and (**B**, **C**) para-axial T2-weighted FSE/TSE with fat suppression at different levels. **D**. Axial post-contrast-enhanced T1-weighted gradient echo with fat suppression.

Case 117 Endometrioid adenocarcinoma of the uterus

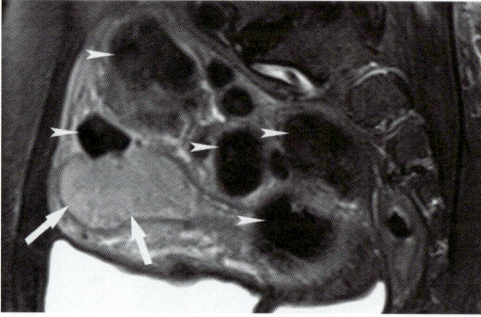

E

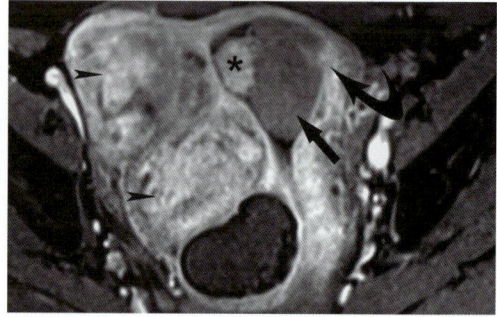

F

Findings

▶ A large polypoid mass (*arrows* in **E, F**) is present within the uterine canal arising from the left endometrial lining and distending the uterine cavity.

▶ Intramural masses (*arrowheads* in **E, F**) displaying low signal intensity on T2-weighted images are diagnostic of leiomyomas. The leiomyomas show variable contrast enhancement.

▶ The thin-section dynamic post-contrast-enhanced images optimally show superficial myometrial invasion (*curved arrow* in **F**) as a discontinuity of subendometrial enhancement with focal spiculation. Part of the mass demonstrates more avid enhancement (*).

Differential diagnosis

▶ Large endometrial polyp with or without malignancy

▶ Endometrial hyperplasia is unlikely given the focality of the mass and age of the patient.

Teaching points

▶ A large intraendometrial mass with myometrial invasion favors endometrial neoplasm. A higher-grade neoplasm is more likely given the patient's age and the degree of distention of the uterine canal. A large intraendometrial mass with only superficial invasion favors endometrioid adenocarcinoma or uterine papillary serous carcinoma.

▶ Diagnosis of leiomyomas is made on their typical low-signal-intensity appearance on T2-weighted images, not their appearance on post-contrast-enhanced images.

▶ Dynamic contrast-enhanced imaging demonstrates differential enhancement between the cancer and myometrium and can better detect subtle myometrial invasion. Necrosis and fluid are also better delineated.

Management

▶ The clear cell and papillary serous carcinomas are tumors with aggressive cell types, spread like ovarian cancer, and are commonly metastatic when detected. The papillary serous carcinoma is likely to have extrauterine spread with little myometrial invasion, and therefore imaging for metastases is important for management.

Further reading

1. Faratian D, Stillie A, Busby-Earle RM, et al. A review of the pathology and management of uterine papillary serous carcinoma and correlation with outcome. Int J Gynecol Cancer 2006;16:972–978.

History

▶ 45-year-old woman with AIDS presents to the emergency department with right upper quadrant pain. Ultrasound showed marked thickening of the gallbladder wall. Cluster of differentiation (CD4) T-lymphocyte count was 12 cells/mm³. MR was requested for further evaluation.

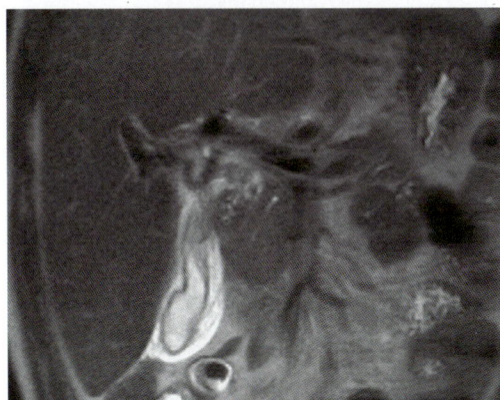

A

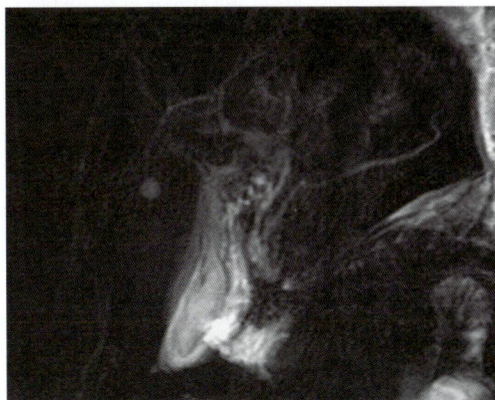

B

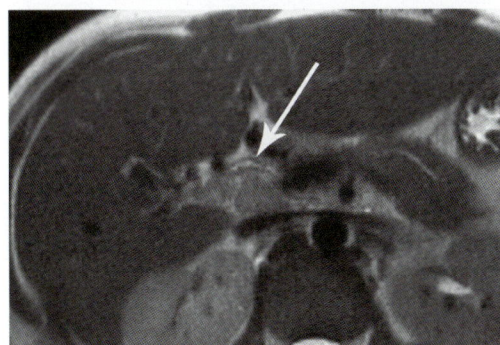

C

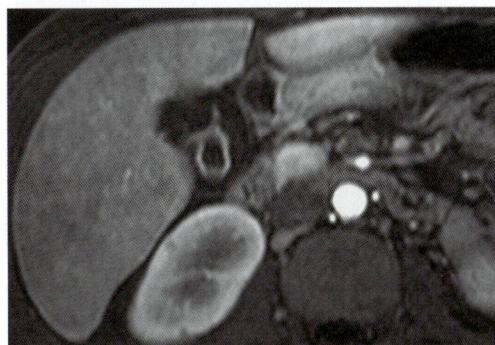

D

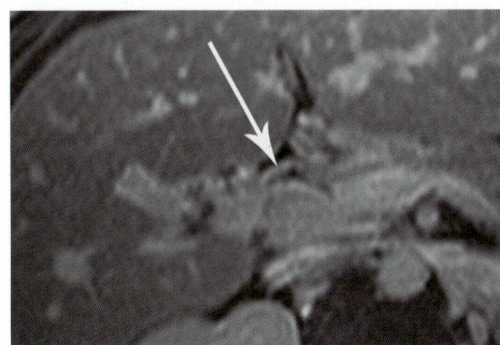

E

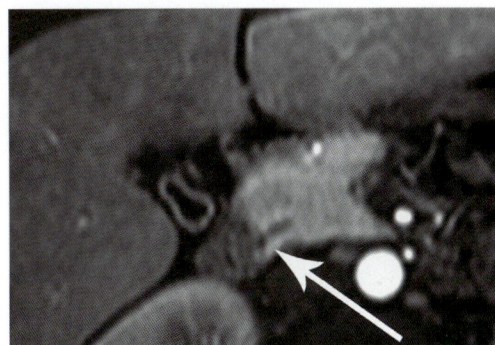

F

A. Coronal T2-weighted single-shot FSE/TSE**. B**. Thick-slab MRCP using single-shot FSE/TSE. **C**. Axial T2-weighted single-shot FSE/TSE. **D**. Axial arterial-phase T1-weighted post-gadolinium contrast-enhanced T1-weighted gradient echo with fat saturation. **E**. Axial late-phase contrast-enhanced image obtained at same level as **C**. **F**. Axial early-phase contrast-enhanced image. Arrows indicate the common bile duct.

Case 118   Acalculous Cholecystitis and AIDS Cholangiopathy

Findings

- ▶ Marked pericholecystic edema with thickening of the gallbladder wall and compression of the gallbladder lumen
- ▶ No evidence of gallstones
- ▶ Mild nodular thickening and enhancement of the wall of the common bile duct
- ▶ Cytomegalovirus was obtained from biliary washings.

Differential diagnosis

- ▶ Sclerosing cholangitis
- ▶ Pyogenic cholangitis

Teaching points

- ▶ HIV infection commonly involves the liver, biliary tree, and pancreas with complicating opportunistic infections. Manifestations include acalculous cholecystitis, papillary stenosis, biliary strictures, periportal lymphadenopathy, and acute and chronic pancreatitis. Opportunistic infections involve a broad array of fungal, protozoan, bacterial, and viral organisms. Common organisms include *Cryptosporidium parvum*, cytomegalovirus, *Mycobacterium avium* complex, and herpes simplex virus. HIV cholangiopathy occurs most frequently when the patient's CD4 T-lymphocyte count is below 100/mm^3. Additional complications include Kaposi sarcoma and peliosis hepatis.
- ▶ MR findings of HIV/AIDS cholangiopathy resemble those of sclerosing cholangitis. Findings include irregular thickening and enhancement of the wall of the common bile duct and the intrahepatic bile ducts, acalculous cholecystitis with thickening and enhancement of the gallbladder wall, long-segment strictures of the extrahepatic bile duct, and papillary stenosis.

Management

- ▶ Treatment options include sphincterotomy, dilation of biliary strictures, and bile duct stent placement. Ganciclovir is used to treat cytomegalovirus infection. Antiretroviral protocols are used to treat HIV infection.

Further reading

1. Bilgin M, Balci NC, Erdogan A, et al. Hepatobiliary and pancreatic MRI and MRCP findings in patients with HIV infection. AJR Am J Roentgenol 2008;191:228–232.

History

► 75-year-old woman with abdominal and back pain

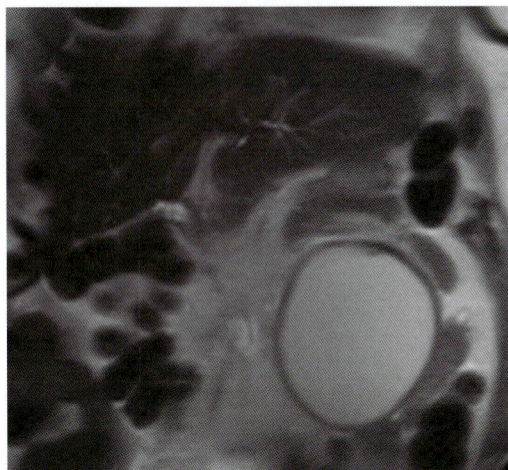

A

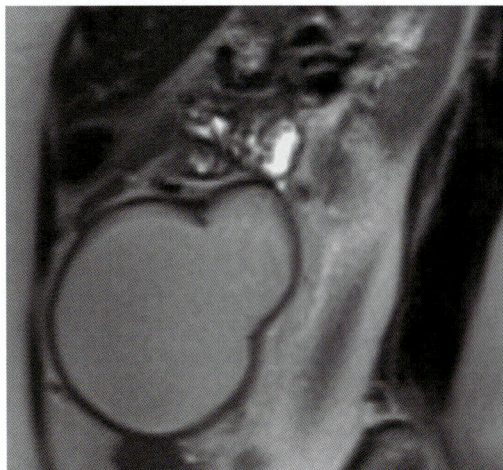

B

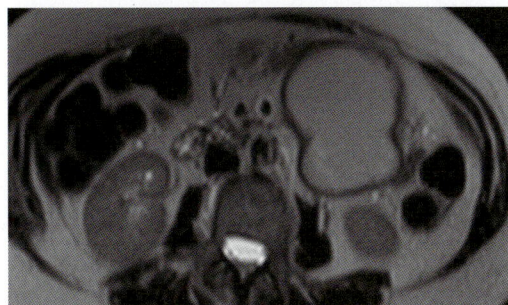

C

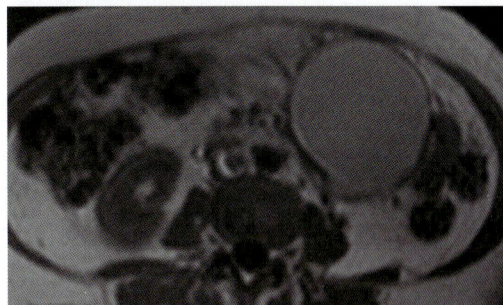

D

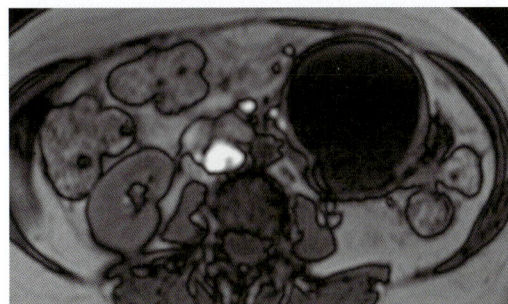

E

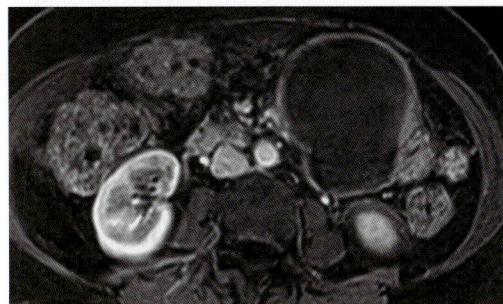

F

A. Coronal, (**B**) sagittal, and (**C**) axial T2-weighted single-shot FSE/TSE. **D**. Axial in-phase and (**E**) out-of-phase T1-weighted gradient echo. **F**. Axial T1-weighted gradient echo with fat saturation.

Case 119 Enteric Duplication Cyst

Findings

▶ Well-defined cystic mass with uniform wall thickness displaces small bowel, consistent with location in the small bowel mesentery.

▶ The mass shows intermediate high internal signal intensity on T1-weighted image (**D**) and high internal signal intensity on T2-weighted images (**A–C**).

▶ Post-contrast-enhanced image (**F**) shows enhancement of the wall of the cyst but no internal enhancement.

▶ Marked loss of signal is seen on out-of-phase image (**E**) compared to in-phase image (**D**), indicating that the cyst fluid contents consist of both water and fat.

▶ The diagnosis was confirmed at surgery.

Differential diagnosis

▶ Mesenteric cyst or cystic lymphangioma of the mesentery
▶ Lymphocele
▶ Abscess
▶ Cystic mesothelioma

Teaching points

▶ Enteric duplication cysts contain all the layers of the normal intestinal wall, including mucosa, circular and longitudinal muscle, serosa, and mesenteric plexus. Ectopic gastric mucosa is present in 24% and ectopic pancreatic tissue is present in 8% of enteric duplication cysts.

▶ The cysts are typically unilocular and thick-walled. Contents are most commonly serous but may be chylous or hemorrhagic.

▶ The cysts most commonly involve the small bowel and are intimately attached to the bowel on the mesenteric side. The ileum and ileocecal region are involved more commonly than the jejunum (4:1). Surgical resection of the lesion shown in this case required en bloc resection of attached small bowel as well as the cystic mass and mesentery.

▶ Enteric duplication cysts may cause bowel obstruction (especially in the neonatal period), intussusception, and abdominal pain.

▶ Enteric cysts differ from enteric duplication in that the cysts are lined by enteric mucosa but not all the layers of the intestinal wall.

Management

▶ Surgical resection is curative and confirms the diagnosis.

Further reading

1. de Perrot M, Brundler M, Totsch M, et al. Mesenteric cysts. Toward less confusion? Dig Surg 2000;17:323–328.
2. Stoupis C, Ros PR, Abbitt PL, et al. Bubbles in the belly: imaging of cystic mesenteric or omental masses. RadioGraphics 1994;14:729–737.

History

▶ 65-year-old man underwent MRI for echogenic lesion seen at the right renal cortex during ultrasound examination.

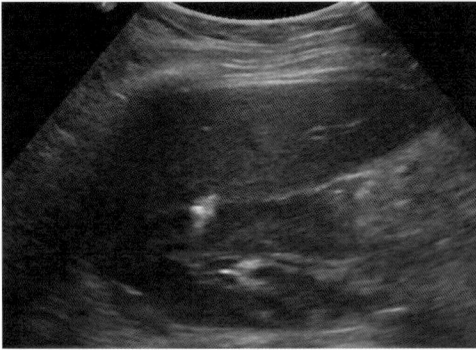
A

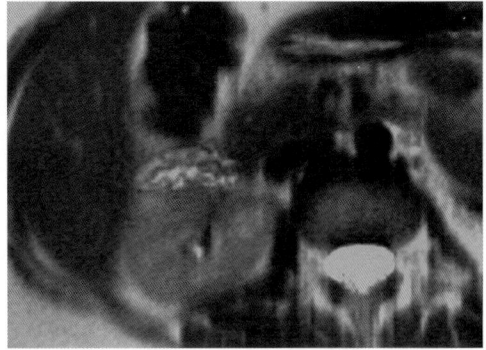
B

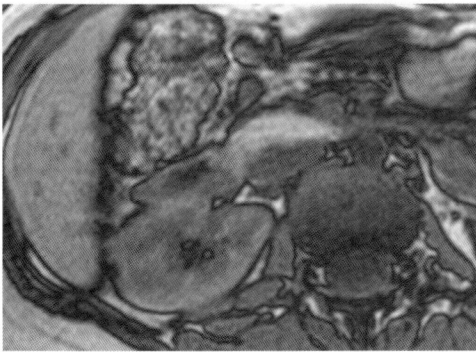
C

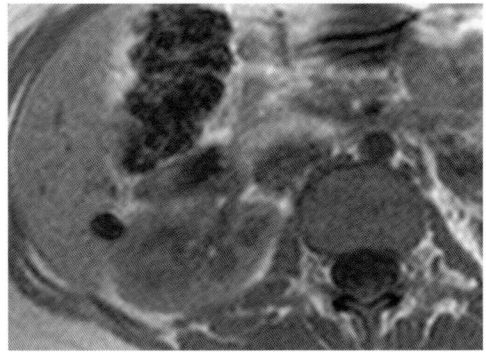
D

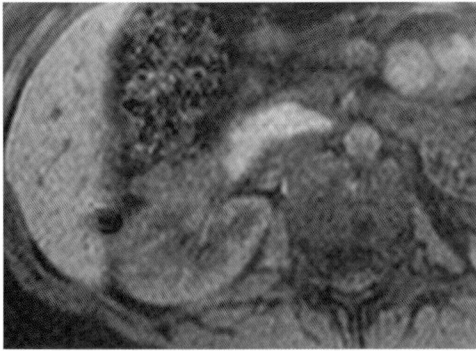
E

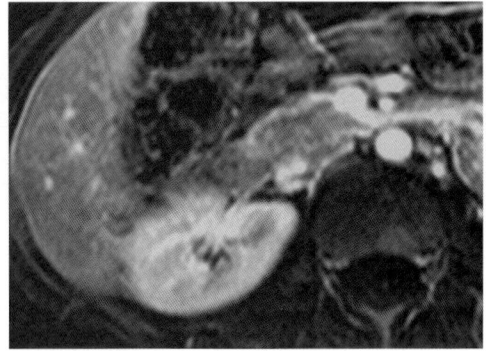
F

A. Oblique sagittal ultrasound. **B**. Axial single-shot FSE/TSE. **C**. Axial opposed-phase (TE 2.3 ms) and (**D**) in-phase (TE 4.6 ms) gradient echo. **E**. Axial pre-contrast-enhanced and (**F**) post-gadolinium contrast-enhanced gradient echo with fat saturation.

Case 120 Susceptibility Artifact from Surgical Clip Mimicking Mass

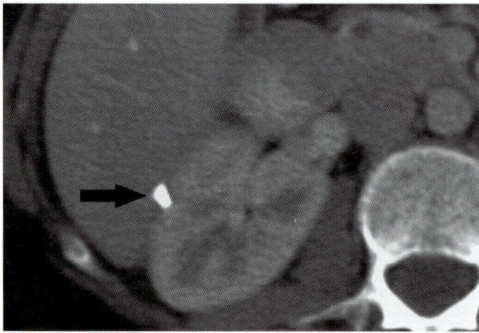

G

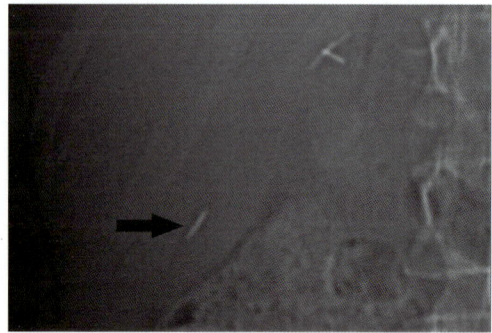

H

Findings

► The hyperechoic focus is seen on ultrasound image (**A**).
► No definite lesion is seen on single-shot FSE/TSE image (**B**).
► On opposed-phase gradient-echo image (**C**), obtained with short TE, a small focus with low signal intensity is seen at the renal margin adjacent to the liver.
► On in-phase gradient-echo image (**D**), obtained with longer TE than **C**, the focus is much more pronounced and appears larger.
► On gadolinium contrast-enhanced image (**F**), there appears to be enhancement compared to the unenhanced image (**E**), suggestive of a renal mass.
► Susceptibility artifact from surgical clip (*arrows*) trapped between kidney and liver shown on CT (**G**) and radiograph (**H**). The clip detached from the cystic duct stump after cholecystectomy.

Teaching points

► The lesion was incorrectly interpreted as a renal mass because of the suggestion of contrast enhancement. However, overlooked on gradient-echo images was that, with increase of the TE from 2.3 ms (**C**) to 4.6 ms (**D**), there was increased signal loss and apparent increase in size of the lesion, indicating magnetic-susceptibility effect.
► The magnetic-field gradients that occur in the immediate vicinity of metal, such as a surgical clip, accelerate dephasing of the transverse magnetization and subsequent signal loss.
► A gradient-echo sequence is relatively sensitive to susceptibility effects because it lacks the 180° refocusing RF pulse that is used in a spin-echo pulse sequence such as FSE/TSE to compensate for the effects of magnetic-field inhomogeneities.
► Increasing the TE in a gradient-echo pulse sequence makes susceptibility effects more visible.
► The dual-echo gradient-echo technique routinely used in most abdominal MR imaging protocols can be used for determining susceptibility effects by comparing the long-TE images to the short-TE images. This is easiest done when the short TE provides opposed-phase images and the long TE in-phase images, as for most 1.5T scanners. Detection of susceptibility effects may be more difficult when the long TE of a dual-echo sequence provides opposed-phase images (which may be the case on some 3T scanners), because in this case the signal loss can also be the result of the cancellation of the signals from fat and water.

Further reading

1. de Lange EE, Mugler JP. MR Acquisition techniques & practical considerations for abdominal imaging. In: Brant WE, de Lange EE (Eds), Essentials of Body MR Imaging. New York: Oxford University Press, 2012.

History

▶ 80-year-old man presented with vague abdominal pain.

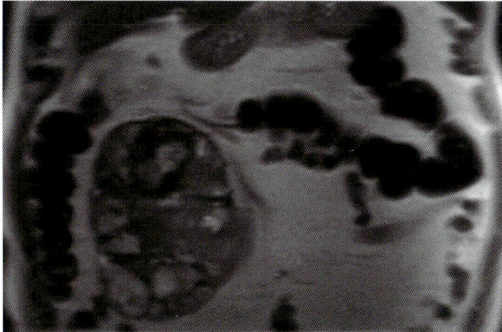

A

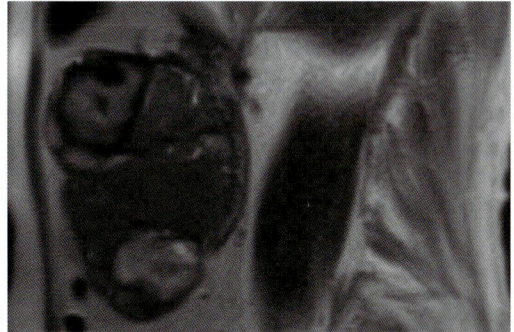

B

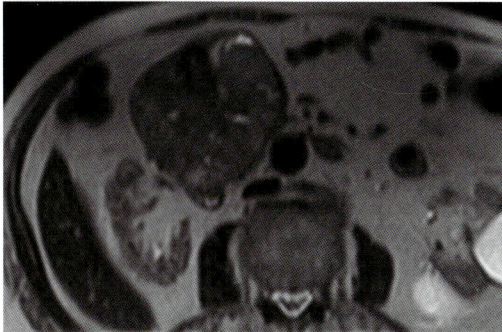

C

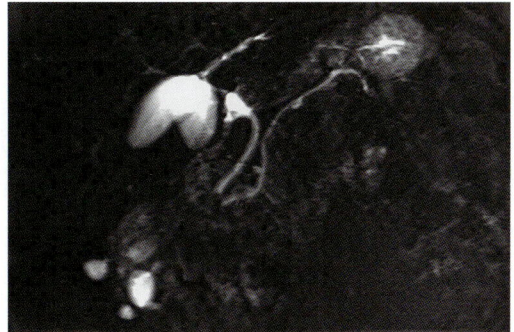

D

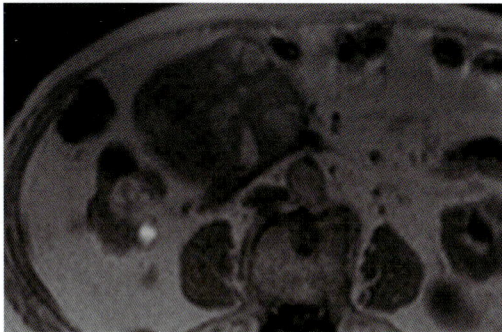

E

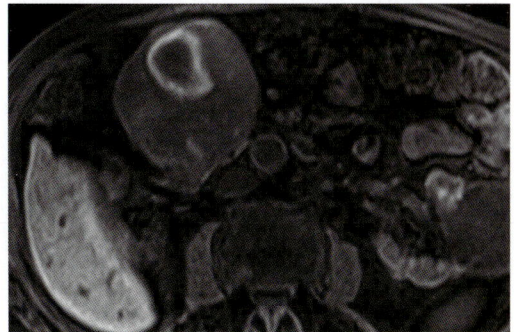

F

A. Coronal, (**B**) sagittal, and (**C**) axial T2-weighted single-shot FSE/TSE. **D**. Thick-slice MRCP using single-shot FSE/TSE.
E. Axial T1-weighted gradient echo. **F**. Axial post gadolinium contrast-enhanced gradient echo with fat saturation.

Case 121 Neuroendocrine Carcinoma Arising from the Pancreas

Findings

► Heterogeneous mass in the right mid-abdomen shows areas of hemorrhage and necrosis as well as foci of avid ring-like enhancement on post-gadolinium contrast-enhanced images.

Differential diagnosis

► Leiomyosarcoma of the duodenum
► Enteric duplication cyst
► Pancreatic neoplasm

Teaching points

► Pancreatic neuroendocrine neoplasms have diverse clinical presentations but share common imaging features. Most are well-differentiated tumors that are composed of cells that resemble pancreatic islet cells. Tumors may be functional, producing endocrinologic syndromes, or nonfunctional. All have malignant potential.
► Small tumors are homogeneous and well defined. Large tumors show necrosis, cystic change, and calcification, often with vascular invasion and metastases.
► On MR small tumors are round and generally well circumscribed, and are relatively low in signal intensity compared to normal pancreatic parenchyma on T1-weighted images. They may show significant high signal intensity on T2-weighted images. Some tumors contain abundant collagen, which is associated with intermediate to low signal intensity on T2-weighted images. Post-gadolinium contrast enhancement is usually intense on arterial- and venous-phase images but may be homogeneous or heterogenous in appearance. Larger lesions show hemorrhage, necrosis, cystic change, and typically ring-like enhancement.

Management

► Treatment is surgical resection. Clinical staging classification of neuroendocrine tumors is the same as that used for pancreatic adenocarcinoma.

Further reading

1. Asa SL. Pancreatic endocrine tumors. Mod Pathol 2011;24:S66–S77.
2. Joseph S, Wang YZ, Boudreaux JP, et al. Neuroendocrine tumors: current recommendations for diagnosis and surgical management. Endocrinol Metab Clin North Am 2011;40:205–231.
3. Lewis RB, Lattin GE Jr, Paal E. Pancreatic endocrine tumors: radiologic-clinicopathologic correlation. RadioGraphics 2010;30:1445–1464.

History

▶ 69-year-old man with right hepatic mass

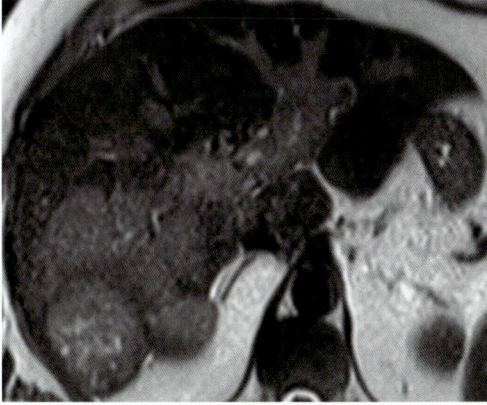

A

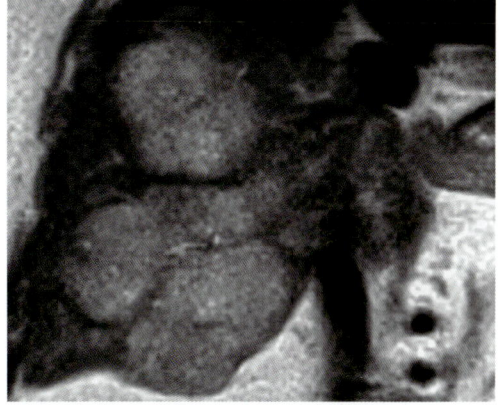

B

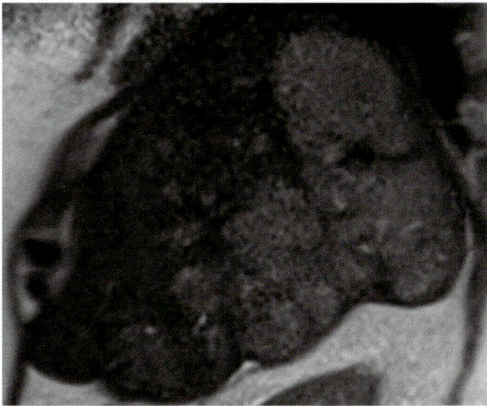

C

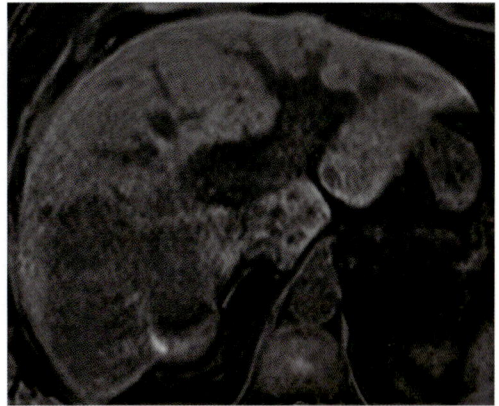

D

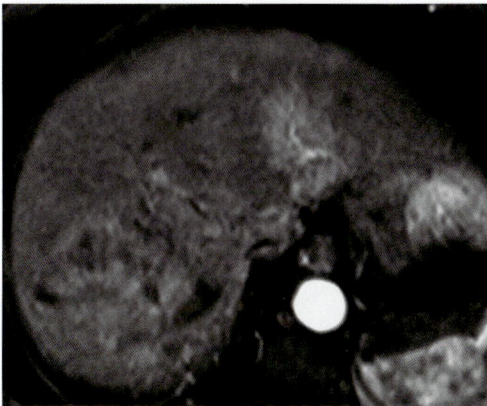

E

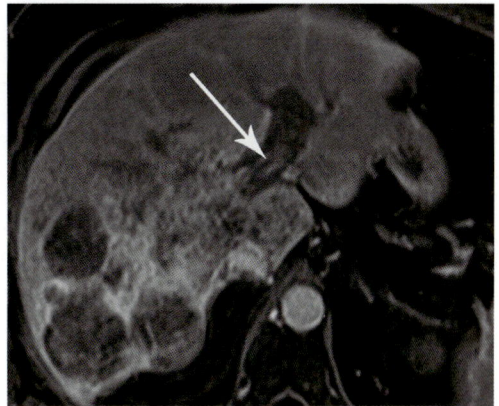

F

A. Axial, (**B**) coronal, and (**C**) sagittal T2-weighted single-shot FSE/TSE. **D**. Axial pre-contrast-enhanced, (**E**) arterial-phase post-gadolinium contrast-enhanced, and (**F**) delayed-phase contrast-enhanced T1-weighted gradient echo with fat saturation.

Case 122 Hepatocellular Carcinoma (HCC) with Portal Vein Invasion

Findings

- Multicentric hepatic mass demonstrating intermediate high signal intensity on T2-weighted images
- Tumor signal extends within the portal veins, well shown on T2-weighted images.
- The mass shows heterogeneous early contrast enhancement and relatively decreased enhancement on delayed-phase contrast-enhanced images.
- The left portal vein shows also relative decreased enhancement (*arrow*) on the delayed-phase contrast-enhanced image.
- Findings are consistent with HCC with tumor invasion of the portal vein.

Differential diagnosis

- Liver metastases, most commonly from colorectal primary. Metastases are less likely to invade the portal vein.
- Cholangiocarcinoma: often cause biliary obstruction and dilatation.
- Focal nodular hyperplasia: homogeneous mass with central scar; often becomes iso-intense to liver on delayed-phase contrast-enhanced imaging.

Teaching points

- HCC is the most common visceral malignancy in the world, accounting for ~90% of adult primary liver tumors. Most HCCs arise in the setting of cirrhosis.
- The most common presentation is a large heterogeneous mass, often with vascular invasion, as in this case.
- Other growth patterns: (1) multifocal, (2) diffusely infiltrating, (3) metastases to lung, adrenal glands, lymph nodes, and bone
- MRI signal characteristics on T1- and T2-weighted images can be quite variable.
- Theory of stepwise progression in cirrhosis: large regenerative nodules/low-grade dysplastic nodules → high-grade dysplastic nodules → carcinoma.

Management

- Definitive treatment is liver transplant.
- Multimodal treatment strategies are evolving, and include chemo- and radioembolization as well as radiofrequency ablation.

Further reading

1. Anders RA, Yerian LM, Tretiakdova M, et al. cDNA microarray analysis of macroregenerative and dysplastic nodules in end-stage hepatitis C. Am J Path 2003;162:991–1000.
2. Winston CB, Schwartz LH, Fong Y, et al. Hepatocellular carcinoma: MR imaging findings in cirrhotic livers and noncirrhotic livers. Radiology 1999;210:75–79.

History

▶ 59-year-old woman who had radical hysterectomy for adenosquamous cervical carcinoma 21 months ago presents with vaginal bleeding and palpable vaginal mass.

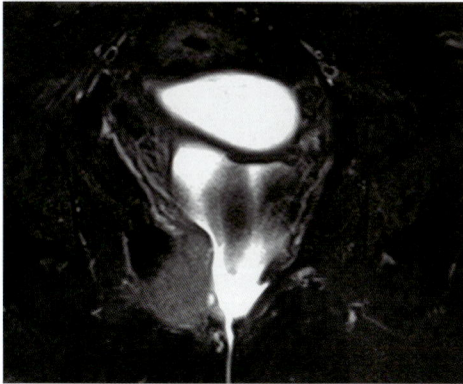

A

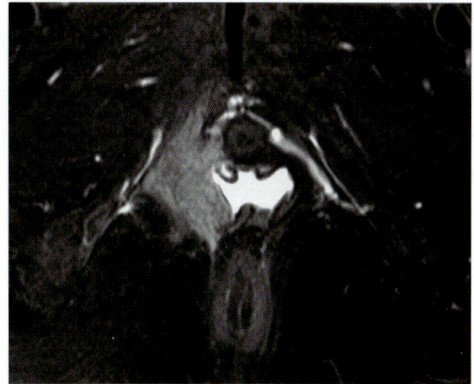

B

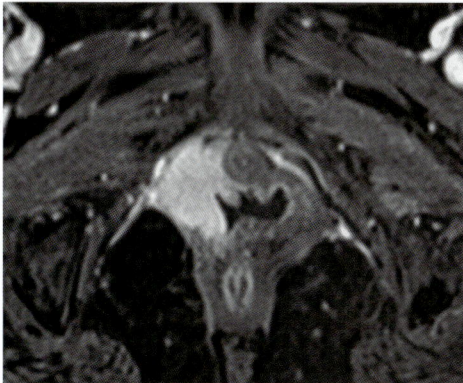

C

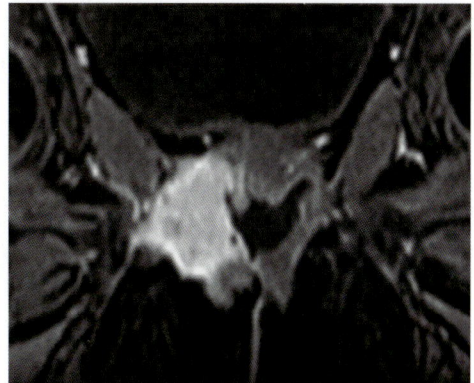

D

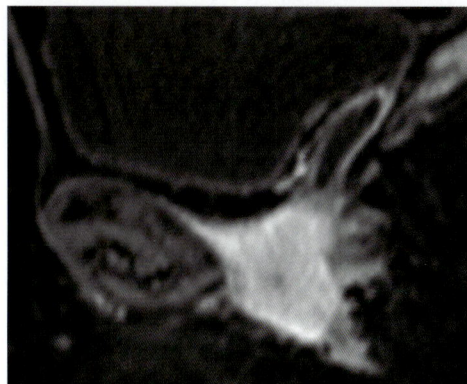

E

A. Coronal and (**B**) axial T2-weighted FSE/TSE with fat saturation. **C**. Axial contrast-enhanced T1-weighted gradient echo with fat saturation, and (**D**) coronal and (**E**) sagittal multiplanar reformatted images generated from the axially acquired 3D contrast-enhanced T1-weighted gradient-echo images with fat saturation.

Case 123 Recurrent Carcinoma of the Cervix

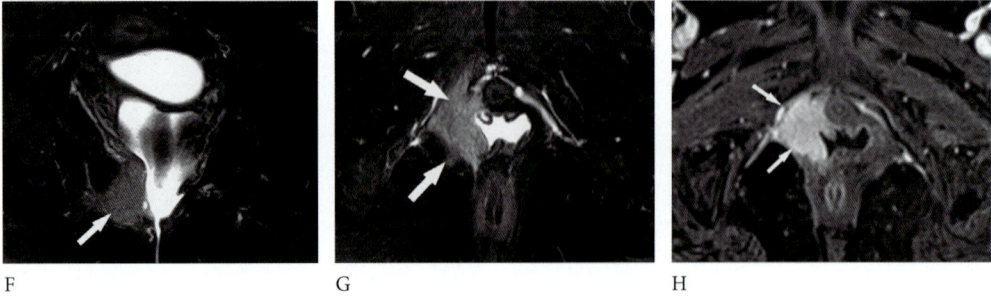

F   G   H

Findings

► An intermediate-high-signal-intensity mass (*arrows* in **F, G, H**) is seen along the right vaginal wall on T2-weighted images. High-signal-intensity vaginal gel is within the vagina, outlining the fornices.

► The margins and extent of the mass are more clearly distinguished from edema on the contrast-enhanced image. The avidly enhancing mass involves the right levator ani muscle, the serosa of the urethra, the periosteum of the symphysis pubis, and the obturator internus.

Differential diagnosis

► Direct local spread or tumor recurrence from malignancies of the cervix, uterus, or rectum

► Primary vaginal malignancy: adenocarcinoma, melanoma, sarcoma

Teaching points

► Recurrence of cervical cancer is most common in the first few years following treatment. In patients with tumor recurrence, 60% occur within the first 2 years and 90% within the first 5 years.

► The vaginal cuff, cervix, parametrium, and pelvic side wall are the most common sites of recurrence.

► Nodules or masses exhibiting high signal intensity on T2-weighted images may represent recurrent tumor, edema, necrosis, or inflammation. The finding of early enhancement on dynamic post-contrast MR imaging is highly indicative of tumor.

► Early radiation change may also show contrast enhancement on MR. PET-CT shows high sensitivity and specificity for tumor recurrence.

Management

► Careful staging by MR imaging allows for planning of surgery, chemotherapy, external beam radiotherapy, or interstitial brachytherapy.

Further reading

1. Kaur H, Silverman PM, Iyer RB, et al. Diagnosis, staging, and surveillance of cervical carcinoma. AJR Am J Roentgenol 2003;180:1621–1632.
2. Parikwwh JH, Barton DPJ, Ind TEJ, Sohaib SA. MR imaging features of vaginal malignancies. RadioGraphics 2008;28:49–63.

History

▶ 63-year-old man with history of sarcoma of the pelvis has follow-up MRI

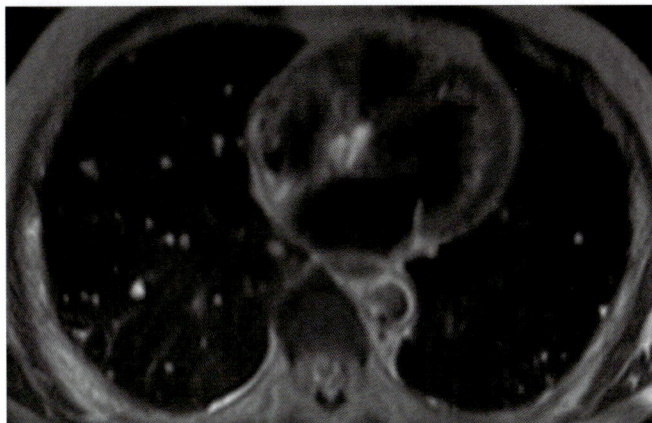

A

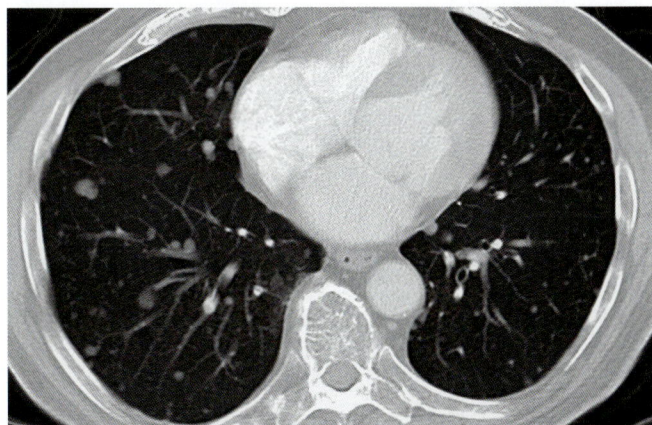

B

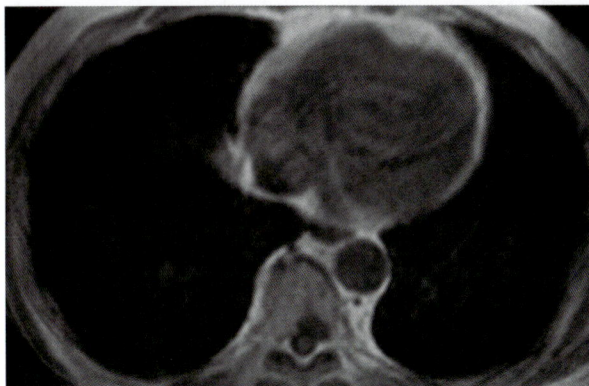

C

A. Axial T2-weighted single-shot FSE/TSE. **B**. Axial contrast-enhanced CT. **C**. Axial T1-weighted gradient echo.

Case 124 Pulmonary Metastases from Sarcoma

Findings

- ▶ Innumerable small lung nodules indicative of metastatic disease
- ▶ Compare to corresponding images from CT of the thorax obtained on the same day as MR of the abdomen and pelvis, which included the lung bases.
- ▶ The lung nodules are poorly demonstrated on the T1-weighted image.

Differential diagnosis

- ▶ Granulomatous disease
- ▶ Infection

Teaching points

- ▶ While the lung is seldom the primary organ of interest for MR imaging, the lung bases are typically included in an abdominal study and must be examined for diagnostic information.
- ▶ T2-weighted single-shot FSE/TSE MR offers an advantage over most other pulse sequences used in abdominal MRI in demonstrating lung metastases because the images are relatively free of motion artifacts from breathing and the beating heart. Using this technique, the nodules appear as high-signal-intensity foci in a background of very low signal intensity of the air-filled lung. Also the pulmonary vessels display low signal intensity, providing easy differentiation from nodules.
- ▶ Diffusion-weighted MR imaging (not shown) offers promise of providing information to distinguish benign from malignant large lung nodules.
- ▶ In general, however, CT is the preferred imaging technique for assessing the lung.

Management

- ▶ Palliative treatment for widespread metastatic disease

Further reading

1. Bruegel M, Gaa J, Woertler K, et al. MRI of the lung: value of different turbo spin-echo, single-shot turbo spin-echo, and 3D gradient-echo pulse sequences for the detection of pulmonary metastases. J Magn Reson Imaging 2007;25:73–81.
2. Knopp MV, Hess T, Schad LR, et al. MR tomography of lung metastases with rapid gradient echo sequences. Initial results in diagnostic applications. Radiologe 1994;34:581–587. (Original in German)
3. Satoh S, Kitazume Y, Ohdama S, et al. Can malignant and benign pulmonary nodules be differentiated with diffusion-weighted MRI? AJR Am J Roentgenol 2008;191:464–470.

History

▶ 42-year-old woman with abdominal pain

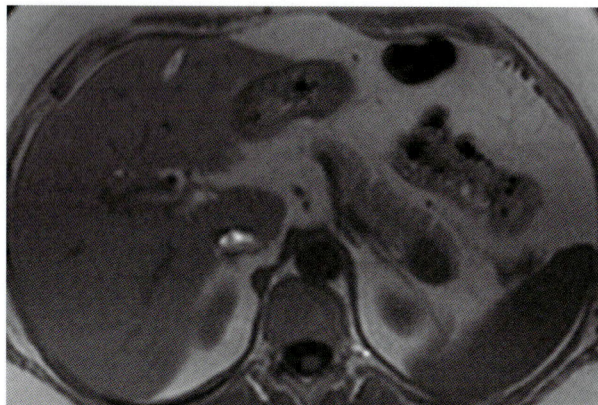

A

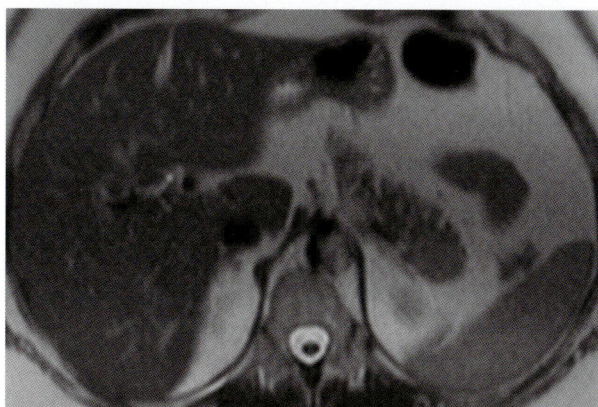

B

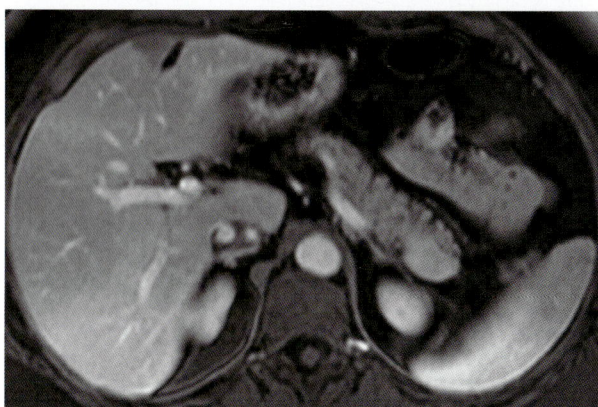

C

A. Axial T1-weighted gradient echo. **B**. Axial T2-weighted single-shot FSE/TSE. **C**. Axial gadolinium contrast-enhanced T1-weighted gradient echo with fat saturation.

Case 125 Ectopic Splenic Tissue or Intrapancreatic Accessory Spleen Mimicking a Pancreatic Mass

Findings

▶ A well-circumscribed mass is present in the pancreatic tail.
▶ The lesion is iso-intense to the spleen on all sequences and enhances the same as the spleen.
▶ Note that the pancreatic parenchyma wraps around the lesion anteriorly.

Differential diagnosis

▶ Neuroendocrine tumor of the pancreas

Teaching points

▶ Splenic variants, such as accessory spleen or splenosis, may mimic a pancreatic mass.
▶ Accessory spleens occur in approximately 10% of the population. Intrapancreatic accessory spleens are found in the pancreatic tail in roughly 16% of these patients.
▶ Technetium 99m (^{99m}Tc) sulfur colloid, radiolabeled heat-damaged red blood cells, and indium 111–labeled autologous platelets may be used to differentiate splenic from pancreatic tissue.
▶ In addition, MR imaging with small iron particles containing intravenous contrast agents such as ferumoxides (Feridex®; Berlex, Wayne, NJ) may be used to demonstrate preferential uptake in hepatic and splenic tissue, with their rich reticuloendothelial composition.

Management

▶ Accessory spleens are generally asymptomatic and are often incidental findings on images obtained for unrelated symptoms. No treatment is needed in asymptomatic patients.
▶ Ectopic splenic tissue may cause persistent, recurrent anemia or thrombocytopenia following surgical splenectomy for idiopathic thrombocytopenic purpura.
▶ Ectopic splenic tissue can also rarely cause abdominal pain from torsion, rupture, or infarction. In these patients, surgical resection may be necessary.

Further reading

1. Bidet AC, Dreyfus-Schmidt G, Mas J, et al. Diagnosis of splenosis: the advantages of splenic scintiscanning with Tc 99m heat-damaged red blood cells. Eur J Nucl Med 1986;12:357–358.
2. Hayward I, Mindelzun RE, Jeffrey RB. Intrapancreatic accessory spleen mimicking pancreatic mass on CT. J Comput Assist Tomogr 1992;16:984–985.

History

▶ 63-year-old woman referred for MR imaging to evaluate a right upper quadrant mass found incidentally on CT

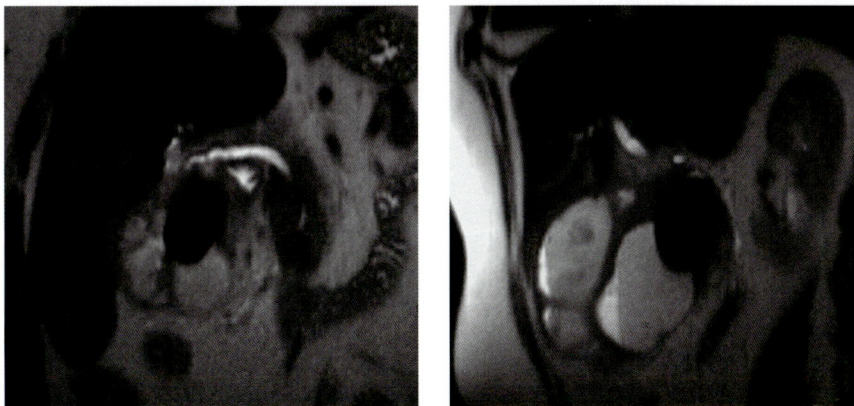

A   B

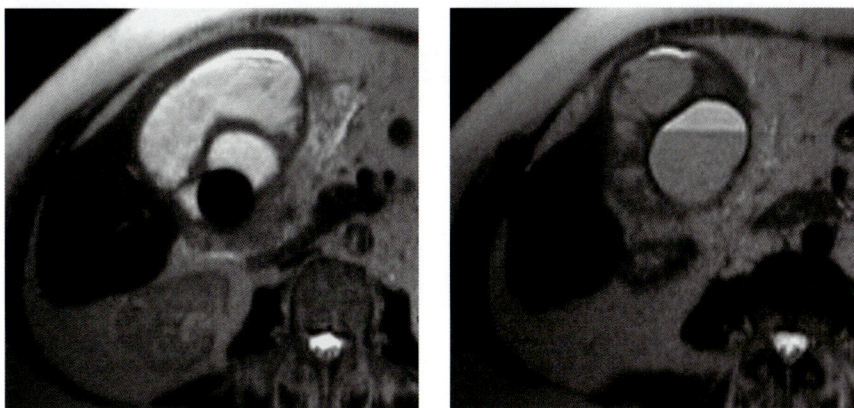

C   D

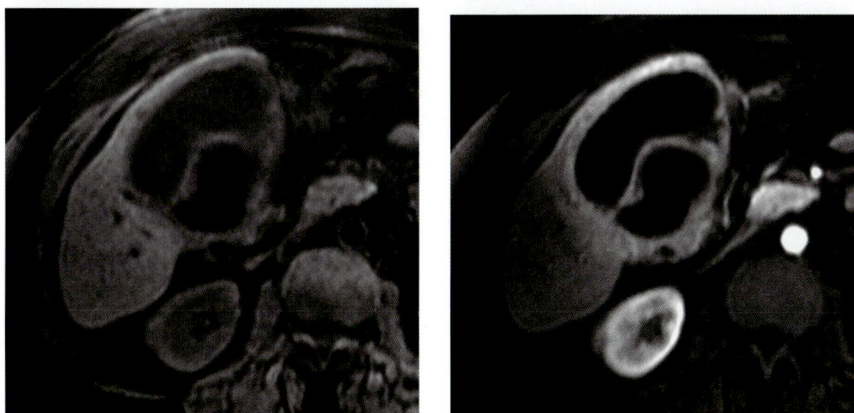

E   F

A. Axial, (**B**) sagittal, and (**C**, **D**) axial T2-weighted single-shot FSE/TSE (**D** at lower level than **C**). **E**. Axial pre- and (**F**) post-gadolinium contrast-enhanced gradient echo with fat saturation.

Case 126   Xanthogranulomatous Cholecystitis

Findings

▶ Marked gallbladder wall thickening with cystic changes containing fluid–fluid levels
▶ Areas of high signal intensity within the gallbladder on T2-weighted images
▶ Avid gallbladder wall enhancement, most prominent at the luminal surface
▶ Large gallstone within the gallbladder neck with luminal distention
▶ Hyperemia of the liver parenchyma adjacent to the inflamed gallbladder

Differential diagnosis

▶ Gallbladder carcinoma
▶ Cholangiocarcinoma
▶ Acute cholecystitis

Teaching points

▶ Xanthogranulomatous cholecystitis is a rare form of chronic cholecystitis that typically presents with right upper quadrant pain, leukocytosis, and positive Murphy sign.
▶ The appearance is often difficult to distinguish from gallbladder carcinoma.
▶ Histologically, the lesion shows chronic inflammatory cells, foamy histiocytes, and bile pigment.
▶ Markedly thickened gallbladder wall, which may be asymmetric
▶ Enhancement of the gallbladder wall, more pronounced at the luminal surface on contrast-enhanced imaging
▶ Areas of marked hyperintensity on T2-weighted images that do not show enhancement compatible with abscesses or areas of necrosis

Management

▶ Cholecystectomy

Further reading

1. Levy AD, Murakata LA, Abbott RM, et al. From the archives of the AFIP. Benign tumors and tumorlike lesions of the gallbladder and extrahepatic bile ducts: radiologic-pathologic correlation. RadioGraphics 2002;22: 387–413.
2. Shuto R, Kiyosue H, Komatsu E, et al. CT and MR findings of xanthogranulomatous cholecystitis: correlation with pathologic findings. Eur Radiol 2004;14:440–446.

History

▶ 48-year-old woman with history of recurrent urinary infections now presents with hematuria.

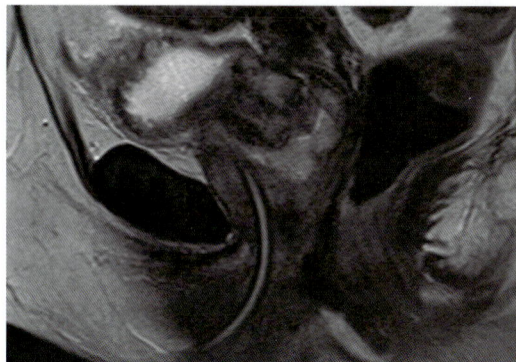
A

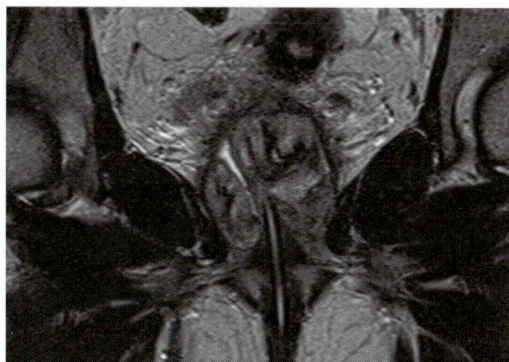
B

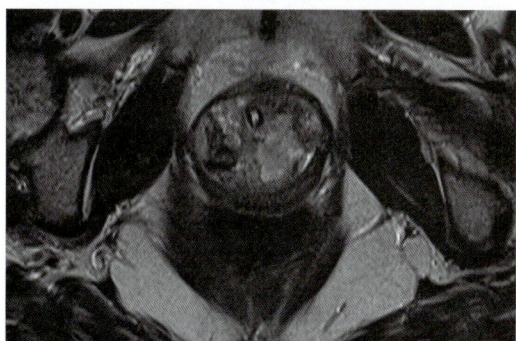
C

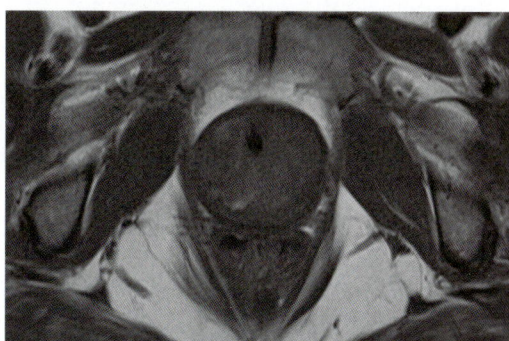
D

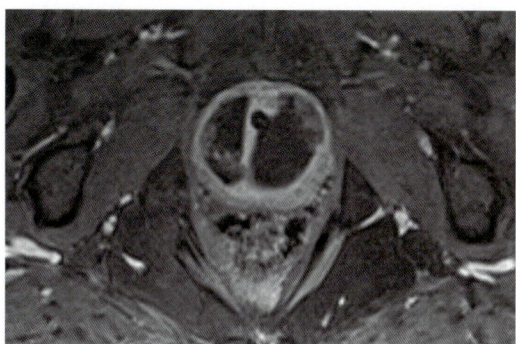
E

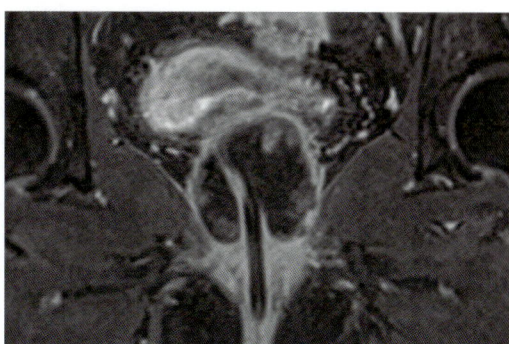
F

A. Sagittal, (**B**) coronal, and (**C**) axial T2-weighted FSE/TSE. **D**. Axial T1-weighted spin echo. **E**. Axial and (**F**) coronal post-gadolinium contrast-enhanced T1-weighted gradient echo with fat saturation.

Case 127 Adenocarcinoma Arising in a Urethral Diverticulum

Findings

▶ Irregular enhancing soft tissue within a cystic dilatation of the urethra
▶ The mass demonstrates relatively low signal intensity on T1-weighted images, intermediate high signal intensity on T2-weighted images, and moderate enhancement on gadolinium contrast-enhanced T1-weighted images.
▶ There is a catheter in the urethra.

Differential diagnosis

▶ Inflamed urethral diverticulum
▶ Urethral leiomyoma

Teaching points

▶ A urethral diverticulum is a localized outpouching of the urethra into the periurethral tissues. The lining mucosa of the diverticulum is identical to that of the urethra and communication with the urethra is maintained. The presence of the diverticulum results in urinary stasis, which commonly leads to recurrent urinary infections, urinary frequency, urgency, and dysuria. Stasis and chronic inflammation may lead to calculi and urethral carcinoma.
▶ Congenital urethral diverticulum is rare. Most diverticula originate from obstruction of periurethral glands and ducts. Other causes of diverticula include trauma or surgery.
▶ Adenocarcinoma is the most common type of urethral cancer associated with a urethral diverticulum.
▶ MRI, particularly with endoluminal coil (endorectal, endovaginal, endourethral), provides excellent visualization of the female urethra and periurethral soft tissues. Endoluminal coil was not used in the case shown here. Urethral diverticula are seen best on T2-weighted images as high-signal-intensity structures adjacent to or wrapping around the mid-urethra.
▶ Intravenous gadolinium-based contrast agent can help distinguish between inflammatory changes and malignancy of a urethral diverticulum.

Management

▶ Optimal treatment is currently in debate in the literature. Treatment has varied from local excision to anterior pelvic exenteration with neoadjuvant chemoradiation.

Further reading

1. Ahmed K, Dasgupta R, Vats A, et al. Urethral diverticular carcinoma: An overview of current trends in diagnosis and management. Int Urol Nephrol 2010;42:331–341.
2. Chou CP, Levenson RB, Elsayes KM, et al. Imaging of female urethral diverticulum: An update. RadioGraphics 2008;28:1917–1930.
3. Hahn WY, Israel GM, Lee VS. MRI of female urethral and periurethral disorders. AJR Am J Roentgenol 2004;182:677–682.

▶ 45-year-old woman had pelvic MRI. Explain irregularly shaped low-intensity areas in the posterior aspect of the bladder.

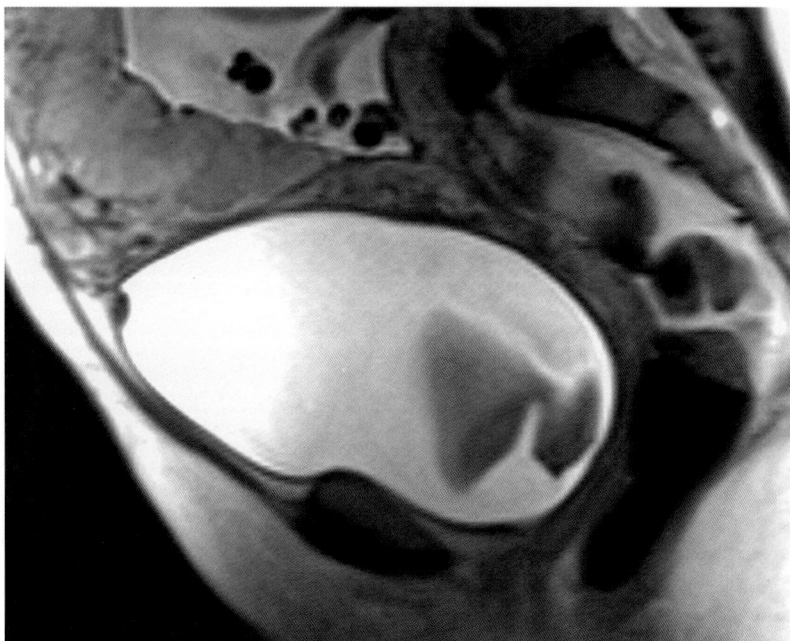

A

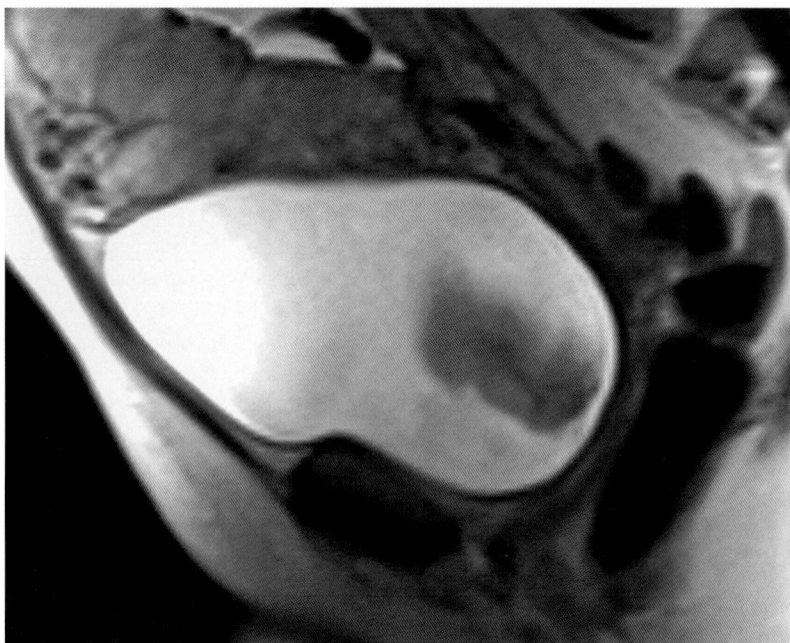

B

A, **B**. Contiguous sagittal single-shot FSE/TSE images.

Case 128 Flow Artifact

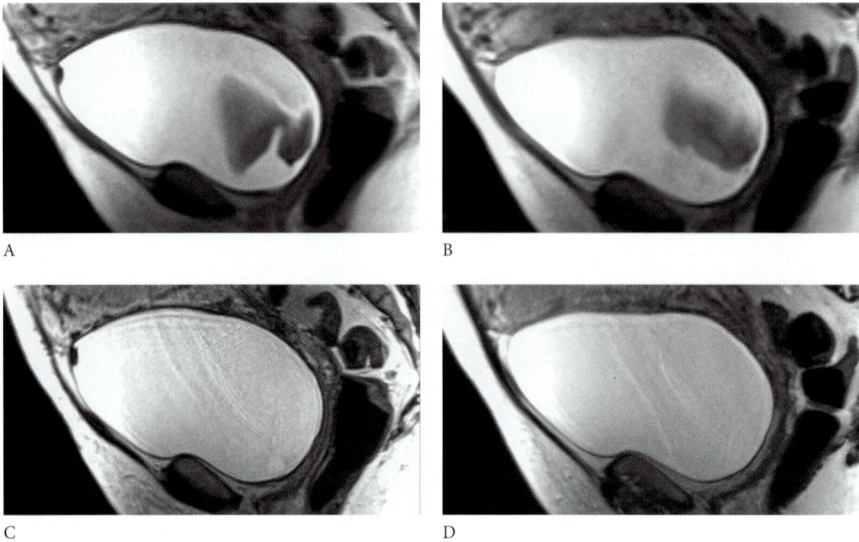

A

B

C

D

Findings

▶ Irregularly shaped low-intensity areas of varying extent in the fluid-filled bladder, without apparent anatomical relationship to each other, are seen on contiguous single-shot FSE/TSE images (**A**, **B**).

▶ The low-intensity regions are not seen on corresponding sagittal images reconstructed from a 3D FSE/TSE acquisition (**C**, **D**).

▶ These irregular regions represent signal-intensity variations caused by fluid moving into or out of the slice during the echo train of the single-shot FSE/TSE acquisition.

Differential diagnosis

▶ Blood products or proteinaceous material within urine

▶ Urine containing high concentration of gadolinium-based contrast material

▶ Bladder mass

Teaching points

▶ With a 2D single-shot FSE/TSE pulse sequence, a single 90° excitation radiofrequency (RF) pulse is followed by a large number of refocusing RF pulses to generate the echoes (echo train), and hence the data, required to fill k-space for a complete single slice.

▶ Bladder fluid that moves into the slice *during* the echo train provides no signal contribution because it does not experience the 90° excitation RF pulse that initiates the echo train. Similarly, fluid that does experience the excitation RF pulse but only a fraction of the refocusing RF pulses, because it subsequently moves out of the slice, also provides reduced signal.

▶ No artifacts from fluid moving during the echo train appeared in the 3D FSE/TSE acquisition because the entire bladder was included in the image slab, and hence all fluid experienced all RF pulses.

▶ Artifacts from moving fluid in a 2D single-shot FSE/TSE acquisition can be reduced by increasing the slice thickness so that the amount of fluid moving into or out of the slice is relatively small compared to the total volume of fluid within the slice. Conversely, the artifact increases when the slice thickness is decreased.

Further reading

1. de Lange EE, Mugler JP. MR acquisition techniques & practical considerations for abdominal imaging. In: Brant WE, de Lange EE (Eds), Essentials of Body MR Imaging. New York: Oxford University Press, 2012.

History

▶ 47-year-old woman with menorrhagia

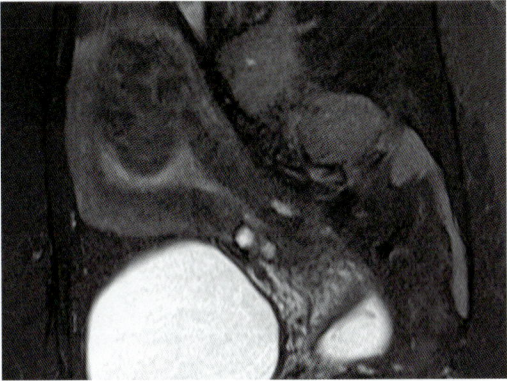

A

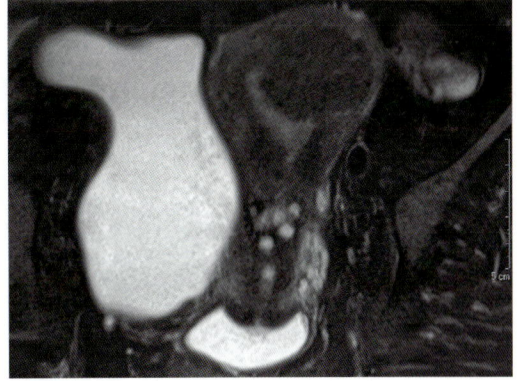

B

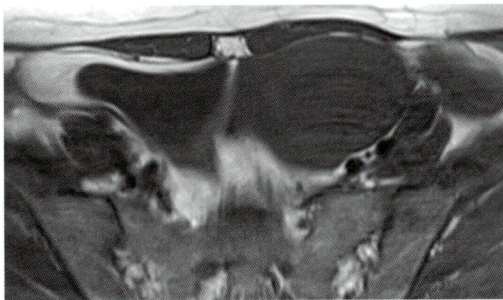

C

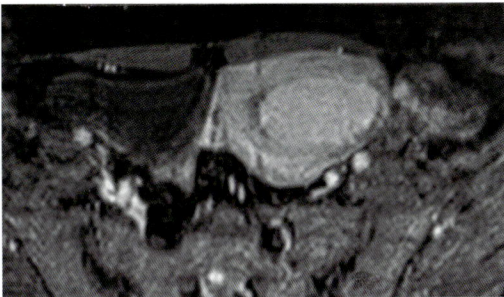

D

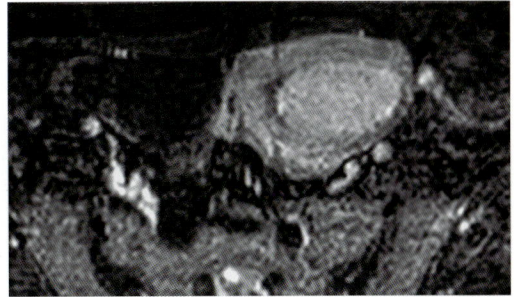

E

A. Sagittal and (**B**) oblique coronal T2-weighted FSE/TSE. **C**. Axial T1-weighted spin echo. **D**. Axial post-gadolinium contrast-enhanced T1-weighted gradient echo with fat saturation, and (**E**) subtraction image derived from **D**.

Case 129 Submucosal Leiomyoma

Findings

▶ Subendometrial (submucosal) mass in the fundus of the uterus demonstrating iso-intensity to the myometrium on T1-weighted images and mild hypointensity on T2-weighted sequences. The mass demonstrates uniform contrast enhancement and occupies the endometrial cavity.

▶ The mass protrudes into the uterine cavity.

Differential diagnosis

▶ Endometrial polyp
▶ Adenomyosis
▶ Endometrial carcinoma

Teaching points

▶ Leiomyomas are benign neoplasms of smooth muscle. Uterine leiomyomas occur in 20% to 30% of women above age 35. Submucosal leiomyomas are commonly associated with abnormal vaginal bleeding, especially heavy bleeding between menstrual cycle bleeding. As the leiomyoma protrudes into the uterine cavity it stretches the endometrium and makes it thin, which may lead to ulceration of the endometrium. The lesions are also associated with infertility by impairing implantation, causing spontaneous abortion or obstruction of the fallopian tube.

▶ Leiomyomas can degenerate or hemorrhage, producing a heterogeneous appearance of the mass and leading to the patient's symptoms of pain.

▶ MR typically shows a sharply marginated subendometrial myometrial mass that displays signal intensity lower than that of myometrium on T2-weighted images.

▶ Pedunculated lesions can become detached and move freely within the uterine cavity.

▶ Leiomyomas are estrogen responsive and, as a result, may enlarge during pregnancy and regress with menopause.

▶ Bulky disease from multiple large leiomyomas may result in urinary urgency or dyspareunia.

Management

▶ Treatment of uterine leiomyomas may include medical hormonal therapy, hysteroscopic or surgical myomectomy, uterine artery embolization, magnetic resonance-guided focused ultrasound, or hysterectomy.

Further reading

1. Imaoka I, Wada A, Matsuo M, et al. MR imaging of disorders associated with female infertility: use in diagnosis, treatment, and management. RadioGraphics 2003;23:1401–1421.
2. Murase E, Siegelman ES, Outwater EK, et al. Uterine leiomyomas: histopathologic features, MR imaging findings, differential diagnosis and treatment. RadioGraphics 1999;19:1179–1197.
3. Ruuskanen AJ, Hippelainen MI, Sipola P, Manninen HI. Association between magnetic resonance imaging findings of uterine leiomyomas and symptoms demanding treatment. Eur J Radiol May 16, 2011. Epub ahead of print.

History

▶ 57-year-old woman presents with heart failure.

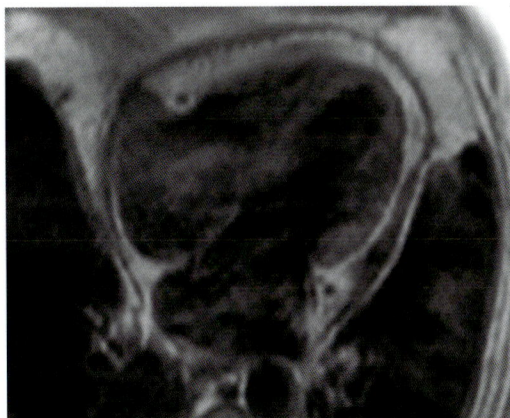

A

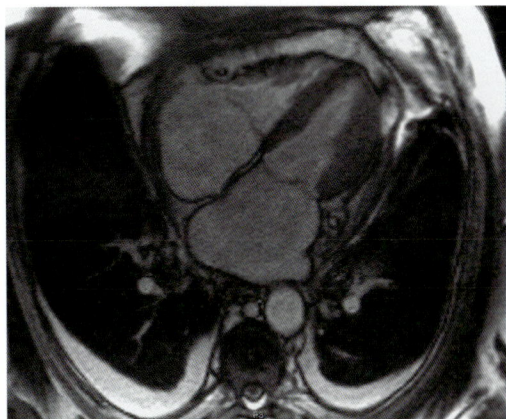

B

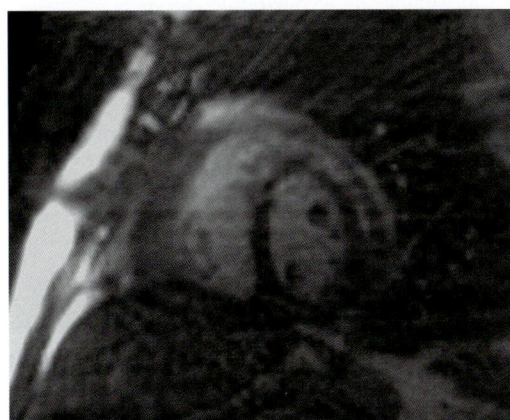

C

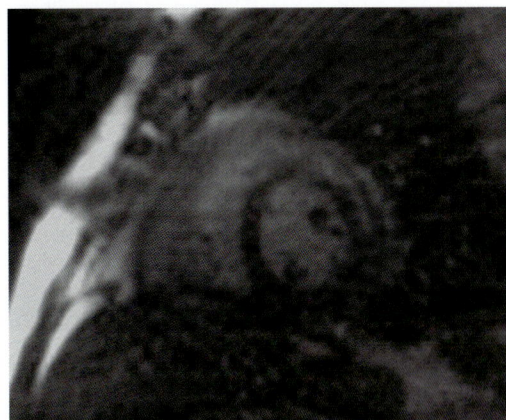

D

A. Four-chamber T1-weighted FSE/TSE. **B**. Four-chamber steady-state free precession (SSFP). **C**. Short-axis SSFP real-time image during inspiration and (**D**) expiration.

Case 130 Constrictive Pericarditis

Findings

▶ Thickening of the pericardium >4 mm (T1-weighted imaging)
▶ Biatrial enlargement
▶ Flattening of the interventricular septum towards the left ventricle during inspiration, with a normal appearance during expiration (SSFP real-time imaging)
▶ Small bilateral pleural effusions

Differential diagnosis

▶ Restrictive cardiomyopathy
▶ Acute pericarditis without constriction
▶ Pericardial neoplasm

Teaching points

▶ The key physiologic feature of constrictive pericarditis is decreased compliance of the pericardium resulting in reduced ventricular filling. The noncompliant pericardium causes ventricular interdependence such that diastolic filling of each ventricle is limited by the other. Thus, as the volume returning to the right ventricle increases during inspiration, there is a compensatory decrease in left ventricular filling; the reverse occurs during expiration. Ventricular interdependence can also be identified on cine MR as septal bounce present during early diastole.
▶ Normal pericardium is <2 mm thick. Pericardial thickening >4 mm is suggestive and >6 mm is highly specific of the diagnosis; however, a normal pericardial thickness is reported in up to 5% of patient with constrictive pericarditis.
▶ Causes of constrictive pericarditis include infection, mediastinal radiation treatment, acute myocardial infarction, uremia, metastatic disease, and idiopathic.
▶ Restrictive cardiomyopathy and constrictive pericarditis both can present with heart failure and demonstrate reduced ventricular filling at cardiac catheterization. MR is 93% accurate at distinguishing between restrictive cardiomyopathy and constrictive pericarditis.
▶ Pericarditis without constriction also presents with a thickened pericardium; however, this is usually an acute process and therefore is associated with pericardial enhancement.
▶ Focal pericardial thickening from a mass is usually associated with enhancement and a known malignancy.

Management

▶ Some patients may benefit from pericardial stripping.

Further reading

1. Norton P. Cardiac MR imaging. In: Brant WE, de Lange EE (Eds), Essentials of Body MR Imaging. New York: Oxford University Press, 2012.
2. Wang ZJ, Reddy GP, Gotway MB, Yeh BM, Hetts SW, Higgins CB. CT and MR imaging of pericardial disease. RadioGraphics 2003;23:S167–S180.

History

▶ 46-year-old woman presents with abdominal pain and unintentional weight loss.

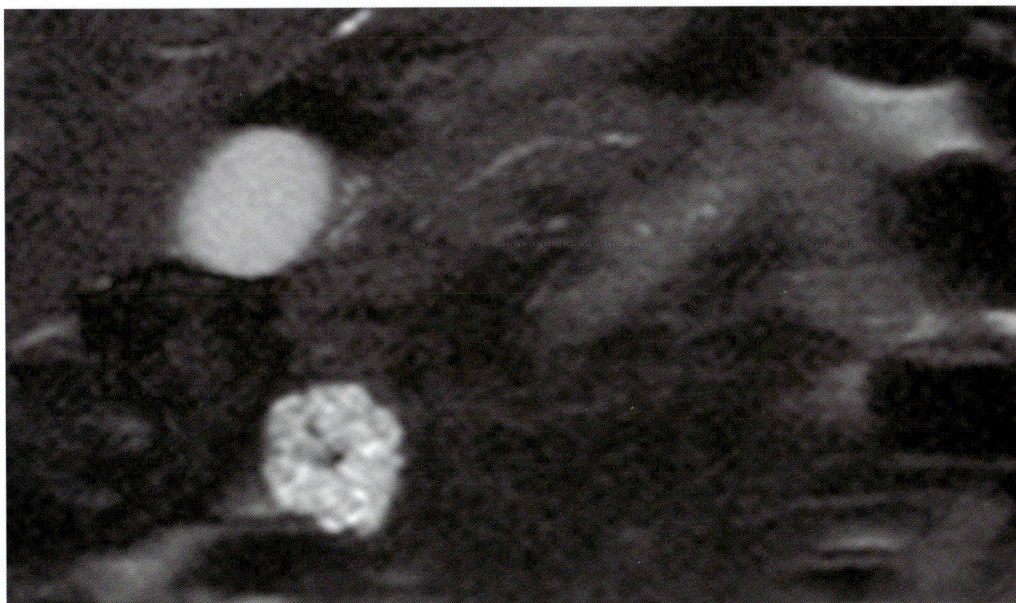

A

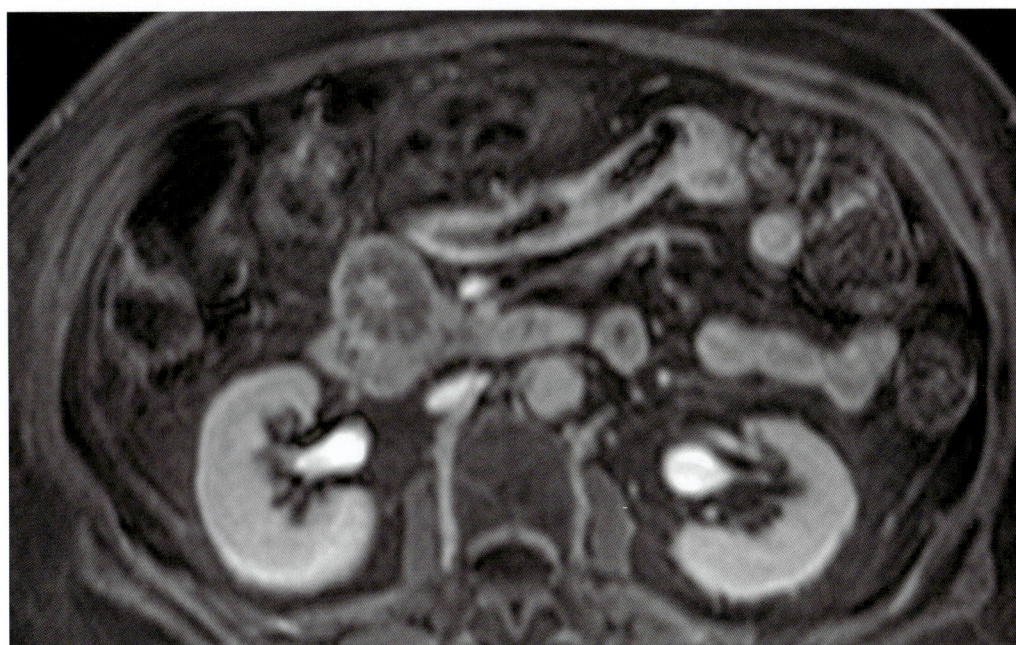

B

A. Coronal T2-weighted single-shot FSE/TSE. **B**. Axial delayed-phase contrast-enhanced T1-weighted gradient echo with fat saturation.

Case 131   Serous Cystadenoma of the Pancreas

Findings

- ▶ A mass with honeycomb appearance in the uncinate process of the pancreas
- ▶ Note the enhancement of the capsule and septa delineating small cysts.
- ▶ The central scar demonstrates enhancement on delayed contrast-enhanced images.

Differential diagnosis

- ▶ Pseudocyst
- ▶ Mucinous cystic neoplasm (mucinous cystadenoma) of pancreas
- ▶ Intraductal papillary mucinous neoplasm
- ▶ Congenital pancreatic cysts

Teaching points

- ▶ Serous cystadenoma, previously referred to as microcystic cystadenoma, is typically found in middle-aged and elderly women with nonspecific complaints of abdominal pain or weight loss or more commonly as an incidental finding.
- ▶ Typical serous cystadenoma is composed of innumerable small cysts (1 to 20 mm). The overall size of the lesions varies, averaging 5 to 10 cm. A central stellate scar with calcifications, which is known to be characteristic of serous cystadenoma, may sometimes be observed. Most commonly found in the head of the pancreas, serous cystadenomas can be seen in any part of the pancreas. Multiple serous cystadenomas may occur in von Hippel-Lindau disease.
- ▶ At MR imaging, serous cystadenomas appear as a cluster of small cysts with signal intensity of simple fluid on T2-weighted images and thin intervening fibrous septa, which enhance on delayed contrast-enhanced MR images. There is no communication between the cysts and the pancreatic duct. As the lesion grows, fibrous tissue retraction produces the pattern of a central scar. When coarse calcifications are present in the central scar, a corresponding signal void is seen on MR images.

Management

- ▶ Asymptomatic serous cystadenomas do not require surgical excision because of the extremely low potential for malignancy.

Further reading

1. Kalb B, Sarmiento JM, Kooby DA, et al. MR imaging of cystic lesions of the pancreas RadioGraphics 2009;29:1749–1765.
2. Sarti M. Pancreas MR imaging. In: Brant WE, de Lange EE (Eds), Essentials of Body MR Imaging. New York: Oxford University Press, 2012.

History

▶ Premature neonate with a large presacral mass seen on fetal ultrasound

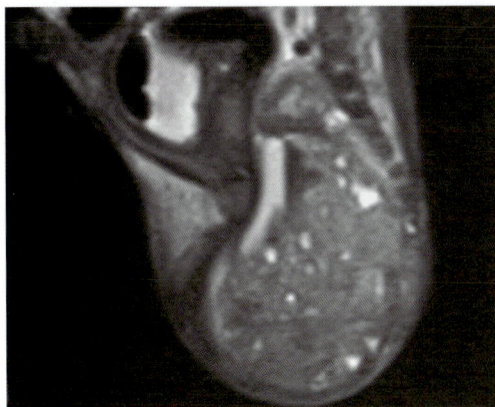

A

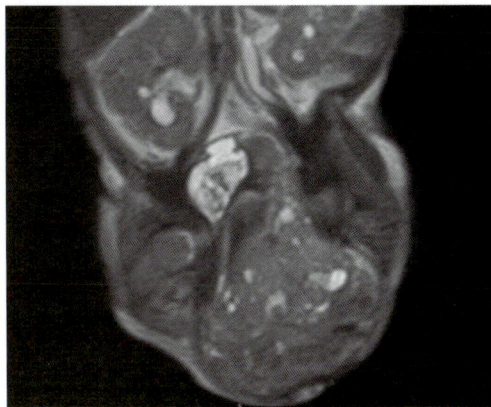

B

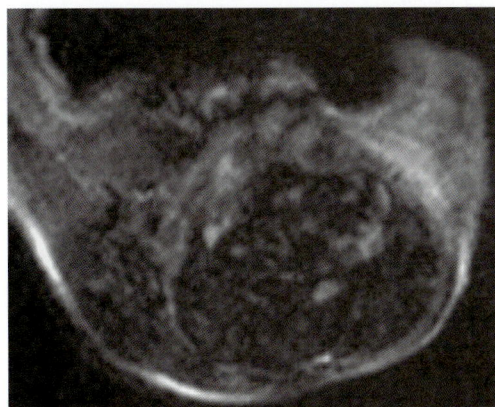

C

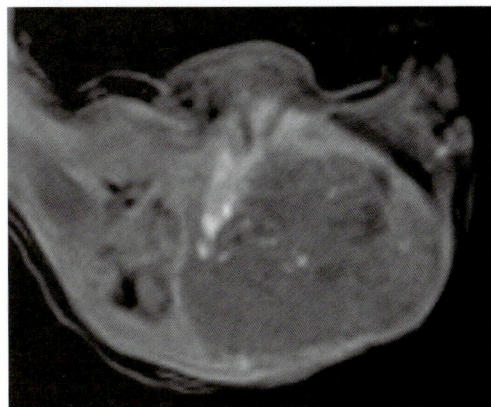

D

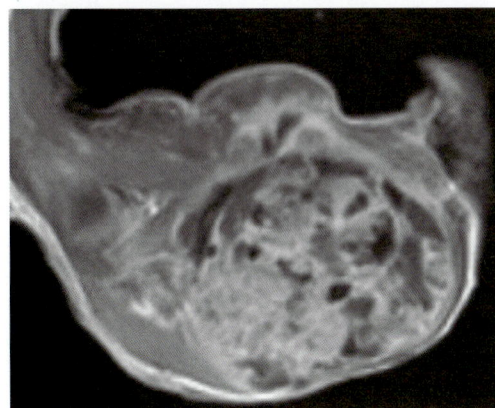

E

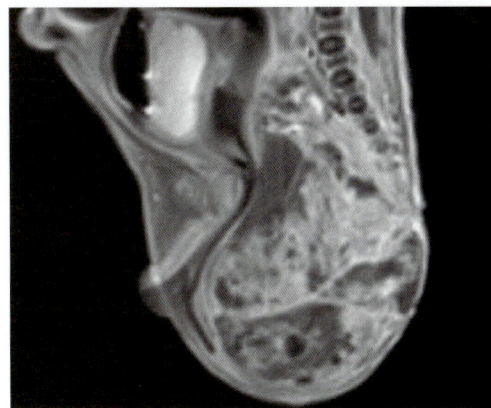

F

A. Sagittal, (**B**) coronal, and (**C**) axial T2-weighted single-shot FSE/TSE with fat saturation. **D**. Axial pre-contrast-enhanced and (**E**) axial and (**F**) sagittal post-gadolinium contrast-enhanced T1-weighted gradient echo with fat saturation.

Case 132 Sacrococcygeal Teratoma, Type III

Findings

▶ Complex large, highly vascular heterogeneous presacral mass that contains scattered solid and cystic components with a hemorrhage fluid level
▶ There is left-to-right displacement of the bladder. There is no involvement posterior to the sacrum, no osseous invasion, and no spinal involvement.

Differential diagnosis

▶ Myelomeningocele
▶ Neurogenic tumor—neuroblastoma
▶ Hemangioma

Teaching points

▶ Sacrococcygeal teratomas (SCTs) have an incidence of 1 in 25,000 to 30,000 live births and represent 70% to 80% of all neonatal teratomas, with a 4:1 female preponderance. Diagnosis can be made in utero on ultrasound or fetal MRI.
▶ SCTs are classified by the American Academy of Pediatric Surgery as follows:
  - Type I: Predominantly external mass with little to no internal components
  - Type II: Predominantly external mass with internal extension
  - Type III: Mixed internal/external mass with extension to abdominal cavity
  - Type IV: Internal with no external component
▶ MRI is the imaging modality of choice for assessing the lesions as it allows excellent visualization of the pelvic musculature, vascular structures, abdominal extent, and spinal invasion. A more cystic component on MR imaging reflects a more favorable prognosis, whereas a more solid component renders a poorer prognosis. Half of these tumors have calcification. The majority of SCTs are benign at birth, but the rate of malignancy rises quickly with the age of the patient. Thus, early diagnosis and resection are important. However, malignant recurrence can occur even after total resection of a benign SCT.
▶ Imaging cannot reliably distinguish benign from malignant tumors, although some features, such as destruction of the sacrum, suggest malignancy. Metastatic deposits are most likely found in bone, lungs, or brain.

Management

▶ Complete surgical resection with coccygectomy

Further reading

1. Keslar PJ, Buck JL, Suarez ES. Germ cell tumors of the sacrococcygeal region: radiologic-pathologic correlation. RadioGraphics 1994;14:607–620.
2. Rescorla FJ, Sawin RS, Coran AG, et al. Long-term outcome for infants and children with sacrococcygeal teratoma: a report from the Children's Cancer Group. J Pediatr Surg 1998;33:171–176.
3. Woodward PJ, Sohaey R, Kennedy A, Koeller KK. A comprehensive review of fetal tumors with pathologic correlation. RadioGraphics 2005;25:215–242.

History

▸ 78-year-old woman with labile hypertension on multiple antihypertensive medications

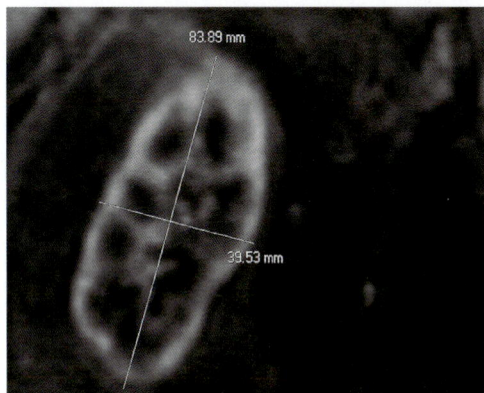

A

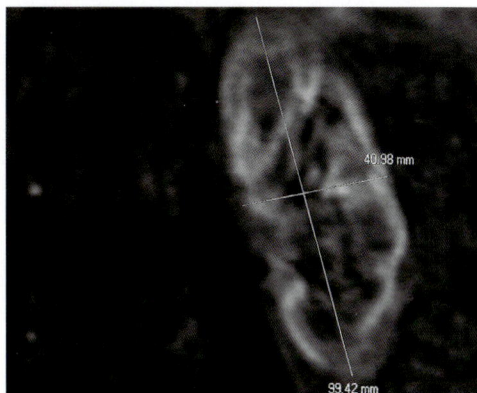

B

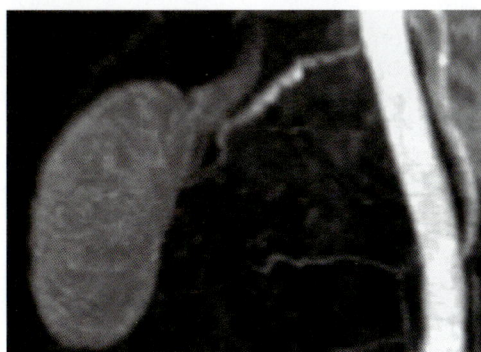

C

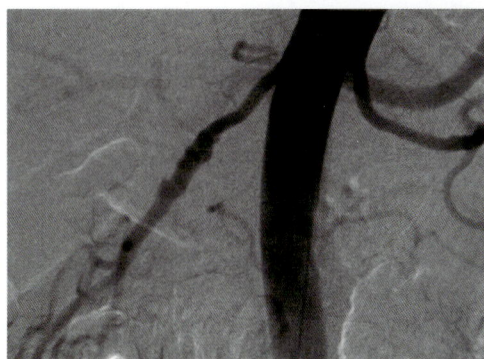

D

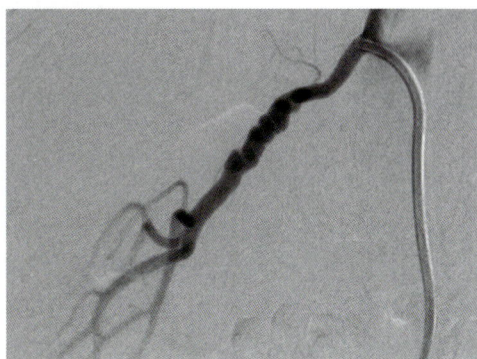

E

A. Measurement of right and (**B**) left kidney using the source images of gadolinium contrast-enhanced 3D T1-weighted gradient echo for MRA. **C**. Full-volume MIP from contrast-enhanced MRA of the abdominal vasculature. **D**. Digital subtraction angiogram (DSA) of renal vasculature. **E**. DSA with selective injection of right renal artery.

Case 133 Fibromuscular Dysplasia (FMD)

Findings

- ▶ Diffuse, irregular narrowing of the middle of right renal artery
- ▶ Decreased size of the right kidney compared to the non-affected left kidney
- ▶ Digital subtraction angiography (DSA) images confirm "string of pearls" appearance of the right renal artery. Note the normal left renal artery in **C**.

Differential diagnosis

- ▶ Atherosclerosis
- ▶ Vasculitis
- ▶ Collagen vascular disease
- ▶ Segmental arterial mediolysis

Teaching points

- ▶ Most common locations of FMD, in order of occurrence, are renal arteries, carotid arteries, and iliac arteries.
- ▶ FMD is categorized by pathological involvement of layers of the arterial wall as intimal, medial, or adventitial.
- ▶ The most common subtype of FMD is medial fibroplasia, which has the classic "string of pearls" appearance, with areas of alternating narrowing and aneurysm.
- ▶ Decrease in kidney size suggest chronic ischemia due to restriction of blood flow.
- ▶ FMD may present with hypertension refractory to multiple medications, although many patients are asymptomatic.
- ▶ FMD is more common in young or middle-aged women (three to five times more frequent than in men).

Management

- ▶ Percutaneous transluminal angioplasty without stenting
- ▶ Antihypertensive medications
- ▶ Surgical revascularization

Further reading

1. Leiner T, Michaely H. Advances in contrast-enhanced MR angiography of the renal arteries. Magn Reson Imaging Clin North Am 2008;16:561–572.
2. Norton P, Hagspiel K. Vascular MR imaging. In: Brant WE, de Lange EE (Eds), Essentials of Body MRI. New York: Oxford University Press, 2012.
3. Olin JW, Sealove BA. Diagnosis, management, and future developments of fibromuscular dysplasia. J Vasc Surg 2011;53:826–836.
4. Willoteaux S, Faivre-Pierret M, Moranne O, et al. Fibromuscular dysplasia of the main renal arteries: Comparison of contrast-enhanced MR angiography with digital subtraction angiography. Radiology 2006;241:922–929.

History

▶ 57-year-old man presenting with atypical chest pain

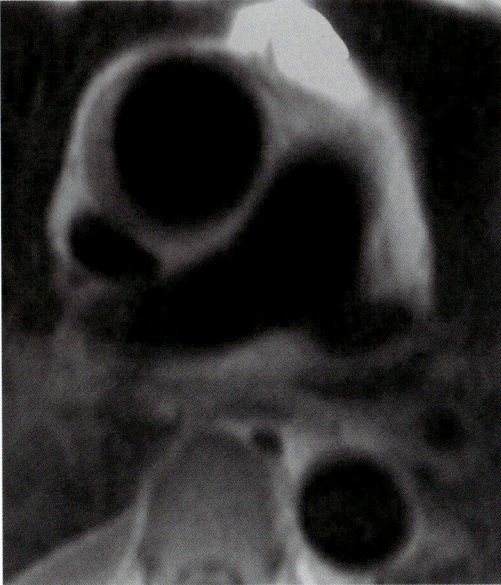

A

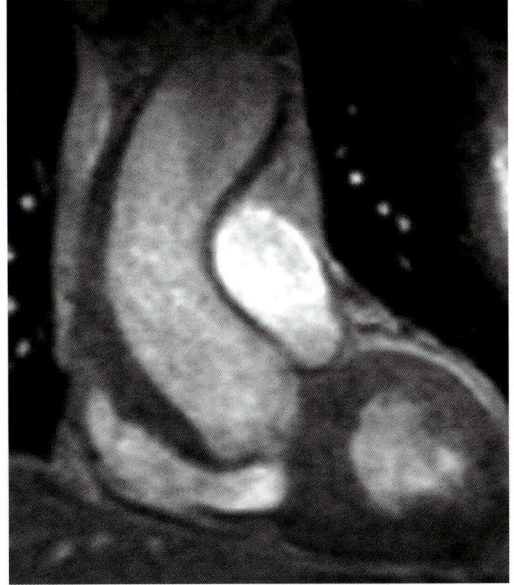

B

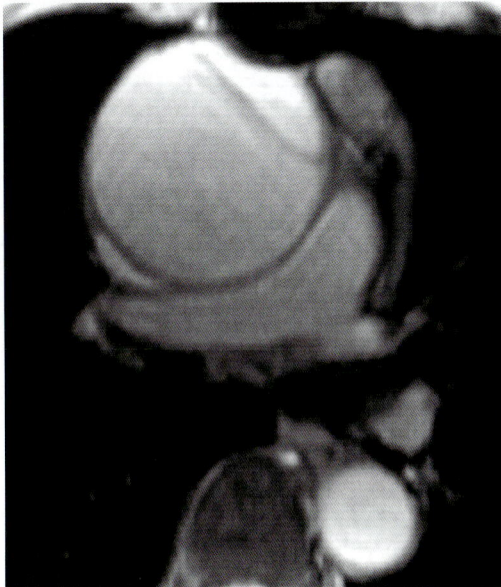

C

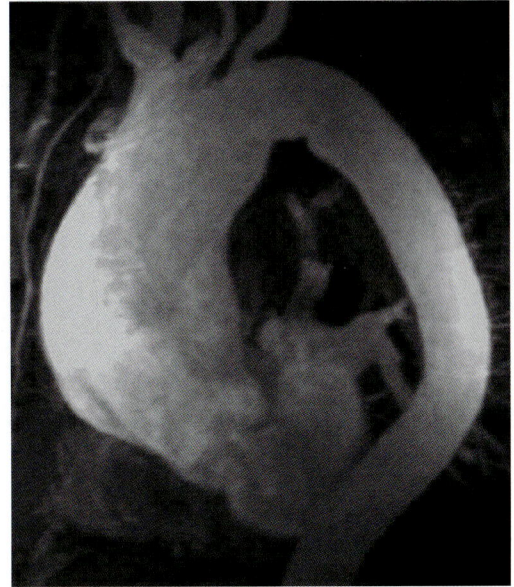

D

A. Axial ECG-gated double inversion-recovery T1-weighted FSE/TSE. **B**. Coronal and (**C**) axial T1-weighted gradient echo.
D. Parasagittal MRA generated from gadolinium contrast-enhanced 3D T1-weighted gradient echo.

Case 134   Aortic Intramural Hematoma (IMH)

Findings

- ▶ Crescent-shaped area of intermediate signal within the wall of the ascending aorta on T1-weighted imaging (**A**)
- ▶ Intermediate signal within the ascending aortic wall without evidence of defect in the intimal layer of the aorta (**B**)
- ▶ Progression of type A intramural hematoma to aortic dissection (**C**) with significant aneurysmal dilatation of the ascending aorta (**D**)

Differential diagnosis

- ▶ Aortic dissection
- ▶ Aortic mural thrombus
- ▶ Penetrating atherosclerotic ulcer

Teaching points

- ▶ IMH classically is seen as thickening of the aortic wall, typically less than 15 mm in thickness, caused by hemorrhage into the media from rupture of the vasa vasorum.
- ▶ IMH may also present in the setting of penetrating aortic ulcer.
- ▶ The most significant risk factor for IMH is hypertension.
- ▶ For classification purposes, Stanford type A IMH involves the ascending aorta, whereas Stanford type B IMH excludes the ascending aorta.
- ▶ Progression from Stanford type A IMH to aortic dissection occurs in approximately 25% of patients and is often treated with emergent surgical repair.

Management

- ▶ Emergent surgical repair is typically performed in patients with hemodynamic instability, signs of impending rupture, cardiac tamponade, significantly dilated ascending aorta, persistent pain, or large hematoma thickness. In the absence of these features, an individualized strategy may include operative repair or medical management.

Further reading

1. Bolger AF. Aortic intramural haematoma. Heart 2008;94:1670–1674.
2. Evangelista A, Eagle KA. Is the optimal management of acute type A aortic intramural hematoma evolving? Circulation 2009;120:2029–2032.
3. Ma X, Zhang A, Fan Z, et al. Natural history of spontaneous aortic intramural hematoma progression: Six years follow-up with cardiovascular magnetic resonance. J Cardiovasc Magn Reson 2010;12:27–29.
4. Norton P, Hagspiel K. Vascular MR imaging. In: Brant WE, de Lange EE (Eds), Essentials of Body MRI. New York: Oxford University Press, 2012.

History

▶ 34-year-old woman with abdominal pain and a questionable pancreatic mass on ultrasound examination.

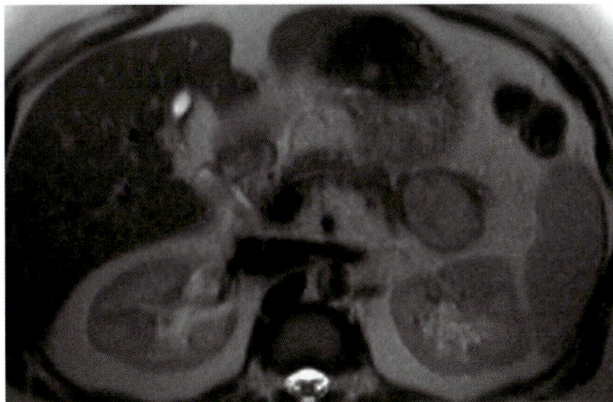

A

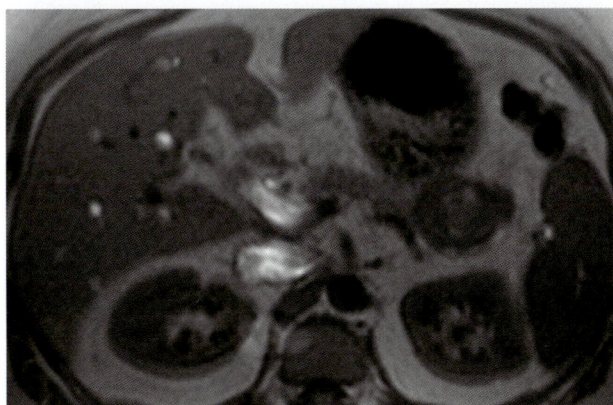

B

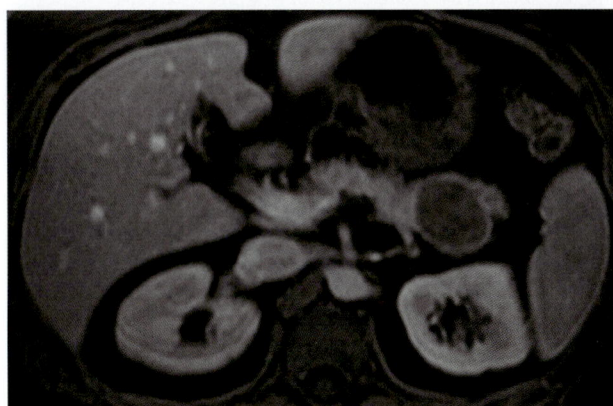

C

A. Axial T2-weighted single-shot FSE/TSE, (**B**) axial T1-weighted gradient echo, and (**C**) axial gadolinium contrast-enhanced T1-weighted gradient echo with fat saturation.

Case 135 Solid Pseudopapillary Tumor of the Pancreas

Findings

▶ A predominantly solid tumor in the tail of the pancreas with heterogeneous, increased signal intensity on the T2-weighted image and heterogeneous decreased signal intensity on the T1-weighted image

▶ Note several foci of increased signal intensity within the tumor on the T1-weighted image, corresponding to hemorrhage, a common feature secondary to tumor degeneration.

▶ Contrast-enhanced image shows a well-circumscribed mass with mild peripheral enhancement of the soft-tissue components.

Differential diagnosis

▶ Mucinous pancreatic tumor
▶ Serous cystadenoma of pancreas
▶ Pseudocyst
▶ Adenocarcinoma
▶ Neuroendocrine tumor

Teaching points

▶ Solid pseudopapillary tumors of the pancreas are uncommon and primarily occur in women (mean age, 28 years) and have low-grade malignant potential. In many cases, these tumors are predominately solid and contain small cystic components that are secondary to tumor degeneration.

▶ On MR images, solid pseudopapillary tumors are well circumscribed. T2-weighted images show mildly increased signal intensity. Those with increased tumor degeneration are mostly cystic, showing signal intensity closer to that of fluid. Enhancing soft-tissue components are uniformly present. The tumor may demonstrate a gradual accumulation of contrast material on delayed contrast-enhanced images, helping differentiate solid pseudopapillary tumors from other pancreatic neoplasms such as neuroendocrine tumors, which show early arterial enhancement.

Management

▶ Solid pseudopapillary tumors of the pancreas have low malignant potential. Surgical resection of the tumor is associated with long-term survival.

Further reading

1. Choi Y-J, Kim M-J, Kim JH, et al. Solid pseudopapillary tumor of the pancreas: typical and atypical manifestations. AJR Am J Roentgenol 2006;187:W178–W186.
2. Yu MH, Lee JY, Kim MA, et al. MR features of small solid pseudopapillary tumors: retrospective differentiation from other small solid pancreatic tumors. AJR Am J Roentgenol 2010;195:1324–1332.

History

▶ 46-year-old man with cardiac conduction abnormalities

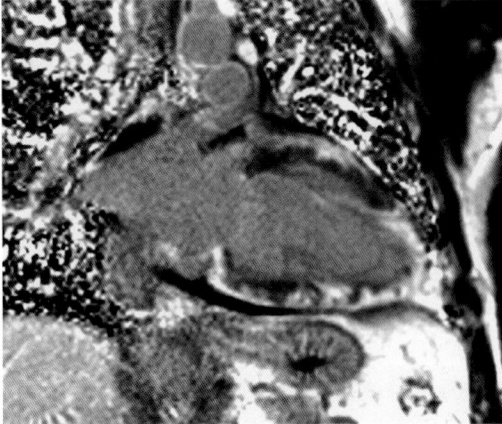

A

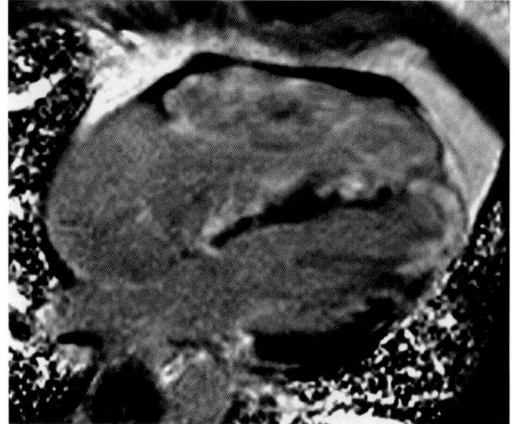

B

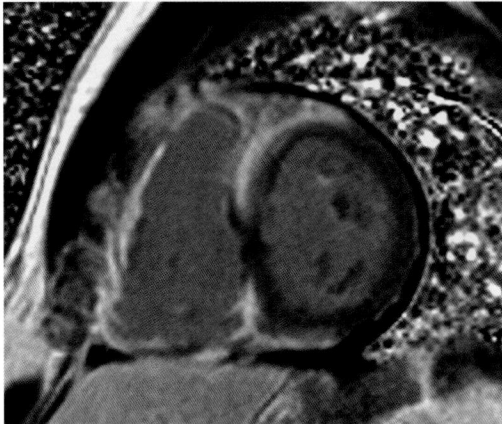

C

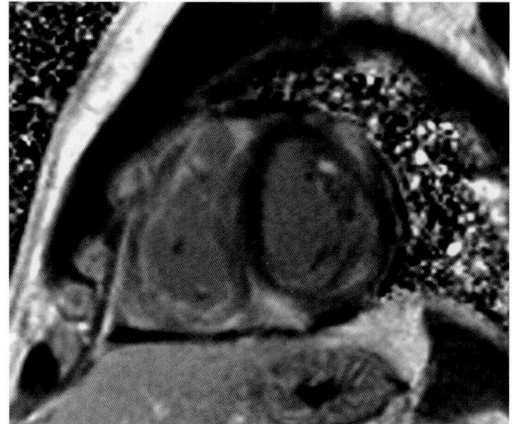

D

A. Two-chamber phase-sensitive inversion recovery (PSIR) gradient-echo late-phase gadolinium-enhanced (LGE) imaging .
B. Four-chamber PSIR LGE imaging. **C**. Short-axis PSIR LGE imaging at the ventricular base. **D**. Short-axis PSIR LGE imaging at the mid-ventricle.

Case 136   Cardiac Sarcoidosis

Findings

- ▶ Transmural late gadolinium enhancement (LGE) of the LV apex on two- and four-chamber views
- ▶ Subepicardial LGE throughout the inferior wall of the LV as well as the mid-anterior wall of the LV on the two-chamber view
- ▶ Subepicardial LGE involving the basal anteroseptum and basal and mid-inferoseptum on the short-axis views
- ▶ Transmural LGE of the entire RV wall on short-axis views

Differential diagnosis

- ▶ Sarcoidosis
- ▶ Myocarditis
- ▶ Chagas disease

Teaching points

- ▶ Approximately 25% of patients with sarcoidosis have cardiac involvement at autopsy, with 5% of all patients demonstrating clinical cardiac disease.
- ▶ Cardiac sarcoidosis may lead to heart failure due to wall-motion abnormalities or heart block and sudden death due to conduction abnormalities
- ▶ Late-phase gadolinium enhancement images are most important for identifying cardiac sarcoidosis with characteristic subepicardial, mid-wall, or transmural enhancement. The most common location for LGE is the basal portion of the septal wall. Myocarditis is rarely transmural in extent.
- ▶ The condition may be distinguished from ischemic heart disease by identifying sparing of the subendocardium on late-phase gadolinium enhancement images
- ▶ T2-weighted images will demonstrate increased signal intensity when inflammatory edema is present.
- ▶ Cine images may demonstrate segmental motion abnormalities.
- ▶ Wall thickening may be present in areas of inflammation.
- ▶ Differentiation between cardiac sarcoidosis, myocarditis, and Chagas disease often relies on clinical findings, including history and laboratory tests.

Management

- ▶ Corticosteroid therapy

Further reading

1. Serra JJ, Monte GU, Mello ES, et al. Cardiac sarcoidosis evaluated by delayed-enhanced magnetic resonance imaging. Circulation 2003;107:188–189.
2. Vignaux O. Cardiac sarcoidosis: spectrum of MRI features. AJR Am J Roentgenol 2005;184:249–254.
3. Vignaux O, Dhote R, Duboc D, et al. Clinical significance myocardial magnetic resonance abnormalities in patients with sarcoidosis: a one-year follow-up study. Chest 2002;122:1895–1920.

History

▶ 45-year-old man had MRI prior to liver transplant for assessment of hepatoma.

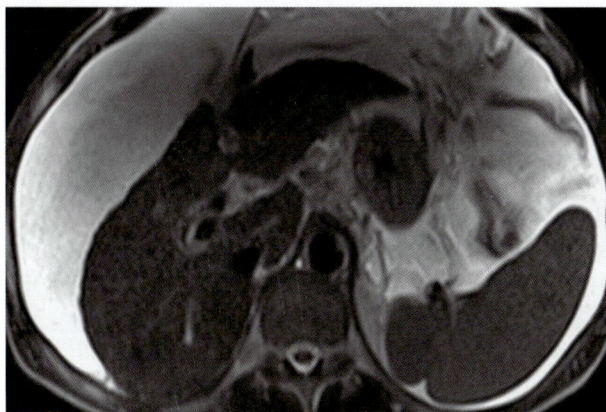

A

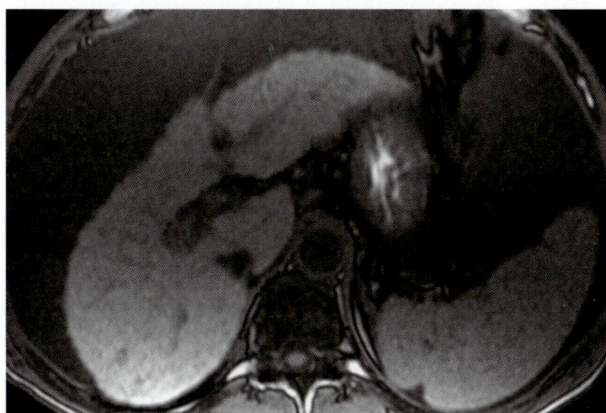

B

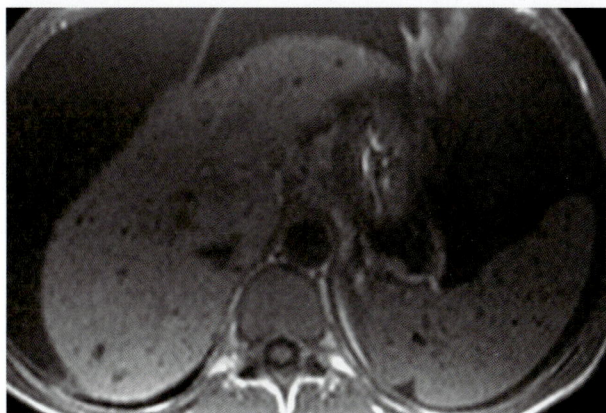

C

A. Axial T2-weighted single-shot FSE/TSE. **B**. Axial opposed-phase (TE = 2.3 ms) and (**C**) in-phase (TE = 4.6 ms) T1-weighted gradient echo.

Case 137   Siderotic Nodules

Findings
- ▶ Shrunken and nodular liver, with large amount of ascites and splenomegaly
- ▶ Multiple tiny foci of low signal intensity are seen on T1-weighted imaging throughout the liver and spleen.
- ▶ These foci become more conspicuous and lower in signal intensity on gradient-echo images as the echo time (TE) increases. Note that the overall liver and spleen signal also decreases which is from hemochromatosis.
- ▶ The diagnosis is advanced cirrhosis with siderotic nodules in the liver. Gamna-Gandy bodies are seen in the spleen.

Differential diagnosis
- ▶ Sarcoidosis
- ▶ Treated metastatic disease, such as breast cancer
- ▶ Microabscesses

Teaching points
- ▶ Cirrhosis is the end-stage response of the liver to insult, such as alcohol, virus, steatosis, primary sclerosing cholangitis, hemochromatosis, and biliary atresia, and is characterized by bridging fibrosis, micro- and macronodules, and arteriovenous shunting.
- ▶ Iron deposition occurs during cirrhosis, both diffusely in hepatocytes and in certain regenerating nodules, also known as siderotic nodules. The susceptibility effect of iron results in low signal intensity on T1- and T2-weighted images. This effect is more pronounced using gradient-echo imaging and is therefore better appreciated on these images than on spin-echo images.
- ▶ Portal hypertension in the spleen results in microhemorrhage, which leads to siderotic nodules showing similar MR signal characteristics as those in the liver. In the spleen these are called Gamna-Gandy bodies.

Management
- ▶ Dysplastic nodules are associated with an increased risk of hepatocellular carcinoma. It is less certain whether siderotic nodules cause increased risk for developing hepatocellular carcinoma.
- ▶ Definitive treatment for cirrhosis is liver transplantation.

Further reading
1. Hussain SM, Zondervan PE, IJzermans JNM, et al. Benign versus malignant hepatic nodules: MR imaging findings with pathologic correlation. RadioGraphics 2002;22:1023–1036.
2. Krinsky GA, Lee VS, Nguyen MT, et al. Siderotic nodules in the cirrhotic liver at MR imaging with explant correlation: no increased frequency of dysplastic nodules and hepatocellular carcinoma. Radiology 2001;218:47–53.

History

▶ 42-year-old woman with a long history of recurrent pancreatitis with multiple pancreatic fluid collections and multiple fluid drainage procedures

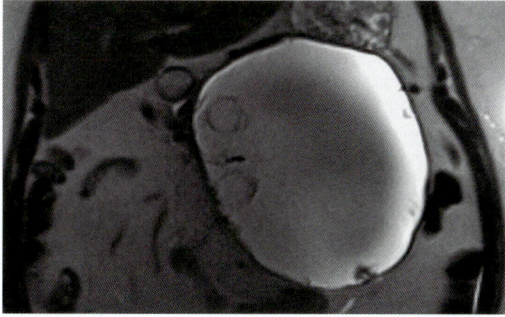

A

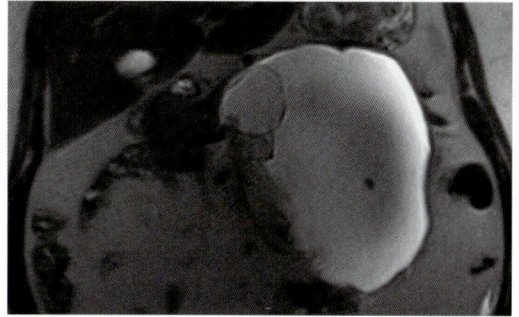

B

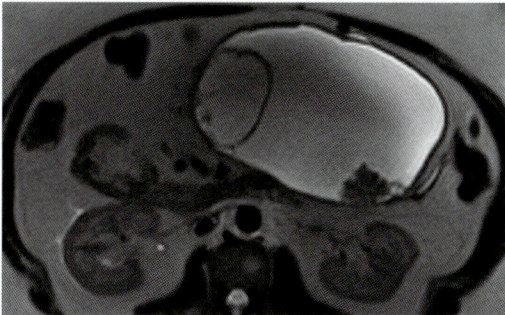

C

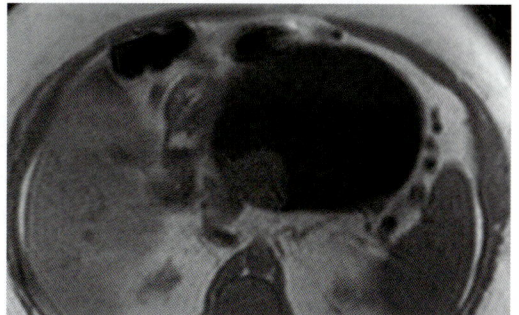

D

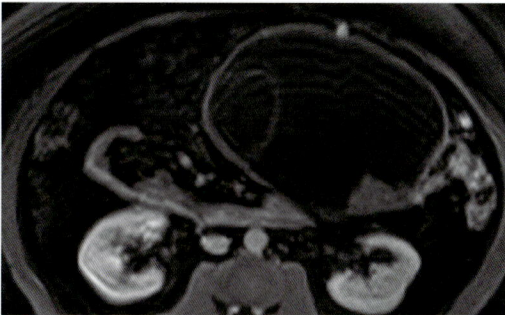

E

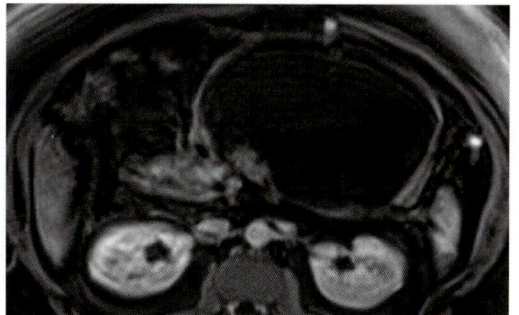

F

A, B. Coronal, and (**C**) axial T2-weighted FSE/TSE. **D**. Axial T1-weighted gradient echo. **E, F**. Axial post-gadolinium contrast-enhanced T1-weighted gradient echo with fat saturation (**F** obtained at slightly higher level than **E**).

Case 138 Mucinous Cystic Adenocarcinoma

Findings

- ► A large multiseptated cystic mass arises from the pancreas.
- ► The mass contains multiple enhancing, papillary, solid nodules projecting from its wall.
- ► Diagnosis: Adenocarcinoma arising in mucinous cystic neoplasm of the pancreas. At surgery, this patient also had cystic metastases from this tumor implanted on the ovaries.

Differential diagnosis

- ► Pancreatic pseudocyst with debris
- ► Serous cystadenoma
- ► Cystic neuroendocrine neoplasm

Teaching points

- ► The term "mucinous cystic neoplasm of the pancreas" encompasses both slow-growing mucinous cystadenomas (two thirds of cases) and invasive mucinous cystadenocarcinomas (one third of cases). The walls of these lesions are usually thick and lined by mucin-producing columnar epithelium. In distinction with intraductal papillary mucinous neoplasms, these tumors do not communicate with the pancreatic duct. The benign mucinous cystadenoma can undergo malignant transformation at any time; thus, surgical removal is recommended for all of these tumors.
- ► The majority (>95%) of these tumors occur in women and they usually arise in the body or tail of the pancreas. Most are clinically silent, allowing growth to large size (10 cm or more).
- ► The presence of mural nodules, nodular wall or septal thickening, or calcification is strong evidence of malignancy.
- ► The mucinous content of the tumor often has MR signal characteristics of simple fluid, displaying high signal intensity on T2-weighted images and low signal intensity on T1-weighted images. The thick walls, septa, and nodules usually show best with contrast enhancement.
- ► While pancreatic pseudocysts represent up to 85% of all cystic pancreatic lesions, cystic neoplasms of the pancreas should always be considered in the differential diagnosis, whether or not the patient has a history of pancreatitis.

Management

- ► Because of malignant potential, surgical resection is recommended for all mucinous cystic neoplasms of the pancreas.

Further reading

1. Kalb B, Sarmiento JM, Kooby DA, et al. MR imaging of cystic lesions of the pancreas. RadioGraphics 2009;29:1749–1765.
2. Khan A, Khosa F, Eisenberg RL. Cystic lesions of the pancreas. AJR Am J Roentgenol 2011;196:W668–W677. Web-exclusive article.
3. Kim YH, Saini S, Sahani D, et al. Imaging diagnosis of cystic pancreatic lesions: pseudocyst versus nonpseudocyst. RadioGraphics 2005;25:671–685.

History

▶ 25-year-old man presents with elevated liver function tests discovered on routine screening. Ultrasound demonstrated a mass in the right hepatic lobe.

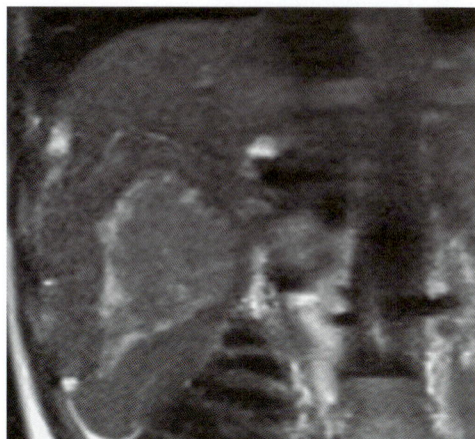

A

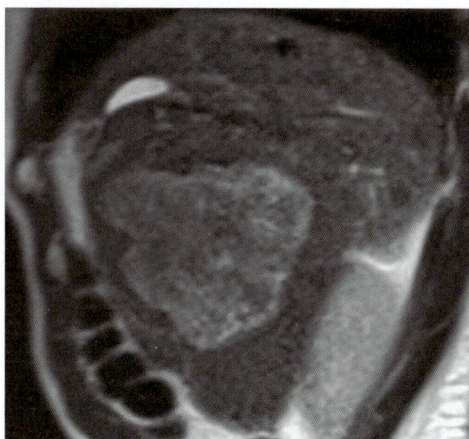

B

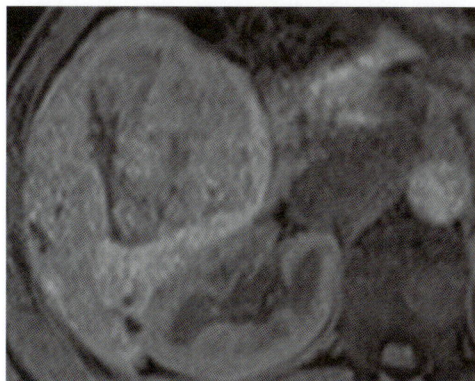

C

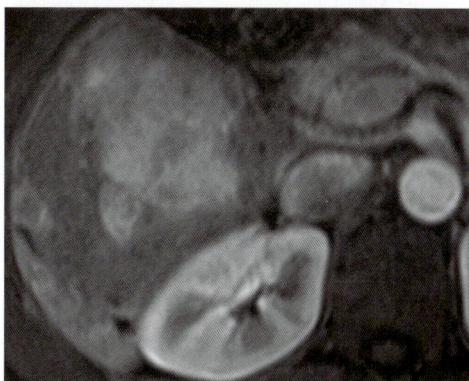

D

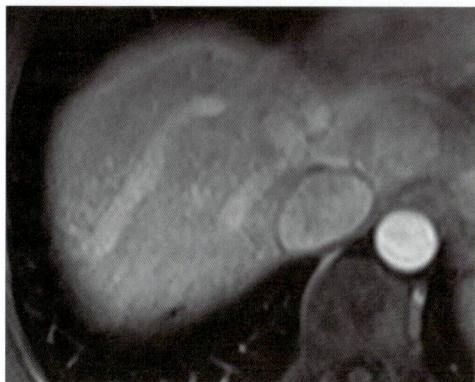

E

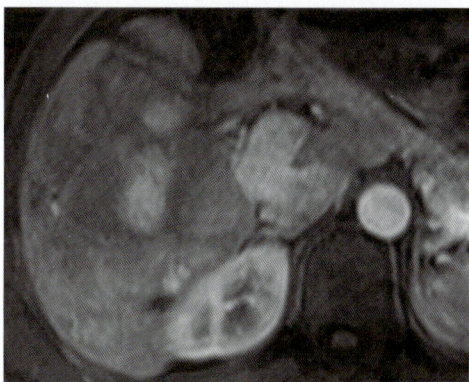

F

A. Coronal and (**B**) sagittal T2-weighted single-shot FSE/TSE. Axial pre-contrast-enhanced (**C**) and early-phase gadolinium contrast-enhanced T1-weighted gradient echo with fat saturation at three different anatomic levels.

Case 139 Hepatic Arteriovenous Malformation (AVM), Congenital Portosystemic Shunt

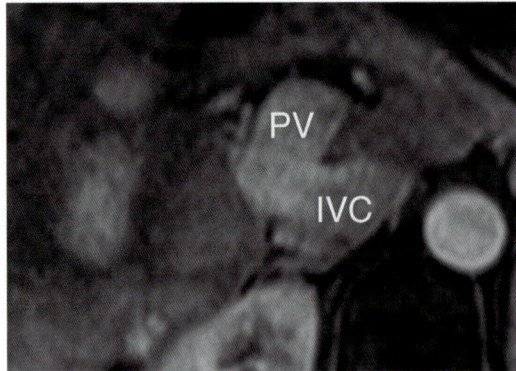

G

Findings

▶ A large, lobulated mass is present in hepatic segments 5 and 6 showing avid but heterogeneous contrast enhancement in the early arterial phase, then becoming iso- to hypo-intense to hepatic parenchyma on later phases (not shown).
▶ Early filling in arterial phase of dilated tortuous hepatic veins (**E**)
▶ A spontaneous shunt between the dilated portal vein (*PV*) branch and the inferior vena cava (*IVC*) is evident **G** which is a cropped and magnified view of **F**.

Differential diagnosis

▶ Hemangioma or hypervascular hepatic neoplasm

Teaching points

▶ Hepatic AVM is associated with hereditary hemorrhagic telangiectasia.
▶ Only 3% to 5% are symptomatic. When symptomatic, patients most often present with high-output heart failure, biliary ischemia, or portal hypertension.
▶ AVMs can be classified as high-flow and low-flow lesions. High-flow lesions such as this one demonstrate early and avid enhancement, whereas low-flow lesions enhance late or not at all. Enlarged supplying arteries are invariably present as well.
▶ Congenital intrahepatic portosystemic shunts are abnormal intrahepatic connections between the branches of the portal vein and the hepatic veins or inferior vena cava.

Management

▶ Asymptomatic lesions do not need intervention and can be followed clinically.
▶ When symptomatic, medical management aimed at the presenting symptom is the first-line therapy. If medical management fails, liver transplant is the definitive therapy. Embolization of the arterial supply, particularly when involving large AVMs, increases the risk of biliary ischemia.

Further reading

1. Gallego C, Miralles M, Marin C, et al. Congenital hepatic shunts. RadioGraphics 2004;24:755–772.
2. Garcia-Tsao, G. Congenital hepatic vascular malformations. In: DeLeve LD, Garcia-Tsao G (Eds), Vascular Liver Disease: Mechanisms and Management. New York: Springer-Verlag, 2011.
3. Khalid SK, Garcia-Tsao G. Hepatic vascular malformations in hereditary hemorrhagic telangiectasia. Semin Liver Dis 2008;28:247–258.

History

▶ 62-year-old woman with small mass of the right kidney found during renal ultrasound examination

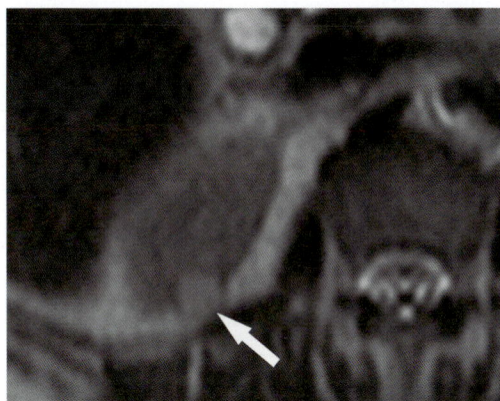

A

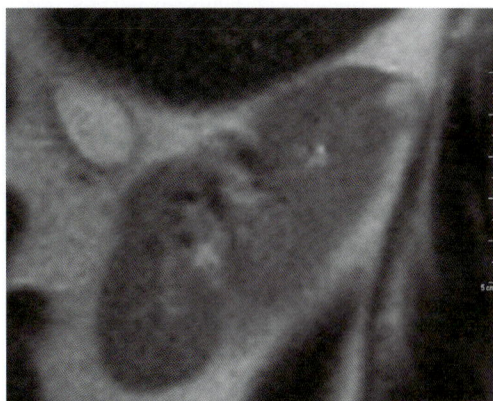

B

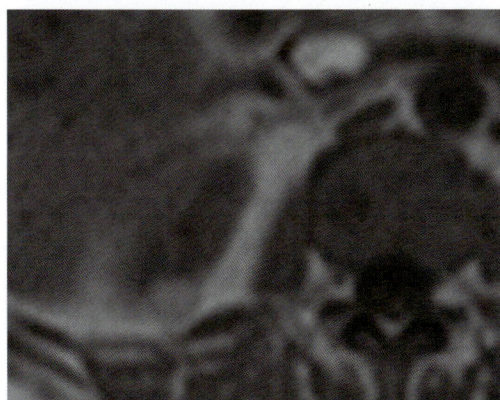

C

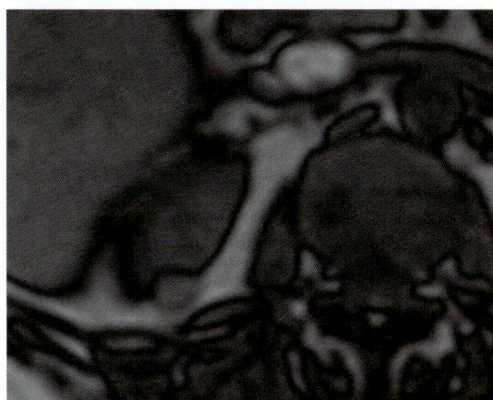

D

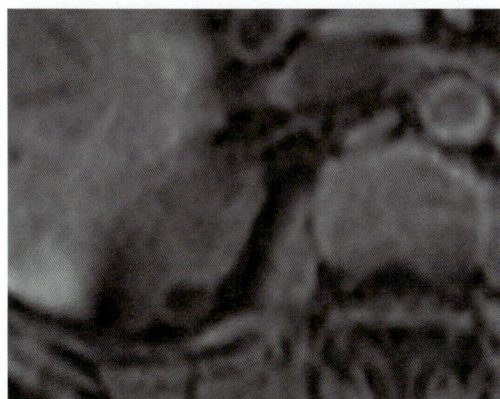

E

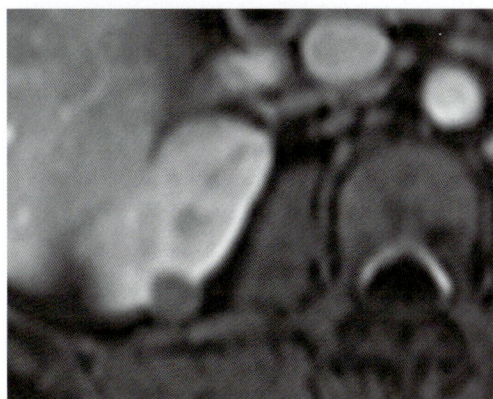

F

A. Axial and (**B**) coronal T2-weighted single-shot FSE/TSE. **C**. Axial in-phase and (**D**) opposed-phase T1-weighted gradient echo.
E. Axial pre- and (**F**) post-gadolinium contrast-enhanced T1-weighted gradient echo with fat saturation.

Case 140 Angiomyolipoma (AML)

Findings

▶ T2-weighted images show a small upper-pole right renal mass (*arrow*) that is slightly lower in signal intensity than the adjacent perinephric fat.

▶ On the opposed-phase gradient-echo image the lesion shows no significant decrease in signal intensity. Note that the India ink artifact, resulting from signal cancellation in voxels that contain the signal from both water and fat, is present between the mass and the renal parenchyma but is absent between the mass and the perinephric fat. This finding indicates that the renal mass contains fat.

▶ On the pre-contrast-enhanced fat-suppressed T1-weighted image the mass shows low signal intensity similar to that of perinephric fat, confirming the presence of macroscopic fat within the mass. The post-contrast-enhanced image shows minimal enhancement.

Differential diagnosis

▶ Renal cell carcinoma
▶ Renal cyst

Teaching points

▶ AML is the most common benign renal tumor, being discovered with increased frequency by the expanded use of routine diagnostic imaging. The lesion is a hamartoma with varying concentrations of thick-walled blood vessels (*angio*), smooth muscle cells (*myo*), and fat (*lipoma*).

▶ Diagnosis of AML is based upon equivocal demonstration of fat within the lesion. CT without intravenous contrast can be used in most instances to make the diagnosis. Bulk (adipose) fat is demonstrated by showing distinct signal loss on images obtained with an MR sequence that includes fat suppression. In-phase/opposed-phase gradient-echo imaging may provide definitive diagnosis when the AML is lipid-poor and the CT diagnosis is equivocal.

Management

▶ Although AML is a benign lesion and an incidental finding in most patients, hemorrhage and rarely catastrophic rupture may occur in tumors larger than 4 cm. In these cases prompt tumor embolization is needed to control the bleeding and save the kidney.

Further reading

1. Halpenny D, Snow A, McNeill G, Torreggiani WC. The radiological diagnosis and treatment of renal angiomyolipoma–current status. Clin Radiol 2010;65:99–108.
2. Israel GM, Hindman N, Hecht E, Krinsky G. The use of opposed-phase chemical shift MRI in the diagnosis of renal angiomyolipomas. AJR Am J Roentgenol 2005;184;1868–1872.
3. Pedrosa I, Sun MR, Spencer M, et al. MR imaging of renal masses: Correlation with findings at surgery and pathologic analysis. RadioGraphics 2008;28:985–1003.

History

▶ 21-year-old woman noted a firm mass in the left lower quadrant of the abdomen.

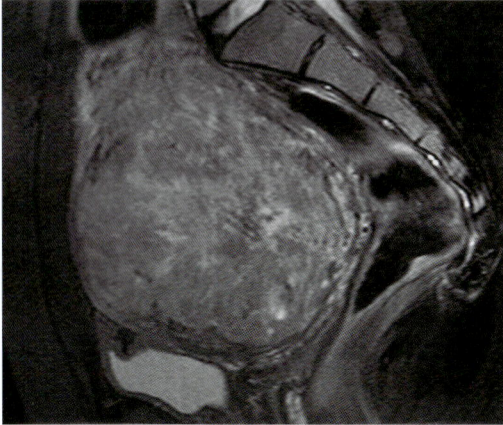
A

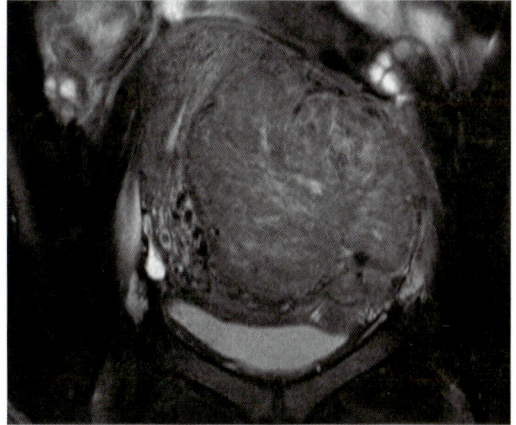
B

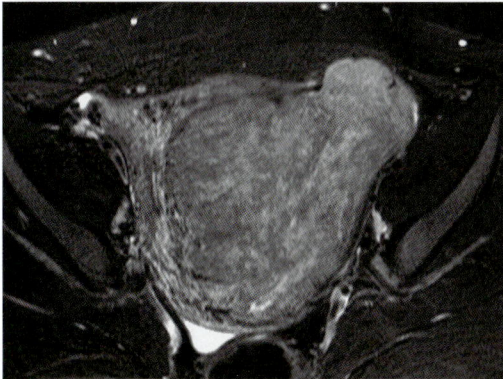
C

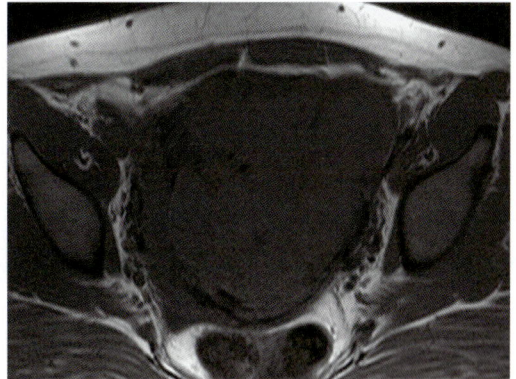
D

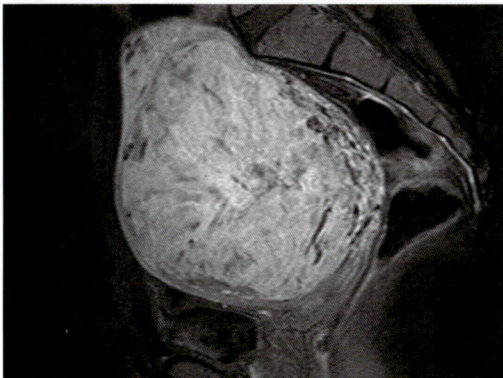
E

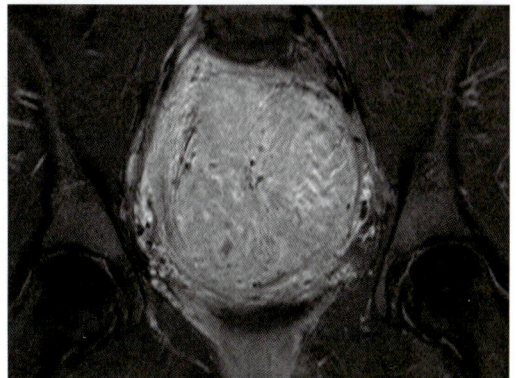
F

A. Sagittal, (**B**) coronal, and (**C**) axial T2-weighted FSE/TSE with fat saturation. **E**. Sagittal and (**F**) coronal post-gadolinium contrast-enhanced T1-weighted spin echo with fat saturation.

Case 141 Smooth Muscle Tumor of Uncertain Malignant Potential (STUMP Tumor)

Findings

▶ A very large solid mass arises from the left side of the uterus, displacing the endometrial cavity rightward.
▶ The mass displays heterogeneous intermediate-high signal intensity on T2-weighted images and low signal intensity equal to that of muscle on T1-weighted images.
▶ The uterine mass enhances avidly.
▶ Normal ovaries are present bilaterally.

Differential diagnosis

▶ Leiomyoma
▶ Uterine sarcoma

Teaching points

▶ The World Health Organization classification of uterine tumors indicates that a uterine smooth muscle tumor that cannot be histologically diagnosed as unequivocally benign or malignant should be called a "smooth muscle tumor of uncertain malignant potential" (STUMP).
▶ STUMPs constitute a heterogeneous group of rare tumors with histological features of atypical mitotically active leiomyomas. Moderate to severe cellular atypia is present. Extended follow-up indicates that most tumors have a benign course, but with risk of recurrence years after hysterectomy has been performed. A recurrence rate of 7% has been reported.

Management

▶ Long-term surveillance for evidence of tumor recurrence following hysterectomy is indicated.

Further reading

1. Guntupalli SR, Ramirez PT, Anderson ML, et al. Uterine smooth muscle tumor of uncertain malignant potential: a retrospective analysis. Gynecol Oncol 2009;113:324–326.
2. Ip PP, Cheung A, Clement PB. Uterine smooth muscle tumors of uncertain malignant potential (STUMP): a clinicopathologic analysis of 16 cases. Am J Surg Path 2009;33:992–1005.
3. Kido A, Togashi K, Koyama T, et al. Diffusely enlarged uterus: evaluation with MR imaging. RadioGraphics 2003;23:1423–1439.

History

▶ 40-year-old woman with left adnexal mass incidentally discovered on CT

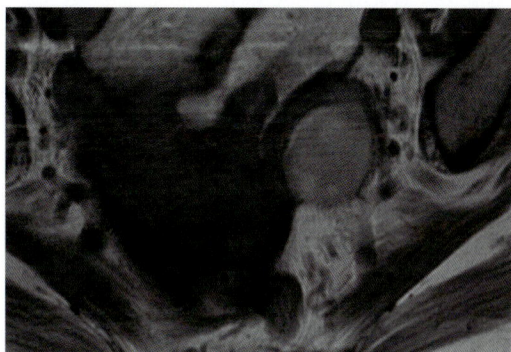

A

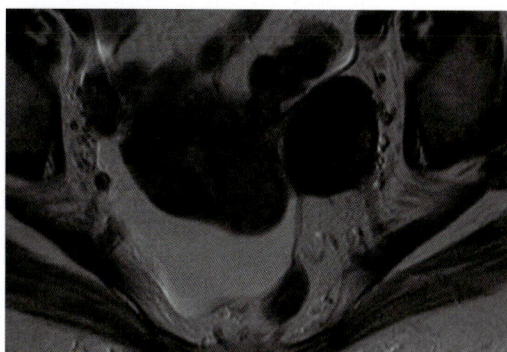

B

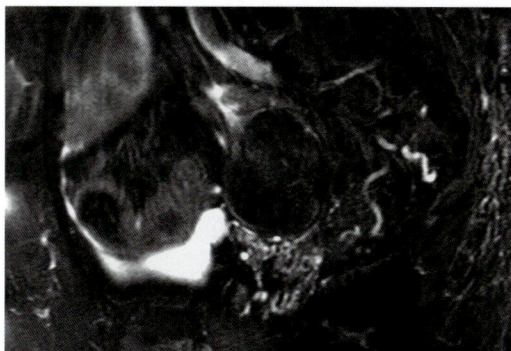

C

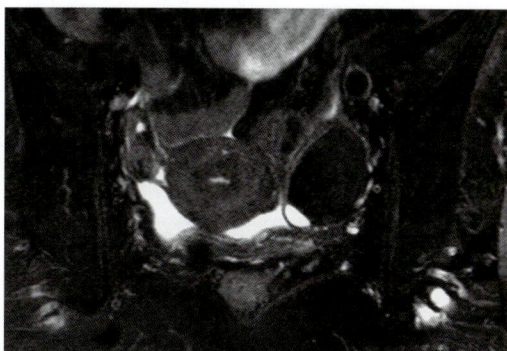

D

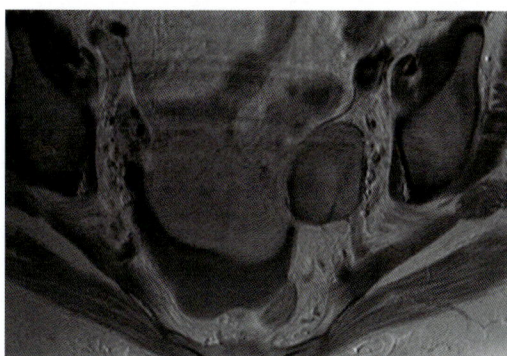

E

A. Axial T1-weighted spin echo. **B**. Axial T2-weighted FSE/TSE. **C**. Sagittal and (**D**) axial T2-weighted FSE/TSE with fat suppression.
E. Post-gadolinium contrast-enhanced axial T1-weighted spin echo.

Case 142 Cystic Endometrioma

Findings

▶ A left adnexal mass shows high signal intensity on T1-weighted images and markedly low signal intensity on T2-weighted images. Fluid is present in the cul-de-sac.

▶ No enhancement of the mass is evident on delayed post-contrast-enhanced images.

▶ Fat-saturated images were obtained with T2 weighting. Fat content of the mass could not be assessed because the mass was already very low in signal intensity on T2-weighted images without fat saturation. T1-weighted fat-saturated images would have been a better choice to assess for fat content characteristic of mature cystic teratomas; however, these images were not obtained in this case.

▶ A preoperative diagnosis of endometrioma was made based on high signal intensity on T1-weighted images and low signal intensity on T2-weighted images (T2-shading). The diagnosis of cystic endometrioma was confirmed at surgery.

Differential diagnosis

▶ Hemorrhagic ovarian cyst
▶ Mature cystic teratoma
▶ Ovarian neoplasm

Teaching points

▶ Endometriomas are thick-walled cysts partially lined by ectopic endometrial tissue and containing degenerated blood products. The physical appearance of degenerated blood products results in the name "chocolate cysts." They may be solitary or multiple and are bilateral in half of the cases. Endometriomas are commonly implanted on the ovary. The cysts contain blood in various stages of breakdown, including clots. On MR images fluid–fluid layers can be seen, with the freshest blood showing at the non-dependent layer and old degenerated blood at the dependent layer. Multiple contiguous endometriomas may form a multilocular appearance. Endometriomas of any size are prone to cyst rupture. The presence of endometriomas is a marker for severe deep pelvic endometriosis.

▶ MR is the best imaging modality from which to make a specific diagnosis of endometrioma. Endometriomas commonly show a classic appearance of high signal intensity on T1-weighted images and low signal intensity on T2-weighted images, the "T2-shading effect." T2 shading is caused by the high iron concentration that results from multiple episodes of hemorrhage. This is in distinction to acute hemorrhagic ovarian cysts, which display high signal intensity on both T1- and T2-weighted images. The T2-shading effect is variable from faint low signal to complete signal void. Solid components, fluid–fluid levels, and septa show variable signal intensity.

Management

▶ Laparoscopic removal of all ectopic endometrial tissue is the treatment of choice.

▶ Medical therapy includes hormone contraceptives, gonadotropin-releasing hormone agonists and antagonists, medroxyprogesterone (Depo-Provera®), and aromatase inhibitors.

Further reading

1. Chamie LP, Blasbalg R, Mendes Alves Pereira R, et al. Findings of pelvic endometriosis at transvaginal US, MR imaging, and laparoscopy. RadioGraphics 2011;31:E77–E100.
2. Choudhary S, Fasih N, Papadatos D, Surabhi VR. Unusual imaging appearances of endometriosis. AJR Am J Roentgenol 2009;192:1632–1644.

History

▶ 80-year-old man with a history of chronic lymphocytic leukemia had a CT scan showing a left renal mass.

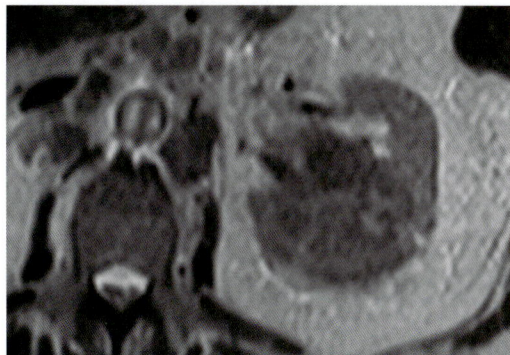
A

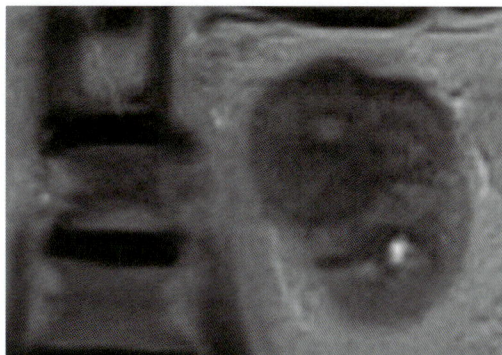
B

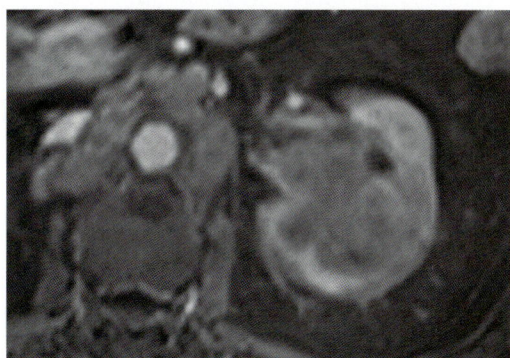
C

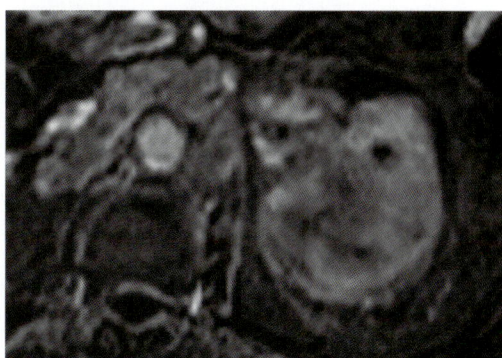
D

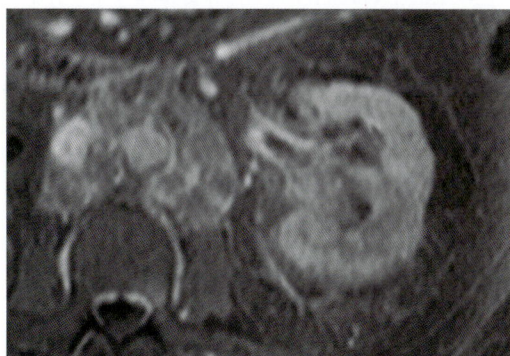
E

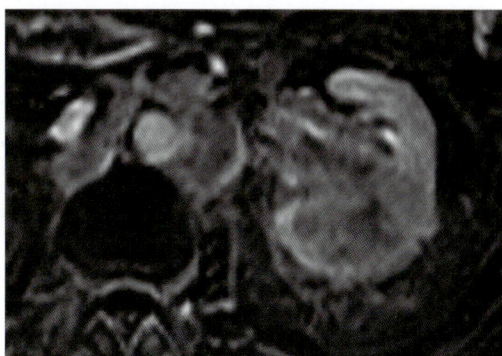
F

A. Axial and (**B**) coronal T2-weighted single-shot FSE/TSE. **C**. Axial post-gadolinium contrast-enhanced T1-weighted gradient echo with (**D**) subtraction image. **E**. Axial post-contrast-enhanced T1-weighted gradient echo with (**F**) subtraction image.

Case 143 Urothelial Carcinoma

Findings

▶ A large mass invades the upper mid-pole intrarenal collecting system and the adjacent renal parenchyma. Enhancement is clearly evident on post-contrast-enhanced subtraction images.

▶ Extension of tumor into the perinephric fat is suggested by the irregular speculated renal margin in the region of the tumor. Compare to the uninvolved portion of the kidney.

▶ Extensive, enhancing retroperitoneal lymphadenopathy is present.

▶ The diagnosis of poorly differentiated urothelial carcinoma metastatic to periaortic lymph nodes was proven by CT-guided core biopsy.

Differential diagnosis

▶ Renal cell carcinoma invading the collecting system
▶ Renal infection

Teaching points

▶ Urothelial cancers arise from the lining of the urinary tract. Upper-tract tumors involve the calyces, renal pelvis, or ureters. Lower-tract tumors involve the bladder and urethra. Urothelial cancers of the renal pelvis and collecting system account for approximately 10% of all renal tumors, with 90% of these classified as transitional cell carcinoma, 9% as squamous cell carcinoma, and 1% as mucinous adenocarcinoma. Synchronous tumors of the ureter or bladder are present in 2% to 4% of patients.

▶ Early-stage tumors are seen as focal thickening of the wall of the pelvicalyceal system or as intraluminal nodules. Frond-like appearance of the tumor outlined by urine with expansion of the collecting system or pelvis is characteristic. Differential diagnosis includes blood clots, fungal balls, and sloughed papillae.

▶ Infiltrative tumors obliterate renal sinus fat and extend into the renal parenchyma, distorting the renal and pelvicalyceal architecture. Most tumors are solid masses, but a multicystic appearance may occur. The tumors may extend into the perinephric fat and psoas muscle. Invasion of the renal vein is rare. Involvement of retroperitoneal lymph nodes is present in 30% of patients.

Management

▶ Complete surgical excision is the treatment of choice.

Further reading

1. Lee EK, Dickstein RJ, Kamat AM. Imaging of urothelial cancers: what the urologist needs to know. AJR Am J Roentgenol 2011;196:1249–1254.
2. Prando A, Prando P, Prando D. Urothelial cancer of the renal pelvicaliceal system: unusual imaging manifestations. RadioGraphics 2010;30:1553–1566.
3. Vikram R, Sandler CM, Ng CS. Imaging and staging of transitional cell carcinoma: part 2, upper urinary tract. AJR Am J Roentgenol 2009;192;1488–1493

Index of Cases

Index of Topics

General Index